Sexually Transmitted Diseases

Previous Anglo-American conferences:

1971: **Medical Care**

SBN 9501555 1 9

1973: **Drug Abuse**

ISBN 0 9501555 5 1

1974: **Continuing Medical Education**

ISBN 0 9501555 7 8

Reports of these conferences may be obtained from The Publications Department, Royal Society of Medicine, 1 Wimpole Street, London W1M 8AE, or through any bookseller

Sexually Transmitted Diseases

Proceedings of a Conference
sponsored jointly by the
Royal Society of Medicine and the
Royal Society of Medicine Foundation Inc
held at
1 Wimpole Street, London W1M 8AE
23–25 June 1975

Edited by
R D CATTERALL and C S NICOL

1976

Academic Press

London New York San Francisco

A Subsidiary of Harcourt Brace Jovanovich, Publishers

ACADEMIC PRESS INC. (LONDON) LTD
24/28 Oval Road
London NW1

U.S. Edition published by
ACADEMIC PRESS INC.
111 Fifth Avenue
New York
New York 10003

Library of Congress Catalog Card Number 75 46328
ISBN 0 12 164150 3

Printed in Great Britain by
William Clowes & Sons Limited
London, Colchester and Beccles

Foreword

This conference on Sexually Transmitted Diseases is one in the series of annual Anglo-American meetings sponsored in Britain and the USA by the Royal Society of Medicine and the Royal Society of Medicine Foundation, Inc at which subjects of common concern on both sides of the Atlantic are presented by equal numbers of speakers from the two countries, with full participation by the registrants.

The Royal Society of Medicine is well known by reason of its long history and its international membership. The Royal Society of Medicine Foundation, Inc was established in New York in 1967 to promote cooperation between members of the medical profession in the United States and in Britain and also to enable the academic, scientific and practical experience of the profession in both countries to be pooled and shared in a way that will create better doctors, better medicine and better relations between the English-speaking peoples. The funds it collects are being used to organize these Anglo-American conferences; to send young American doctors to the United Kingdom for periods of up to three months, with the opportunity of living at the Society's Domus Medica for part of that time, to see British medicine at work both generally and in areas directly connected with their specialty; to plan Anglo-American symposia, followed by publication and wide distribution, on subjects of outstanding medical importance; to help involve American MDs and PhDs in medical meetings taking place in London; and to strengthen the Society's links with medical organizations in North America and to broaden its membership there.

The affairs of the Royal Society of Medicine Foundation, Inc are in the hands of leading members of the American medical, legal and business professions. Additionally, the President of the Royal Society of Medicine is *ex officio* a member of the Foundation's Board of Directors, and the Society's Executive Director is Vice President of the Foundation.

The President and Council of the Society and the Directors of the Foundation wish to acknowledge donations made specifically in support of this conference by Becton Dickinson Foundation, Bristol Myers Company International Division, The Commonwealth Fund, Hoffman-LaRoche Inc, Prudential Insurance Company of America and William H Rorer Inc; the assistance given by the National Institutes of Health with the travelling expenses of some speakers and registrants from the USA; and a donation by the Wellcome Foundation Ltd to meet the cost of providing the printed report of the conference for those who attended.

They also take this opportunity of thanking those who support their other endeavours in the promotion of Anglo-American relations in medicine, namely the members of the Royal Society of Medicine in the USA and the following corporate donors: Abbot Laboratories Fund, Adair Fund for Cancer Research Inc, Mary Reynolds Babcock Foundation Inc, Becton Dickinson & Co, Bristol Myers Products, Bristol Myers Fund, Burroughs Wellcome Co, Burroughs Wellcome Fund, The Commonwealth Fund, Walter Ames Compton Foundation, Cyanamid International, Dudley Foundation Inc, Endo Foundation Inc, Exxon Corporation, General Telephone and Electronics Foundation, Grant Foundation Inc, Hoffman-LaRoche Inc, Hoffman-LaRoche Foundation, IBM World Trade Corporation, Interim Faculty Club Committee of the University of Alabama Medical Center, Johnson & Johnson Associated Industries Fund, Eli Lilly & Co, Eli Lilly & Co Foundation, William Muir Manger Research Foundation, Inc, Merck & Co Inc, Merck Co Foundation, Merck Sharp & Dohme Postgraduate Program, Merck Sharp & Dohme Research Laboratories, Merrell-National Laboratories, Miles Laboratories Inc, Miles Laboratories Foundation, Mobil Foundation Inc, Mobil Oil Corporation, Parke Davis & Co, SB Penick Foundation, Gustavus & Louise Pfeiffer Research Foundation, Pfizer International Inc, Pfizer Pharmaceuticals, Rockefeller Foundation, Rohlf Memorial Clinic Foundation, Rorer Foundation Inc, Sandoz-Warner Inc, GD Searle & Co, Searle Foundation, Smith Kline & French Foundation, Smith Kline Corporation, ER Squibb & Sons Inc, Sterling Drug Inc, Henry M and Lillian Stratton Foundation, Syntex Corporation, Syntex International, Syntex Pharmaceuticals Ltd, University Associates in Psychiatry, Wallace Pharmaceuticals, Warner-Lambert Co, Warner Lambert Charitable Foundation, Warner Lambert Pharmaceutical Co, William C Whitney Foundation.

John Stallworthy
Harry J Robinson

Members of the Conference Committee
Alexander G Bearn
R D Catterall
Richard M Krause
C S Nicol
Harry J Robinson
Sir John Stallworthy

Contents

Editors' Note: American spelling has been used in all the papers contributed by American members of the Conference, and English spelling in the papers from British speakers. In the general discussions, however, English spelling has been used.

Index of Contributors

Introductory Remarks

Sir John Stallworthy

President, Royal Society of Medicine

It is a special privilege for me to welcome you here to the conference which is about to start. Many of you, both from abroad and from these islands, are already Fellows of the Royal Society of Medicine, and I welcome you back to your own home. Some of you are not Fellows but I can assure you that our welcome for you is just as sincere. I hope you are going to enjoy the next three days here as well as find them very profitable.

There is one mistake in the programme. For once it is a pleasure to admit the mistake. You will see that we are to have the honour this morning of having the Conference opened, according to your programme, by Dr Henry Yellowlees. That is a mistake but not one for which the authors of this guide are responsible, because at the time it was written it was true, but since then Her Majesty has honoured Dr Yellowlees for his work, and we are now to have the proceedings opened by Sir Henry Yellowlees, who is the Chief Medical Officer of the Department of Health and Social Security. We do congratulate you, Sir Henry. We are particularly grateful to you for coming because we know that the pressures on you at present must be quite incredible. I am sure all present join me in thanking you for your kindness in sparing this time to wish this Conference every success. May I call on you to open the proceedings?

Sir Henry Yellowlees

Chief Medical Officer, Department of Health and Social Security

I would like first of all to thank you very much for your kind remarks. They are much appreciated.

I am very happy indeed to have the opportunity of being the opening speaker at this conference. I am sure that one more

Anglo-American conference at the Royal Society of Medicine here in London will carry on the tradition which already exists. These conferences have now established themselves as outstanding professional events of an extremely high standard. In addition, they represent an important and continuing link between our two countries. I am delighted to be here, and thank you for asking me, Sir.

Most countries have reported an increasing incidence of gonorrhoea in recent years and some increases in early syphilis, with the rates in young people tending to rise disproportionately. All this, paradoxically, in spite of our having more knowledge about these diseases and more ability to treat them effectively than ever before. Changes in behaviour and attitude partly account for the paradox. A new environment has appeared, and much more mobile populations, especially of young people, and I am sure these are factors.

The increasing interest in and concern about sexually transmitted diseases is illustrated by the fact that the WHO chose the subject for technical discussions in Geneva this year. I was there. Claude Nicol from this country was there, and perhaps others of you were there also. It was an excellent discussion, and some very helpful points were raised. The European Office of WHO is planning a symposium, including the behavioural aspects of sexually transmitted diseases, in 1977, and the Committee of Ministers for the Council of Europe have also taken the subject on board; in February 1974 they recommended that member states should take into account certain principles and practices with a view to promoting the control of sexually transmitted diseases.

Variations in criteria for diagnosis and in the reporting facilities available, and the extent to which treatment is given by private practitioners, &c., make it difficult to compare statistics from the various countries. In the United Kingdom it is thought that over 90% of diseases such as syphilis and gonorrhoea are seen at National Health Service clinics, and therefore reported in the official statistics. Even so, the incident rates are among the lowest of any of the industrial countries. So we hope this is true.

In recent years there has not only been a great increase in the number of cases seen at these clinics but also a marked change in their type. Nowadays less than a quarter of the cases fall into the old definition of venereal disease, that is to say syphilis, gonorrhoea and chancroid. The remainder of the patients needing treatment are suffering from other sexually transmitted diseases and other genitourinary conditions.

We are proud of the free service in this country, which was started in 1916 and has gradually developed as an almost unique phenomenon. It was incorporated into the National Health Service in 1948, and now there are 230 sexually transmitted disease clinics in the United Kingdom, where all consultations, investigations and treatment are free. Most doctors refer patients to these clinics, or patients go to them direct, so that an accurate diagnosis can be made and confirmed, and appropriate treatment given, follow-up tests and cure carried out and contact-tracing initiated. Good clinical teaching, undergraduate and postgraduate, has thus been facilitated, and it is particularly appropriate on this occasion to recall that many of the post-war generation of British consultants in this subject have owed much to the training received from the late Dr Earl Moore of Johns Hopkins Hospital in Baltimore.

I think there is general agreement that an ideal service for sexually transmitted diseases should be free; it should be easily accessible to patients; it should be situated in the out-patient departments of general hospitals and staffed by doctors and nurses with special training, supported by efficient laboratories and by staff properly trained to carry out contact-tracing and counselling.

Last year my department – the Department of Health and Social Security – issued a design guide for the building of such clinics. Its recommendations were general and adaptable to different circumstances. It is aimed to contribute towards improving working conditions by helping those who have to plan clinics in our district general hospitals.

Improvement in the effectiveness of contact-tracing is, of course, most important. The basic function of the health worker responsible, it now seems to us, is to get information about sex contacts by interviewing patients, mainly those with early infectious syphilis or gonorrhoea. Our aim is to prevent the spread of infection by educating the patient to accept responsibility for ensuring that his or her partner or partners attend the clinic, though visits to contacts in the community will still be necessary from time to time.

At interview information can be given on how to avoid reinfection and the importance of completing treatment and follow up can be stressed. If any social or emotional problem is revealed the patient can be referred for specialized attention. The careful selection and training of contact-tracing staff is essential.

I believe that health education is of prime importance at the moment. More and more the need to focus on "at risk" groups is to be stressed. These groups have to be defined. The educational objectives must be established, and finally a plan of operation, to include an evaluation of results, must be formulated. Long-term multidisciplinary preventive efforts are needed.

The epidemiological situation may well be finely balanced. Big changes in incidence may result from apparently slight changes in control activity.

I think there is every reason to regard the future with hope if we manage to concert our efforts. Progress has been achieved at research centres in various parts of the world, but today I would particularly like to pay special tribute to the outstanding contribution made in the field by the United States of America, where research work of the highest calibre and standard has been carried out, as exemplified by the studies at the Center for Disease Control, Atlanta.

Advances are hoped for on certain points in particular: a serological test for gonorrhoea, immunization for syphilis or gonorrhoea, the causation of nonspecific genital infection, systemic therapy for candidiasis and genital virus infections and, above all, I think, epidemiological studies to investigate social and behavioural factors involved in the assessment of sexually transmitted diseases. We need to know the patterns of behaviour in high-risk groups, and what the attitudes to the problems are within these groups, and whether these can be altered.

Recently in this country, on the recommendation of the Royal College of Physicians of London, the title of the specialty has been changed from venereology to genitourinary medicine. The change seems logical as the new term is less emotive and a more precise description of the present-day tasks of the clinicians who are involved. It is hoped that the recruitment to this specialty will be improved to the benefit of the patients and the family doctors referring them. The change should help to obviate the persisting stigma connected with the VD clinic.

Mr Chairman, I hope and believe that you will have a very profitable and interesting conference here. With so many well-known people in the field gathered together I am certain that this will be in the general tradition of these Anglo-American conferences. I am sorry that I shall not be able to be here very much myself, but I do hope to have the opportunity at various functions of meeting more of the people who are here. In the meanwhile may I wish you a very successful and enjoyable conference.

World Trends in Sexually Transmitted Diseases

Chairman

Dr Ambrose J King

The London Hospital, London E1

The Situation in the United States

Paul J Wiesner, Oscar G Jones
and Joseph H Blount
Department of Health, Education and Welfare,
Center for Disease Control, Atlanta, Georgia 30333

Data Collection

The data sources for this presentation of trends in sexually transmitted infections are: (1) The United States Public Health Service. (2) IMS INC (National Disease and Therapeutic Index). (3) Commission on Professional and Hospital Activities. Each system has its own unique combination of the usual biases which limit interpretation. We hope that these biases vary insignificantly with the passage of time and that the *trends* have validity. The trends are used to assess changes in the relative magnitude of disease problems, to evaluate the impact of control measures, and to allocate resources.

The United States Public Health Service data are based upon State laws requiring reporting of cases of gonorrhea, syphilis, lymphogranuloma venereum, chancroid and granuloma inguinale. The system is biased by underdiagnosis, inaccurate diagnosis and incomplete reporting (particularly by private physicians), but can be considered an accurate reflection of disease incidence trends among patients seeking care in the public sector of medicine.

The IMS System is a national random sample of one in 5000 office-based physician-days, where all diagnoses associated with every patient seen on the sample days are recorded and subsequently coded according to the International Classification of Disease. In addition to diagnostic uncertainties, this system is biased by a large sampling error.

The third data source is a computerized hospital data system, operated by the Commission on Professional and Hospital Activities in Ann Arbor, Michigan. This system samples approximately one in every 80 patients discharged from all United States short-term hospitals. The system lacks diagnostic accuracy and precise criteria for priority diagnoses when multiple conditions afflict a patient.

The relative frequency of sexually transmitted conditions recorded in the IMS Survey of private physicians during the calendar years

Table 1

Ratio x100 of the frequency of selected conditions to the frequency of gonorrhea. Survey of office-based private physicians in the United States, 1970–1974

Condition	*Male*		*Female*		*Total*	
	Ratio x100	*Confidence limits* •	*Ratio x100*	*Confidence limits* •	*Ratio x100*	*Confidence limits* •
Gonorrhea	100.0		100.0		100.0	
Primary and secondary syphilis					3.4	±1.9
Non-gonococcal urethritis	56.4	±14.9				
Acute salpingitis			19.6	±8.5		
Trichomonal vaginitis			203.7	±52.8		
Herpes genitalis					11.3	±6.9
Venereal warts					27.0	±13.1
Pediculosis pubis					9.6	±5.4

•Approximate 95% level.
Source: IMS INC. Sample Surveys of Office-based Private Physicians (National Disease and Therapeutic Index)

1970–1974 is shown in Table 1. We have listed the relative frequency of the other diseases per every 100 cases of gonorrhea, with approximately 95% confidence limits. For every 100 cases of gonorrhea there were: 3.4 ± 1.9 cases of primary and secondary syphilis, 56.4 ± 14.9 cases of nongonococcal urethritis in men and 19.6 ± 8.5 cases of acute salpingitis in women.

Trichomonal vaginitis was about twice as common as gonorrhea in women. Herpes genitalis was recorded in an approximate ratio of

1:10, genital warts 1:5, and pediculosis pubis 1:10. The relative frequency of nongonococcal urethritis is probably underestimated because of the tendency to overdiagnose gonococcal urethritis in the United States. Pediculosis pubis is also probably underestimated because many patients treat themselves with nonprescription remedies.

In order to assess the relative magnitude of these and other sexually transmitted diseases in the United States, the Venereal Disease Control Division has initiated pilot sentinel surveillance systems in 10 geographically distributed venereal disease clinics in the United States. Depending upon the results of such surveillance and the development of practical control measures for these diseases, future plans may include the promotion of State laws for reporting specific diseases. Currently, however, these sentinel clinics function by systematically recording the evaluations of all patients in a manner similar to that undertaken in Great Britain. Additionally, we have set up in two cities a comprehensive, computer-based surveillance of all the sexually transmitted diseases, not unlike that carried out in Sweden as described by Erikson *et al.* (1975).

Syphilis

The United States case rates of reported late latent and late syphilis have steadily decreased from a high of 196 per 100 000 population in fiscal year 1943, to a low of 16 per 100 000 in fiscal year 1974. However, the trends in early syphilis are less consoling.

The reported cases of primary and secondary syphilis for fiscal years 1950–1974 are shown in Fig. 1. From the 18 679 cases in fiscal

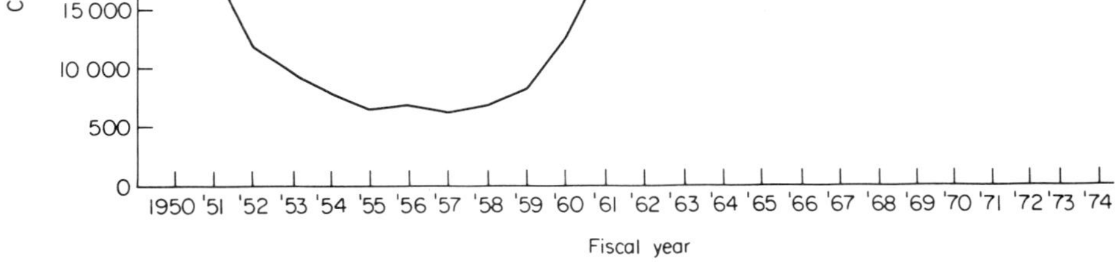

Fig. 1 *Primary and secondary syphilis. Cases reported in the United States, fiscal years 1950–1974*

year 1969, we experienced yearly increases of 3–16% until, in fiscal year 1974, we noted a modest but real decrease of 1.4% – the first decrease in reported cases in the most recent five years. However, the picture is mixed because from fiscal year 1973 to fiscal year 1974, a 9% increase was reported in early latent syphilis.

High reported rates of primary and secondary syphilis tend to be focal. In 1974, 83.9% of the counties reported 4 or fewer cases of primary and secondary syphilis. Sixty-three percent of the nation's infectious syphilis cases were reported by the 63 largest cities, even though these cities encompass only 28% of our population. The highest age-specific rate of primary and secondary syphilis is in the 20–24 year age group, followed by the 25–29, then the 30–39 year old group.

Table 2

Primary and secondary syphilis and gonorrhea – sex distribution of cases reported July 1973–June 1974

	Reported cases		*Ratio*		
	Male	*Female*	*Male*		*Female*
Syphilis P and S	17 079	7 649	2.2	:	1
Early latent (2 years duration)	14 065	10 225	1.4	:	1
Late and late latent	16 617	16 848	1.0	:	1
Gonorrhea	523 298	350 863	1.5	:	1

Source: HSM 9.688. DHEW-PHS-BSS-VDC-Division, Atlanta, Ga. 30333

Recent data on the sex distribution of cases of the various stages of reported syphilis show that for primary and secondary syphilis males predominate, at a ratio of 2.2 : 1 (Table 2). If this were merely evidence of greater ease of diagnosis, a reversal of the ratio might be expected in the later stages, if the missed female cases are to be accounted for. But the ratio never reverses, suggesting an actual increased acquisition of syphilis by men.

At least part of this acquisition results from increased transmission of syphilis between men. According to information based on 10 000–14 000 interviews yearly, the proportion of men with early syphilis who name other men as sexual partners has increased from 23.4% to 36.3% from 1969 to 1974.

Gonococcal Infection

The epidemic of reported cases of gonorrhea in the United States is well known. The 874 161 cases and rate of 420 per 100 000 population in fiscal year 1974 (Fig. 2) are the highest ever reported since the United States Public Health Service started keeping records 55 years ago.

Gonorrhea rates also vary somewhat from State to State, with highest rates (400 and over) in the South. Overall, only one State,

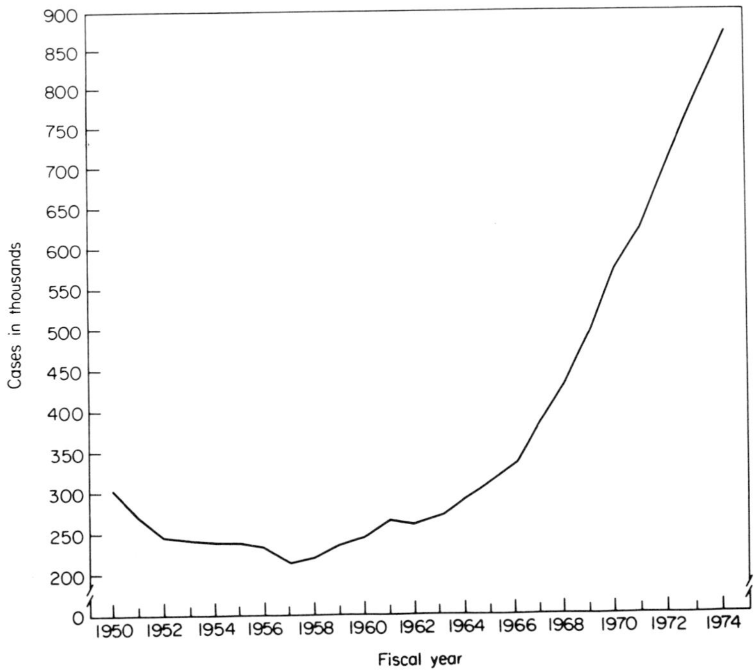

Fig. 2 *Gonorrhea. Cases reported in the United States, fiscal years 1950–1974*

New Hampshire, reported a case rate less than 100 per 100 000 population.

As is generally well known, reported gonorrhea case rates are highest for large urban areas (797), as compared to medium-sized cities (503) and smaller towns and rural areas (173). In the United States, very high age-sex-specific case rates for gonorrhea occur in the 20–24 age group but, in contrast to syphilis, also involve the 15–19 year age group in both sexes. The male : female ratio of reported cases of gonorrhea has dropped from 2.4 : 1 in 1971, to 1.5 : 1 in 1973.

This drop in the male to female ratio of reported cases of gonorrhea resulted in part from a national gonorrhea screening program, initiated in July 1972. The number of cultures performed in women of the sexually active age group undergoing pelvic examination increased dramatically until it leveled off in mid-1973. Since then, between 700 000 and 800 000 culture tests have been performed monthly. The percentage of positive cultures has been between 4% and 5%.

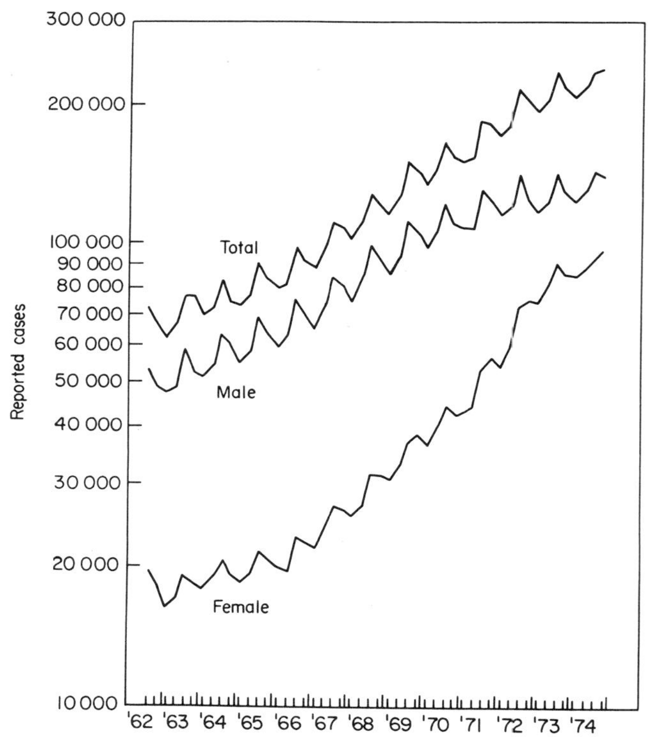

Fig. 3 *Reported cases of gonorrhea in the United States, 1962–1974, by sex and quarter*

Three points can be made from an examination of the quarterly trends of reported cases of gonorrhea in men and women from 1962–1974 (Fig. 3). First, the effect of the screening can be noted in the female trends, evidence by an upturn in 1972–1973. Second, there is a rather marked seasonal variation in reported incidence, with third quarter (July–September) peaks. Third, there is an apparent, and perhaps real, leveling off of the curve in reported male incidence.

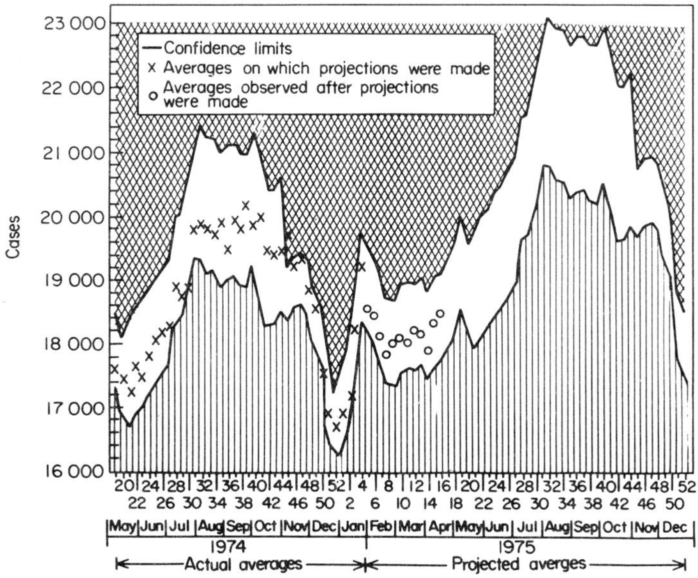

Fig. 4 *Projected 5 week moving average of reported cases of gonorrhea, United States, 1975 (based on 1974 trend and 1972–1974 seasonality)*

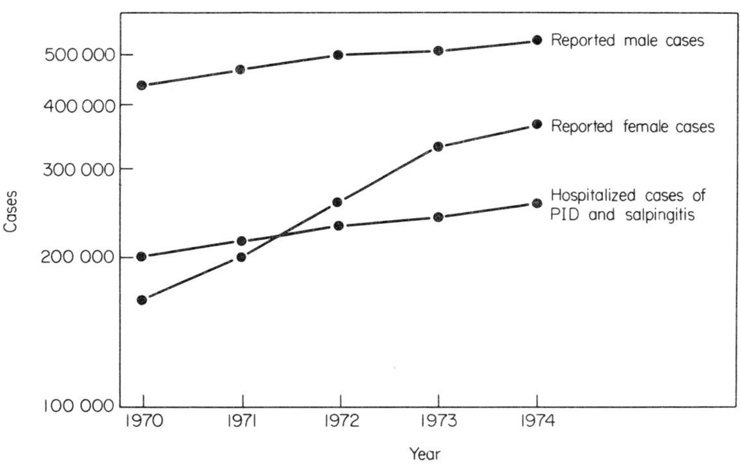

Fig. 5 *Reported cases of gonorrhea and estimated frequency of diagnoses of pelvic inflammatory disease and salpingitis among hospitalized females. United States, 1970–1974*

Based on weekly reports published by the Center for Disease Control in the *Morbidity and Mortality Weekly Report*, we have projected a 5-week moving average of cases, with confidence limits of two standard deviations for calendar year 1975 (Fig. 4). This projection is based upon 1974 trends (depicted by the stars) and seasonality in 1972–1974. The circles are the actual values since the projection. We hope that the reported cases, as indicated by the

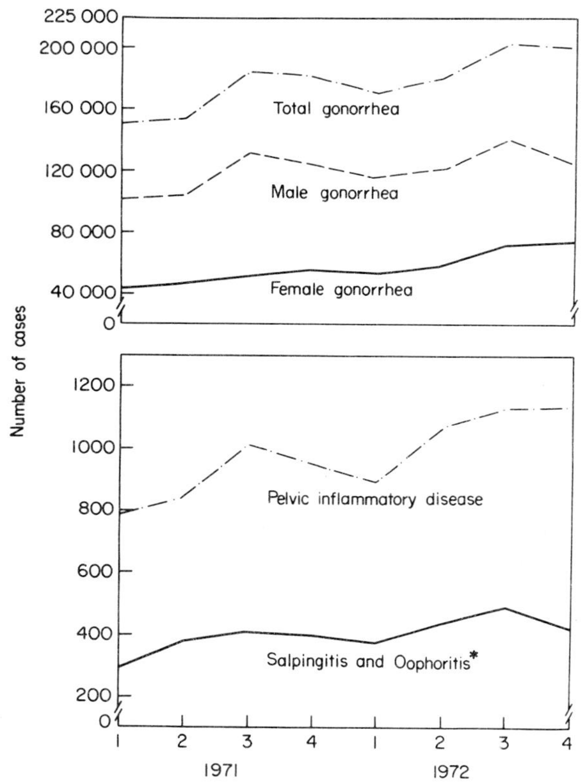

Fig. 6 *Reported gonorrhea cases by sex and quarter; salpingitis and oophoritis and pelvic inflammatory disease by quarter. United States, calendar years 1971–1972*

circles, will soon decline and drop below the lower limits, reflecting a declining trend of gonorrhea in the United States.

Some data show a close correlation between reported cases of male gonorrhea and pelvic inflammatory disease. As shown in Fig. 5, the two trends parallel each other for the period 1970–1974.

This correlation is more dramatically demonstrated in Fig. 6, where diagnosis of pelvic inflammatory disease (PID) follows closely the seasonality of gonorrhea. The close seasonal association between acute gonococcal urethritis in men and pelvic inflammatory disease among women suggests that PID is a relatively early complication of gonorrhea.

Conclusion

We are attempting to assess the real magnitude of several sexually transmitted infections heretofore essentially ignored in the US. We are experiencing focal areas of syphilis transmission and increased awareness of male homosexual transmission. We see some dampening of the gonorrhea epidemic.

Reference

Erikson G., Persson L. and Wessman J. (1975). *British Journal of Venereal Diseases* 51, 104–109

The Situation in the United Kingdom

C S Nicol
St Thomas's Hospital, London SE1 7EH

Two hundred and thirty clinics providing care for patients with sexually transmitted diseases (STD) are distributed throughout the United Kingdom. There are 30 in Greater London, 154 in the provinces, 2 in the Channel Islands, 1 in the Isle of Man, 14 in Wales, 18 in Scotland and 11 in Northern Ireland. (For details of the STD service system in Britain *see* Dr R D Catterall's paper, p 61.)

This report deals with the statistics for England and Wales from the Department of Health and Social Security (DHSS); separate figures are provided from the Scottish Home and Health Department and from the Northern Ireland Department of Health and Social Security.

Physicians in charge of clinics make quarterly returns of cases on Form SBH 60 (Fig. 1) to the Statistics Department at the DHSS. Each year a chapter on STD appears in the Chief Medical Officer's report on the health of the nation. The chapter includes an introduction, details of statistics obtained from SBH 60s and a discussion of the present position of the subject. In more recent years tables showing the number of cases of the various diseases related to 100 000s of population have been introduced (Tables 1 and 2). These figures can be compared with similar figures from

FORM SBH 60

DEPARTMENT OF HEALTH AND SOCIAL SECURITY

Return for the quarter ended 31 MAR 1975 to be made by
Physicians in charge of treatment centres

SEXUALLY TRANSMITTED DISEASES

Name and address of centre: ....
....

	PART A NEW CASES OF SYPHILIS	TOTAL	MALE	FEMALE
A1	Primary			
A2	Secondary			
A3	Latent in the first two years of infection			
A4	Cardio vascular			
A5	Of the nervous system			
A6	All other late and letent stages			
A7	Congenital aged under 2 years			
A8	Congenital aged 2 years and over			
	TOTAL OF LINES A1 to A8			
	PART B NEW CASES OF GONORRHOEA			
B1	Post-pubertal infections			
B2	Pre-pubertal infections			
B3	Ophthalmia neonatorum			
	TOTAL OF LINES B1 to B3			

	PART C NEW CASES OF OTHER GENITAL INFECTIONS			
C1	Chancroid			
C2	Lymphogranuloma Venereum			
C3	Granuloma Inguinale			
C4	Non-specific genital infection			
C5	Non-specific genital infection with arthritis			
C6	Trichomoniasis			
C7	Candidiasis			
C8	Scabies			
C9	Pubic lice (pediculosis pubis)			
C10	Herpes simplex			
C11	Warts (condylomata acuminata)			
C12	Molluscum Contagiosum			
	TOTAL OF LINES C1 to C12			
	PART D NEW CASES OF OTHER CONDITIONS			
D1	Other treponemal diseases			
D2	Other conditions requiring treatment in the centre			
D3	Other conditions not requiring treatment in the centre			
	TOTAL OF LINES D1 to D3			
	GRAND TOTAL OF PARTS A, B, C & D			

Fig. 1 *Form SBH 60 (Parts A–D)*

PART E **AGE GROUPS OF NEW CASES**

		SYPHILIS (lines A1 & A2)			GONORRHOEA (line B1)		
	AGE GROUP	TOTAL	MALE	FEMALE	TOTAL	MALE	FEMALE
1	Under 16						
2	16 and 17						
3	18 and 19						
4	20 to 24						
5	25 and over						
	TOTAL LINES 1 to 5						

PART F **LOCALITIES IN WHICH INFECTIONS TOOK PLACE**

	PRIMARY & SECONDARY SYPHILIS (Lines A1 and A2)	TOTAL	MALE	FEMALE
1	In locality of centre			
2	Elsewhere in Great Britain and Northern Ireland			
3	Outside Great Britain and Northern Ireland			
4	Not known			
	TOTAL OF LINES 1 to 4			
	POST PUBERTAL GONORRHOEA (line B1)			
5	In locality of centre			
6	Elsewhere in Great Britain and Northern Ireland			
7	Outside Great Britain and Northern Ireland			
8	Not known			
	TOTAL OF LINES 5 to 8			

PART G CONTACT ACTION AND DIAGNOSES

		TOTAL	MALE	FEMALE
	SYPHILIS			
1	Contact action taken ie number of contacts sought			
2	Contacts attending with syphilis			
3	Contacts attending, syphilis not diagnosed			
	GONORRHOEA			
4	Contact action taken ie number of contacts sought			
5	Contacts attending with gonorrhoea			
6	Contacts attending, gonorrhoea not diagnosed			

PLEASE REFER TO ACCOMPANYING NOTES

Signed ....

Physician in charge of treatment centre

Fig. 1 *Form SBH 60 (Parts E–G)*

other countries published by the World Health Organization. Trends in diseases such as syphilis, gonorrhoea and nonspecific genital infections can be followed over the years (Figs 2–5).

It is recognized, however, that statistics do not give the full picture of the incidence of sexually transmitted diseases in the whole

Table 1

The Venereal Diseases — new cases per 100 000 population, by age, seen at hospital clinics in England 1969–73

Disease	*1969*			*1973*		
	Male	*Female*	*Total*	*Male*	*Female*	*Total*
Early syphilis						
All ages	5.86	1.28	3.51	7.98	1.39	4.59
Early syphilis (primary and secondary only)						
All ages	4.43	0.87	2.60	5.75	0.90	3.26
Under 16	0.03	0.05	0.04	0.07	0.07	0.07
16 and 17	3.00	3.29	3.14	3.02	2.06	2.56
18 and 19	9.37	6.19	7.79	9.60	4.24	6.99
20–24	14.35	3.22	8.82	15.32	4.51	10.07
25 and over	4.87	0.56	2.59	7.00	0.65	3.64
Late syphilis						
All ages	3.75	2.45	3.08	3.52	1.58	2.52
Congenital syphilis						
All ages	0.38	0.61	0.50	0.27	0.43	0.35
Gonorrhoea (post-pubertal)						
All ages	158.34	60.84	108.26	167.40	87.04	126.10
Under 16	1.36	6.22	3.73	2.53	8.09	5.24
16 and 17	131.11	248.64	188.64	167.40	405.56	283.59
18 and 19	466.05	412.36	439.31	551.55	664.28	606.44
20–24	625.86	290.25	458.98	751.15	450.75	602.41
25 and over	151.23	31.49	88.00	150.80	41.61	93.08
Chancroid						
All ages	0.24	0.01	0.12	0.15	0.01	0.08

country; it is also recognized that improvement in certain details of statistical collection can be made. A meeting on epidemiology was held at the Medical Research Council in 1973 in the course of which Dr Valerie Beral presented a paper in which were listed categories of information not included in the CMO's report. These were: (1) Persons treated outside the clinics. (2) Persons who do not seek a

Table 2

Other sexually transmitted diseases and other conditions – new cases per 100 000 population at all ages and by sex seen at hospital clinics in England, 1969–1973

Disease	*1969*			*1970*			*1973*		
	Male	*Female*	*Total*	*Male*	*Female*	*Total*	*Male*	*Female*	*Total*
Lymphogranuloma venereum	0.13	0.02	0.07	0.18	–	0.08	0.23	0.03	0.13
Granuloma inguinale	0.01	–	0.01	0.03	–	0.01	0.02	0.01	0.02
Non-specific genital infection	178.20	–	–	204.79	–	–	301.70	62.54	178.80
Non-specific genital infection with arthritis	1.61	–	–	1.65	–	–	1.93	0.08	0.98
Trichomoniasis	–	–	–	5.73	61.00	34.12	7.16	73.48	41.22
Candidiasis	–	–	–	–	–	–	21.65	113.20	68.68
Scabies	–	–	–	–	–	–	9.36	1.90	5.53
Pubic lice (pediculosis pubis)	–	–	–	–	–	–	13.97	4.73	9.23
Herpes simplex	–	–	–	–	–	–	14.71	6.48	10.48
Warts (condylomata acuminata)	–	–	–	–	–	–	51.19	26.48	38.50
Molluscum contagiosum	–	–	–	–	–	–	2.13	0.74	1.42
Other treponemal diseases	2.20	1.15	1.82	2.28	1.38	1.81	2.43	1.32	1.86
Other conditions requiring treatment in a centre	–	–	–	–	–	–	111.10	44.00	76.67
Other conditions not requiring treatment in a centre	162.67	85.58	123.08	167.37	89.70	127.48	235.70	126.30	179.50

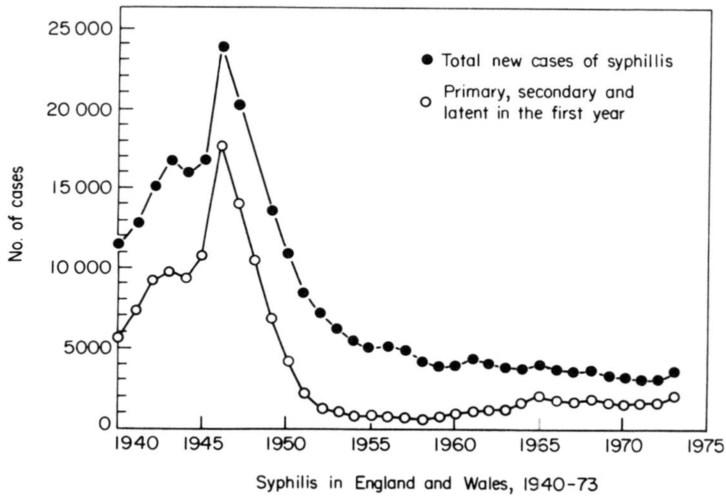

Fig. 2 *Syphilis in England and Wales, 1940–1973*

medical opinion. (3) Reporting numbers of cases *not* patients. (4) Full breakdown by age. (5) Differing diagnostic criteria between clinics. (6) Variations in reporting between clinics.

(*1*) *Treatment Outside Clinics*

SBH 60 returns do not include cases of STD treated by general practitioners under the NHS, or by GPs or specialists in private

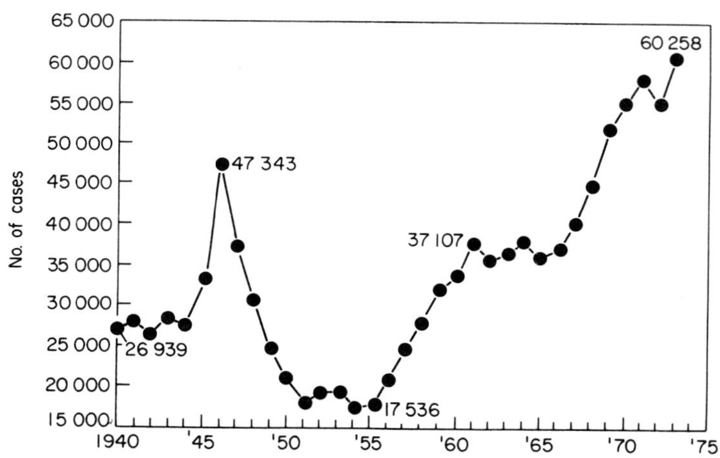

Fig. 3. *Number of cases of gonorrhoea dealt with for the first time in England and Wales from 1940*

practice or by the medical services of the Armed Forces. In 1959, at the request of the DHSS, the BMA, in cooperation with the British Cooperative Clinical Group (BCCG), circularized 1743 doctors in areas of London and the provinces: 562 replies were received concerning 455 STD cases. Of the doctors replying 84.4% were GPs and only 15.6% were specialists. It was estimated that if the cases treated outside the NHS were added to the SBH 60 returns there would have been a rise of one-quarter in figures for syphilis and one-seventh for gonorrhoea and nongonococcal urethritis (which were often not differentiated).

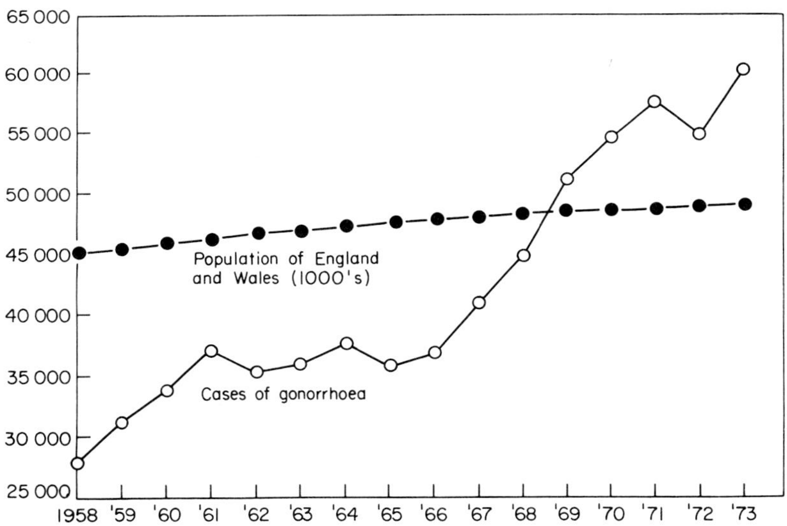

Fig. 4. *Cases of gonorrhoea in England and Wales 1958–1973*

In 1973 diagnostic kits were supplied to over 400 GPs in a certain area of London. In 20 specimens for men returned only 6 showed evidence of gonorrhoea. Eighteen specimens for women were returned unsolicited: none showed evidence of gonorrhoea. During this period of time the GPs referred 154 men and 42 women with gonorrhoea to the main clinic in the area, and it was estimated that 95% of them referred men with urethritis direct to a clinic. These findings suggest that in a country with a free health service providing STD clinics of high standard GPs will tend to refer cases for diagnosis, treatment, surveillance and contact action provided they receive medical reports on their patients from the clinics.

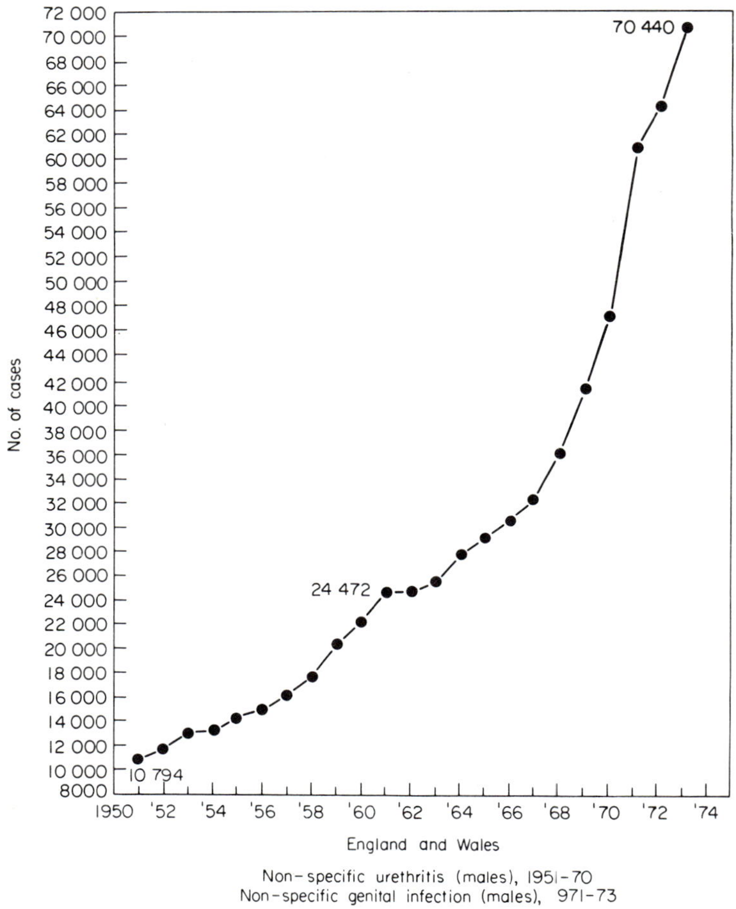

Fig. 5. *Nonspecific urethritis (1951–70) and genital infection (1971–73) in males, in England and Wales*

(2) *Cases in which no Medical Opinion is Sought*

The most likely reason for individuals with STD not seeking a medical opinion is that they are symptomless and therefore unaware of their infection. This situation is far commoner in women, but can occur in men, and can only be rectified by a fully integrated and active contact-tracing service in the clinics, which brings in the group at highest risk. This method is far more efficient and productive and far less expensive than methods of general population screening. In fact it is suggested that the more effective the STD contact-tracing service in any country, the lower the percentage of infections found when screening the public. Another possible reason for individuals not seeking an opinion is that they may be getting drugs for treatment from unauthorized persons. However, in this country the Venereal Diseases Act of 1917 imposes fines or imprisonment on any unqualified person who gives advice or offers facilities for treatment. There is further protection in the UK from the fact that antibiotics can only be dispensed by chemists on a doctor's prescription.

(3) *Reporting Cases not Patients*

Cases of individual diseases in patients are recorded on SBH 60, but patient numbers are returned on forms SH 3 as with other outpatient departments, so that the annual total patient numbers can be obtained from DHSS publications. A study in 1962 involving 7 large clinics was listed in the CMO's report (Ministry of Health 1963); it related to gonorrhoea, 10 323 cases of which were reported in 8694 male patients. However, to include as a matter of routine statistics for patients as well as cases on SBH 60s would impose an intolerable strain on the physicians in charge of clinics, who are reponsible for these returns. As an alternative, further periodic checks could be arranged with the help of the BCCG.

(4) *Breakdown by Age*

Full breakdown by age is not at present available in SBH 60s: rather more information is available on the equivalent form used in Scotland. A recent approach by the Scottish Home and Health

Table 3

Gonorrhoea-definitions

Newborn	: Ophthalmia neonatorum and/or infection of ano-genital orifices.
Pre- and post-pubertal	: Physician's judgement determines pre- or post-pubertal infection.
Lower genito-urinary tract infection	: Urethritis, tysonitis, cervicitis, bartholinitis, vulvitis, proctitis, etc.
Mouth, throat and eye infection	: Stomatitis, pharyngitis, tonsilitis, conjunctivitis, etc.
Upper genital tract complication	: Salpingitis and other pelvic involvement, prostatitis, epididymitis, cowpertitis, etc.
Systemic complications	: Gonococcaemia, septic dermatitis, arthritis, tenosynovitis, anterior uveitis, endocardititis, myositis, meningitis, etc.

Department is being taken up by the DHSS in the hope that forms can be standardized for the whole of the UK, which could also lead to UK statistics being made more readily and more rapidly available. In considering revised forms the suggested reporting form of the recent Council of Europe report by Guthe (1974) on STD must be looked at, particularly in relation to Section B (Tables 3 and 4). R. S. Morton (1975, personal communication) recently suggested that Item 3 in Section D of SBH 60 should be subdivided into cases not requiring treatment and a separate category, perhaps styled "D4", concerning cases requiring investigation and referral for treatment elsewhere. In this way, more accurate information about the time taken up by such cases could be provided in the Chief Medical Officer's annual report.

Table 4

Suggested model for a reporting form of sexually transmitted diseases (STD)

B. Gonorrhoea
Newborn
Pre-pubertal
Post-pubertal
with lower genito-urinary tract infection
with mouth and throat infection
with eye infection
with upper genital tract complications
with systemic complications
Total under B

(5) *Differing Diagnostic Criteria between Clinics*

This was illustrated by the BCCG gonorrhoea survey for 1968 (British Cooperative Clinical Group 1971), which was based on information obtained from 206 STD clinics in the UK. They found that it was the usual practice to report as gonorrhoea those cases with positive smear results. In 2% of clinics, however, gonorrhoea was reported only if smears were confirmed by culture; in addition, 6% of clinics reported gonorrhoea on clinical grounds, 9% on epidemiological grounds and 17% on combined clinical and epidemiological grounds. This survey again shows the value of the BCCG work in demonstrating reporting problems in the STD service. It is to be hoped that physicians in charge of clinics have noted these findings and, when necessary, have conformed with the majority in gonorrhoea reporting.

(6) *Variations in Reporting between Clinics*

Reporting practices may vary between clinics, within clinics, and from patient to patient. These variations can be reduced only if the senior medical staff make the final case note diagnosis for coding. Guidelines for diagnoses are also issued by the DHSS and are reviewed on an annual basis.

A balance must be kept: improving the standard of information provided by the statistical returns will involve extra work — care must be taken not to overburden the busy and often hard-pressed staff of STD clinics.

References

Beral, V. (1973). The Epidemiology of STD. Medical Research Council Sub-Committee on the Epidemiology of Sexually Transmitted Diseases (STD 73/3)

British Co-operative Clinical Group. (1971). *British Journal of Venereal Diseases* 47, 17

Department of Health and Social Security (1974). Annual Report of the Chief Medical Officer on the State of the Public Health for the Year 1973. HMSO, London; pp 48, 55, 56

Guthe, T. (1974). Sexually Transmitted Diseases (STD) — Scope and Control Measures. Council of Europe — European Public Health Committee, Strasbourg

Ministry of Health (1963). Annual Report on the State of the Public Health for the Year 1962. HMSO, London; p 64

Venereologists' Group Committee of the British Medical Association, and the British Cooperative Clinical Group (1959). *British Journal of Venereal Diseases* 35, 111

The World Picture

G M Antal
World Health Organization, Geneva

The World Health Organization has, in numerous articles, drawn attention to the extraordinarily high level and seemingly increasing trend of sexually transmitted diseases (STD) almost everywhere in the world. The latest review by Causse was published only recently in "Today's VD Control Problem" (1975) and was based on official reports received from some 67 countries: 25% of their total population live in countries which reported an increase in VD rates. It

Table 1

Veneral diseases reported to central government in Country "A" 1968–1974

Year	*Syphilis I and II*		*Gonorrhoea*		*Chancroid*	
	Cases	*Rate*	*Cases*	*Rate*	*Cases*	*Rate*
1968	856	9.8	8384	95.9	123	1.4
1969	599	6.8	7795	88.9	129	1.5
1970	598	6.8	7443	84.7	71	0.8
1971	678	7.7	7319	82.7	61	0.7
1972	921	10.4	8666	97.5	54	0.6
1973	503	5.7	3565	40.0	73	0.8
1974	493 ●	5.5	2857 ■	32.0	68	0.8

Rate per 100 000 population
● Male : female 11.6 : 1
■ Male : female 18.4 : 1

should be noted, however, that our information is rather incomplete as a number of countries do not publish data on STD for a variety of reasons. Furthermore, a close look at some of the data we do receive brings to light a completely different epidemiological situation from that indicated at first sight by the raw figures. Here are a few examples:

Country "A" (Table 1) reports a decrease in the number of syphilis cases and gonococcal infections. The disproportionate ratio of male to female cases seen by reporting services would indicate a much higher disease endemicity than the raw data show and it may be assumed that the decrease in the number of reported cases is more likely to have resulted from a shift of patients to non-reporting clinics.

Table 2

Venereal diseases: compulsory notifications in Country "B" 1968–1973

Year	*Early syphilis*		*Gonorrhoea*	
	Cases	*Rate*	*Cases*	*Rate*
1968	217	2.7	243	3.0
1969	296	3.6	239	2.9
1970	440	5.3	238	2.8
1971	757	8.8	374	4.3
1972	1757	20.0	739	8.0
1973	3785 ●	40.0	1784 ■	20.0

Rate per 100 000 population
● Male : female 2.6 : 1
■ Male : female 18.4 : 1
Note: Since 1972 syphilis case-finding programme

The raw statistical data from country "B" (Table 2), on the other hand, indicate a fivefold increase in reported early syphilis and gonorrhoea between 1971 and 1973. Additional information revealed that this increase coincided with the implementation of a VD control programme aimed at the detection of syphilis cases. It appears that the programme, which employed a multidisciplinary approach, had also motivated a large number of gonorrhoea patients to seek treatment at health centres.

In country "C" (Table 3), an organized VD control programme is being carried out over several years. A favourable male/female ratio among early syphilis cases and the virtual disappearance of congenital syphilis lead one to believe that the increase in the number of syphilis cases might be largely the result of intensive case-finding

Table 3

Venereal diseases reported by VD clinics in Country "C" 1968-1974

Year	*Early syphilis*		*Congenital syphilis*	*Gonorrhoea*	
	Cases	*Rate*	*Cases*	*Cases*	*Rate*
1968	448	43.9	5	8720	854.4
1969	443	43.1	—	8303	807.8
1970	464	45.2	—	10149	986.5
1971	501	48.5	1	8546	827.7
1972	448	42.7	—	8939	853.0
1973	523	49.2	1	10 451	982.2
1974	631 ●	57.1	—	7153 ■	647.3

Rate per 100 000 population
● Male : female 1.3 : 1
■ Male : female 11.3 : 1

efforts and may not necessarily represent an increased transmission of the disease. The unfavourable male/female ratio among detected gonorrhoea cases, which has actually deteriorated over recent years, would contradict a decrease in the gonorrhoea problem as indicated by this country's returns.

Considering that, by and large, national data on STD indicate only a fraction of the total extent of the problem, they clearly signify a public health problem of unparalleled magnitude (Table 4). Studies in Africa indicate that 20–40% of females of childbearing age suffer from a sexually transmitted disease, and a close correlation between high rates of infertility and gonococcal endemicity could be demonstrated. In Sri Lanka, both infectious syphilis and gonorrhoea increased by 25% between 1972 and 1973· and recent reports indicate a further significant increase. In New Zealand, the number of syphilis cases decreased by 26% between 1969 and 1973, but over the same period the number of gonococcal infections seen at government hospitals increased by 31% and that of nongonococcal urethritis by as much as 118%.

Large population movements caused by tourism or labour migration as well as socioeconomic changes favouring the transmission of these diseases tend to equalize intercountry differences in disease levels.

Table 4

Venereal diseases: prevalence in different groups (Africa)

Area and group	*N. gonorrh.*		*T. vaginalis*		*Candida*	
	Cases	*%*	*Cases*	*%*	*Cases*	*%*
Nigeria (Ibadan)						
130 symptomless, illiterate market women (Osoba 1972)	7	5	19	15	15	12
282 IUD acceptors (Onifade & Osoba 1972)	13	4.6	75	26.6	47	16.6
208 pregnant women (Osoba & Onifade 1973)	7	3.4	43	20.7	49	33.2
Kenya (Nairobi)						
100 FP clinic, 1st visit (Hopcraft *et al.* 1973)	17	17	22 ●	25	19	19
100 FP clinic users (Hopcraft *et al.* 1973)	22	22	24 ■	27	36	36
Kenya (rural)						
50 FP clinic, 1st visit (Hopcraft *et al.* 1973)	7	14	–▲	–▲	4	8
Uganda (rural)						
269 males, random (Arya *et al.* 1973)	24	8.9	–▲	–▲	–▲	–▲
295 females, random (Arya *et al.* 1973)	54	18.3	–▲	–▲	–▲	–▲

● Out of 88 tested
■ Out of 90 tested
▲ Not tested

Since official morbidity data may, at the most, indicate trends in VD levels, there is an urgent need to supplement these data by epidemiological studies indicating disease levels in representative population groups, and aiming at the delineation of high-risk groups, using acceptable diagnostic techniques and thus permitting international comparison. In addition, we may look for other indicators of endemicity levels in the population (e.g. hospital admissions for ectopic gestation, &c.) to evaluate disease trends and to design and propose relevant and more epidemiologically-based national STD control programmes. With the anticipated intensification of the activities of the World Health Organization in the area of sexually transmitted diseases, and with the knowledge and tools developed by research groups all over the world, we hope that an increasing number of countries will initiate well-organized STD control activities with a built-in self-evaluation mechanism, and that this will automatically lead to an improvement in the relevance of official morbidity data.

The technical discussions on the control of STD which took place in May 1975 during the 28th World Health Assembly were a complete success. In the opinion of the 200 or so participants, sexually transmitted diseases are one of the most important public health problems in the world today. Even though most countries lack epidemiological data of sufficient accuracy to appreciate the full extent of the problem, there was full recognition of an urgent need to take steps to ameliorate the situation. The complexity and magnitude of the problem, lack of trained manpower and financial resources, coupled with the misconception that a specialized highly technical service is a *conditio sine qua non*, have been the main constraints to the implementation of control activities. It was agreed that STD control services should be an integral part of the general health services and should form a part of the overall communicable disease control programme, particularly in developing countries.

While it was the consensus that a multidisciplinary approach should be aimed at in the control of sexually transmitted diseases, discussions centred on the practical measures which have to be taken for the stepwise implementation of a technically sound control programme. The need was stressed for WHO to assist member countries in the evaluation of the disease problem, in the training of health manpower and in giving advice on control techniques relative to resources, the epidemiological situation and level of the health infrastructure. The need for increased basic research with relevance to a public health programme was also stressed and encouraged.

Stimulated by the technical discussions, a resolution (WHA 28.58) was passed by the World Health Assembly requesting member states to collect, disseminate and communicate to WHO epidemiological and statistical information, to strengthen STD control activities, and to increase the training of health workers and medical professionals in STD. At the same time the resolution requests WHO to provide member countries with assistance in the evaluation of the STD problem, to assist and support training and educational activities, to establish guidelines for the organization of control activities, including technical specifications, and to support and coordinate research activities.

It was apparent that member countries expect WHO to concern itself more actively with the practical problems of implementing control programmes in the field, taking into consideration differences in cultural settings and in levels of proficiency in the health infrastructure, and the possible adjustments in well-proven control techniques necessitated by local conditions and resources. New methodologies and organizational patterns for the control of these diseases may need to be sought, particularly so as to permit the optimal use of existing infrastructures, both at the central level and at the level of local health units as a basis for prevention, case-finding and treatment under optimum cost-effectiveness conditions. Thus, while a diagnostic work up may be important in countries with a good and readily available laboratory system, in developing countries with a high disease incidence it may be preferable — as a first step — to treat cases and their contacts on the basis of clinical diagnosis rather than do nothing. The establishment of a central unit for reference, evaluation of the programme and training could form a useful element for the promotion of a national control programme.

Full justification and encouragement is given to fundamental research with the aim of providing the clinician, the laboratory and the epidemiologists with simple, effective and low cost methods of diagnosis and treatment, and of developing specific preventive measures. Research activities deserving equally high priority would be in the field of psychosocial and behavioural factors which promote the spread of STDs, so that preventive measures, e.g. health education, can be better adjusted and improved, as well as operational research, in order to determine and recommend a methodology and an organization of this infrastructure relative to health priorities and economic and health manpower potential of each country.

References

Arya O. P., Nsanzumuhire N. and Taber S. R. (1973). *Bulletin of the World Health Organization* **49**, 587–595

Causse, G. (1975). *In* Today's VD Control Problem. American Social Health Association, New York; pp 47–52

Hopcraft, M., Verhagen, A. R., Ngigi, S. and Haga, C. A. (1973). *Bulletin of the World Health Organization* **48**, 581–585

Onifade, A. and Osoba, A. O. (1972). *Journal of Tropical Medicine and Hygiene* **75**, 213–216

Osoba, A. O. (1972). *British Journal of Venereal Diseases* **48**, 116–120

Osoba, A. O. and Onifade, A. (1973). *West African Medical Journal* **22**, 23–25

Society and High-risk Groups

R R Willcox
St Mary's Hospital, London W2 and
King Edward VII Hospital, Windsor

I. Factors Leading to High-risk Groups

The term "high-risk group" has never been properly defined, and in the same context the meaning of "society" is somewhat different depending on whether it is regarded from a group, local, national or international standpoint. Indeed, all persons who contract a sexually transmitted disease could be considered to be a high-risk group compared with those who do not.

In this paper high-risk groups are defined as groups of persons able to be classified by reasons of age, sex, occupational, geographical, behavioural, psychological or other characteristics who have a higher than average chance of contracting venereal disease as indicated either by a higher yield of positive results by screening tests, a higher annual incidence or more repeated infections per unit of time. The term "higher than average" is a fair one as the average itself is compounded to include the infections of those of higher risk.

These indices are generally related only to syphilis and gonorrhoea as these diseases are more readily diagnosed and reported. Quite a different picture may emerge if other sexually transmitted conditions such as nongonococcal urethritis, trichomoniasis, Type II herpesvirus infections, genital warts, &c., are also included, the picture thus becoming considerably larger and more blurred.

Indeed it may justly be stated that with very few exceptions all society is at risk at some time and that the difference between those who contract no infections in their life and many of those who do so but once may be dictated more by luck than behaviour.

The basic factors which lead to membership of a high-risk group are multiple sex contacts, indiscrimination in the choice of partners, failure to take precautions and the frequency of repetition.

Multiple Sex Contacts

These may be considered to be due to the natural sexual urge associated with greater opportunity, failure to make a lasting relationship, or financial reward.

Natural sexual urge: The young man has always sown his wild oats. Some experimentation, desire for sense of adventure or "trophy hunting" is natural. In the past, in most societies, acceptance of this did not extend to young girls, who were chaperoned to prevent it, and on whom society imposed a number of brakes in terms of religious, family, tribal, group, marital and other influences which were combined with fears of pregnancy and venereal disease.

The latter have been important. It is probably true that if there were no sexually transmitted disease, and if man could be sure that the children he was helping to rear were indeed his own, universal free sex might well have been the norm. After all, it was St Paul who said it is better to marry than burn.

In the present permissive society the brakes have been removed or loosened. With the demand for full sex equality the double standard between the sexes has largely gone and women have their rights to experiences which may lead to the contraction of venereal disease along with the men; as a result the clinics of this country now find their originally smaller facilities for dealing with the female sex under greater strain than those for the males.

With modern channels of communication this greater sexual freedom amongst the young has spread widely within a frame of the more traditional ideas amongst the old in virtually all parts of the world.

The present climate of opinion concerning sex, however desirable it may be thought to be concerning sexual expression, can hardly be conducive to the suppression of venereal disease. This is typified by the advertisement of an institute of sex education which endorses an "aesthetic view of human sexuality emphasizing the value of sexuality and of proficiency, rather than constraint" and offers week-end courses on the sensual and sexual enrichment of couples (which married and single persons can attend at $65.00 per couple). Its brochure states that "seating is on pillows on the floor – informal comfortable clothing is advised" (Mid-West Association 1975).

Greater opportunities for sexual encounter: In this situation, and partly because of it, social and technical progress has provided many more opportunities for the sexes to meet, while the introduction of sexually transmitted diseases into previously "closed" circles of sexual encounter, with the subsequent rapid spread within them, has magnified the situation considerably.

The factors involved here include increased urbanization and industrialization, more female employment, more coeducation and more universities; while greater affluence, or search and hopes for greater affluence, resulted in increased migration of labour and of business and pleasure travel (Causse 1975)

Failure to make a lasting sexual relationship: This may be temporary or long-term. It frequently results from occupational reasons in the male and is sometimes associated with temporary loneliness and consequent mating with high-risk females. However, in its long-term sense there is usually a more deep-seated psychological reason such as, for example, a dislike of accepting the responsibilities and costs of marriage; a desire for anonymity in order to perform certain sexual practices; and – particularly in the female – from a sense of inadequacy, loneliness or rejection combined with an anxiety to please, or of antagonism to parents or society. Such a failure may follow an earlier parental failure in the same situation and a previously unsatisfactory or absent family life. Indeed the increase in venereal diseases inherent to our times has been equated with other indices of social ill health (Morton 1973), including crimes of violence and theft, divorces, abortions, &c., when a similar background may be cited.

Gain: Prostitution has always been with us and doubtless always will be. Although in Europe and North America it now has a relatively minor role in the spread of venereal disease it remains a major cause of infection in India, the Far East, Africa and South America (Willcox 1958). It is fostered by lack of female employment, and the prospect of a financial return impossible to achieve by other means. It accompanies the merchandizing of alcohol and its followers are often exploited by criminal syndicates. Nevertheless, it is also pursued for preference and there are some "happy hookers" (Hollander 1973).

Lack of Discrimination

The possibilities of infection in the partner may differ widely, as has been shown by screening tests for gonorrhoea. In the United States, for example, screening tests for gonorrhoea have shown infection rates of 5% in correction or detention centres, 1.9–3.3% in family planning clinics and 2.8–3.9% amongst hospital in-patients and out-patients (American Social Health Association 1975). However, as it is only certain members of such groups who indulge in repeated multisexual activity the proportion of infections in those who do is much higher.

Although discrimination is a dangerous guide in individual cases ("But she was clean, doctor!" or "She was a nurse, doctor!" being repeatedly heard expressions of incredulity from patients when being presented with a diagnosis of sexually transmitted disease) lack of it may play a significant part in circumstances in which a choice *can* be made of less rather than more promiscuous partners.

Lack of discrimination may result from lack of opportunity of alternative choice, ignorance, poverty, an inherent inability or from the influence of alcohol.

Failure to Take Precautions

This may be due to ignorance of prophylactic techniques or their value; a dislike of available methods; a lack of fear of venereal disease and, in repeaters, a failure to benefit from past experience; a "Russian roulette"-like feeling of piquancy or excitement if they are not used and the very common factor – which already may have led to an indiscriminate choice of contact – alcohol.

Existing method using the condom are frequently individually or socially unacceptable and there is a return to the investigation of chemical techniques for use by the female.

Antibiotic prophylaxis is also effective but carries greater dangers to the community in terms of developing resistance not only of venereally transmitted organisms but of many bacteria which prohibit its widespread use. Vaccines are still far distance and so there is a need for new methods. The possibilities of ion-liberating coils have been considered (Fiscina *et al.* 1973). Nevertheless it has been calculated that if existing methods were used by only a quarter of patients and were only 50% successful a dramatic fall in incidence would ensue (Lee *et al.* 1972).

Number of Exposures per Unit of Time

The most essential factor which leads to inclusion in a high-risk group is the number of exposures per unit of time. This figure may be modified by feasibility, opportunity, inclination or compulsion.

This is a very variable figure and patients attending venereal disease clinics provide a spectrum of admitted previous sexual exposure with different persons which ranges from nil to 200 or more before the age of 30, while figures of 100 or more in a year for some persons have also been quoted (Gebhard 1971).

Mathematical Models

Basic considerations: Basically, therefore, the chances of acquiring infections from multiple sex contacts depend on three factors: (1) The number of exposures per unit of time. (2) The proportion of the sexual contacts who are infected. (3) The chance of acquiring the disease from a single exposure.

Table 1

Average number of new exposures required for infection

Partners infected (%)	*Chance of contraction/single exposure (%)*					
	100	*50*	*25*	*10*	*5*	*2.5*
1	100	200	400	1000	2000	4000
2.5	40	80	160	400	800	1600
5	20	40	80	200	400	800
10	10	20	40	100	200	400
25	4	8	16	40	80	160
50	2	4	8	20	40	80
100	1	2	4	10	20	40

The last depends on sex (chances significantly greater for women than for men), disease (chances greater for gonorrhoea than syphilis), and how far prophylactic measures have been used. On the other hand, because of more frequent asymptomatic infections in the female, the chances of the partner being infected are higher in that sex. The average number of new exposures required to contract infection according to these factors can be readily calculated (Table 1).

Men: Assuming, in heterosexual males, that the chance of acquiring infection from an infected female is 25% (a calculation for gonorrhoea has been made of 22%; Holmes *et al.* 1970), the average duration in years before infection occurs according to the number of exposures per year and likelihood of infection in the partner is shown in Table 2. Thus, a businessman making one overseas trip a year and consorting with prostitutes 100% infected could, if he

Table 2

Men: average duration in years before infection occurs – no precautions (25% risk of infection)

No. of exposures per year	*Likelihood of infection in partner (%)*				
	5	*10*	*25*	*50*	*100*
1	80	40	16	8	4
2	40	20	8	4	2
4	20	10	4	2	1
8	10	5	2	1	0.5
16	5	2.5	1	0.5	0.25
32	2.5	1.25	0.5	0.25	0.13
64	1.25	0.63	0.25	0.13	0.06

With partial precautions (12.5% risk) the duration of time doubles
With complete precautions (2.5% risk) it increases tenfold

indulged on every occasion, be expected to last four years without infection if he used no precautions, and to complete his sexual lifetime in freedom if he wore a condom. Should he make 8 trips a year and wear a condom on half of them he will be infected once yearly. It is the number of exposures which is decisive. Even with only a 5% infection rate in the partners, 64 exposures with different partners in a year will result in infection every $1\frac{1}{4}$ years.

If the male was able to discriminate so as to consort with females only 5–10% of whom were infected he might do so 4 times a year for ten to twenty years without either precautions or infection, and 8 times a year for five to ten years.

Table 2 may also be used to illustrate why nongonococcal urethritis is a greater numerical problem than gonorrhoea if it is assumed that a female with, say, a 5% likelihood of carrying the gonococcus has a 10% chance of carrying chlamydia. The chances of catching nongonococcal urethritis would be twice as great for the same number of exposures.

Women: Women are less fortunate in that the chances of infection with gonorrhoea following intercourse with an infected man are virtually 100% although, as the infected man is more frequently symptomatic, she theoretically has the chance of discrimination by rejecting an infected partner or insisting on precautions. The overall incidence of asymptomatic infections is, however, greater than in the male. A mathematical model for women is presented in Table 3.

Here again the number of exposures is all-important. The sexually unsatisfied but otherwise maritally adjusted or resigned female who takes her holiday abroad for occasional extramarital indulgence twice

Table 3

Women: average duration in years before infection occurs – no precautions (100% risk of infection)

No. of exposures per year	*Likelihood of infection in partner (%)*				
	1	*2.5*	*5*	*10*	*25*
1	100	40	20	10	4
2	50	20	10	5	2
4	25	10	5	2.5	1
8	12.5	5	2.5	1.25	0.5
16	6.25	2.5	1.25	0.63	0.25
32	3.13	1.25	0.63	0.31	0.13
64	1.56	0.63	0.31	0.16	0.06
128	0.78	0.31	0.16	0.08	0.03

With partial precautions (50% risk) the duration of time doubles
With complete precautions (10% risk) it increases tenfold

yearly could on average last for twenty years before becoming infected if she could discriminate so as to confine her favours to those with only a 2.5% risk of being infected – even without precautions. A promiscuous young girl, on the other hand, consorting with those with a 10% chance of infection and switching partners 16 times in a year would become infected every $7\frac{1}{2}$ months.

These are, of course, only theoretical considerations, but they do illustrate clearly that for those who are caught many more escape, and are more likely to do so if they practise moderation, discrimination or prophylaxis – particularly if used in combination. The present methods of prophylaxis have largely been unacceptable, whether individually or socially, but the Tables nevertheless illustrate the reasons behind the motivation of those who seek improved prophylactic methods.

Conclusions

(1) While high-risk groups are composed of those who frequently change their partners, membership of such a group depends on how often the partner is switched, the likelihood of infection in the partner and what, if any, precautions are taken.
(2) Mathematical models for the two sexes in relation to these factors can, to some extent, be used to assess probable sexual activity in venereal disease patients, especially those with known repeated infections, or the prevalance of disease in their partners when the number of exposures is known.
(3) While multiplicity of exposure is all-important, moderation in terms of frequency, discrimination in the choice of partners, and care in the taking of precautions can allow multiplicity to continue for long periods without a person becoming infected and qualifying for inclusion in a high-risk group.
(4) Those who do qualify, therefore, tend to be immoderate, nondiscriminating, ignorant, feckless or careless, but all are influenced by opportunity and by the general attitude of society to such behaviour.

II. Illustrations of High-risk Groups

In this part of the paper illustrations are given of some generally accepted high-risk groups and indications are given of how they are influenced by the factors outlined. Such groups can be broadly classified according to occupation or behaviour.

Those based on occupation include seamen, military personnel, immigrant and other migrant workers including commercial travellers, stage and club entertainers, tourists, peripatetic businessmen and conference attenders, those engaged in the travel business including airline personnel and long-distance lorry drivers. These people are the mobile recipients, often obtaining infections from each other and from the providers, who are locally-based prostitutes and other promiscuous women, hostesses, hotel and bar employees and bath attendants. The essential factors involving these groups are mobility, enhanced opportunities for sexual contact, an absence of their normal sexual outlets and diminished restraint in the receivers and often the prospects of financial or other gain in the providers.

A few occupations are listed as being of high risk to others although not necessarily to themselves. These include blood donors, barbers and those who work in children's institutions – for some of whom obligatory serum tests for syphilis are required in many countries. Glassblowers were at one time at special risk from syphilis (Wilcox 1967*a*).

Those in high-risk groups based on behaviour include those unable to form stable relationships, among whom are the emotionally immature, those with marital breakdown, the psychologically disturbed, the socially deprived, prostitutes, delinquents, prisoners, commune dwellers, vagabonds, free lovers, group sex participators, male homosexuals and above all "repeaters" who really represent an index of a high-risk group rather than a group in themselves.

Obviously, behavioural and occupational factors are interwoven, the two combining to compound the risk. For example, participants at a medical conference may perhaps be a lower risk than attenders at a pop festival, and a heterosexual Turkish bath attendant is at little if any greater than normal risk because of his occupation but a homosexual bath attendant very much more so.

Other factors may be superimposed to increase the risk such as age and domicile.

Young Persons

Persons of the age group 20–24 years in males and slightly less in females are those at the greatest risk. They are followed by those aged 25–29 years in males and 15–19 years in females (Table 4).

Thus a male aged 40–49 years has approximately 18 times less risk of contracting gonorrhoea, and a female nearly 36 times less, than in their early 20s. The differences are related to sexual activity, experimentation before settling down and other factors. Such figures, however, concern only reported infections; since many older males are more able to pay for private treatment a greater proportion of their infections may not appear in the statistics. The young – who

Table 4

Gonorrhoea – USA 1972 – specific case rates per 100 000 by age (American Social Health Association 1974)

Age in years	*Male*	*Female*	*Male : female ratio*
0–14	10.3	25.1	0.41
15–19	1075.6	995.0	1.08
20–24	2593.0	1110.5	2.33
25–29	1416.2	456.0	2.86
30–39	560.8	148.1	3.79
40–49	141.9	31.1	4.56
50+	22.4	5.1	4.39
Total	506.1	246.0	2.06

are maturing earlier – are more closely involved in the changing attitudes and behaviour of present-day society than the old, and in recent years venereal disease rates in a number of countries (e.g. USA and UK) have increased more rapidly amongst the 15–19 year olds than in older persons.

The much higher rates among those aged 20–24 years are enhanced during student life at universities, where high annual infection rates, up to 25–30%, have been reported (Arya & Bennett 1967, Willcox 1967*b*, Juhlin 1968). Travelling students of whom there are increasing numbers, are particularly at risk (Siboulet 1976). This is in spite of the fact that such persons should be better informed than the remainder of the community; nevertheless they are often ignorant concerning venereal disease.

However, age is only one factor and wide regional differences may be found. For example, in the USA in 1973 the gonorrhoea rates for the 20–24 year olds were nearly 7 times higher and amongst the 15–19 year olds 16 times higher in Florida than in the State of Vermont (American Social Health Association 1975).

Table 5

Male : female ratio in gonorrhoea (King Edward VII Hospital, Windsor)

Year	*Total*	*Male*	*Female*	*Male : female ratio*
1962	69	60	9	6.7 : 1
1965	95	77	18	4.3 : 1
1968	136	97	39	2.5 : 1
1969	179	120	59	2.0 : 1
1971	142	91	51	1.8 : 1
1974	195	114	81	1.4 : 1

With the increased emancipation and liberation of women which has accompanied changing behavioural patterns and attitudes, the female is at greater risk from venereal disease than formerly. In spite of the many more known infections in homosexual males, and no counter-balancing equivalent amongst lesbian women, there has been a remarkable shortening of the male:female ratio amongst patients with gonorrhoea (Table 5) – although improved diagnosis and increased willingness to attend must play some part.

Town Dwellers

With technical progress, industrialization and urbanization have vastly expanded in recent years. The resultant large conurbations attract many floating populations and provide greater anonymity, with consequently much greater difficulties in contact tracing. There is, therefore, a much greater concentration of venereal disease in the larger towns and cities (Guthe and Willcox 1971). For example, in the USA in 1972 (American Social Health Association 1973) it was found that 70.5% of the reported cases of gonorrhoea occurred in 55 cities which made up only 33.6% of the population; and 73.2% of the reported cases of primary and secondary syphilis occurred in 63 cities which made up 34% of the population.

Some Occupational Groups

Seamen: Lacking the opportunity for stable relationships and released ashore after long spells at sea to consort with high-risk prostitutes, seamen have traditionally been a high-risk group. In the past, venereal infections have been shown to be 16–20 times more common in water than in land populations (Eng and Jenson 1960, Guthe and Idsøe 1964).

However, in recent decades changes have occurred in the pattern of life of many seafarers with new types of vessels providing improved accommodation and recreational facilities for the crews and sometimes opportunities for wives to accompany their husbands. The flying of crew members from their homeland bases, better port hostels and clubs for seafarers, reduced opportunities for going ashore in many ports as a result of offshore loading and discharging, and quick turnarounds, have also played some part (Cross and Harris 1976). Seamen today would seem to be less at risk than formerly.

Military: Soldiers, like sailors, have always had high rates of infection. They, too, are sexually active and often lack opportunities for stable relationships and, moreover, their only available sexual outlet is with prostitutes and others with a high incidence of infection. Also, in war zones they are subject to very considerable strain, or the prospect of it.

The reported rates are well documented in respect of the US forces. In 1972 (American Social Health Association 1974) the projected incidence per 1000 of venereal disease in the US Army was as follows: for the forces in Europe, 20.64 per 1000; In Japan 28.08; in the continental USA 39.72; in Central and South America 105.84; in Okinawa 116.16; in Thailand 641.16; in Korea 700.08; and in Vietnam 739.56.

In the Far East the rates are indeed very high, the equivalent of 74% being infected in one year in Vietnam. The "excellent showing" in Europe, where the infection rates were virtually half those in the continental USA, has been commented upon by Greenberg (1972) as unlikely to be due to mutual unattractiveness but rather, perhaps, to a greater control of prostitution in Germany and possibly to more treatment by nonmilitary agencies with consequent under-reporting.

Figures in the military must be related to the incidence of disease in the different civilian populations, i.e. to the possibility of infection in the partner. For example, in 1972 the reported incidence of gonorrhoea in the civilian population in the USA (349.7 per 100 000 – American Social Health Association 1974), where four-fifths of the cases are unreported (McKenzie Pollack 1970), was three times higher than in England and Wales (Department of Heath and Social Security 1973) where it is believed the majority of cases are reported. Indeed the military figure for the continental USA (3972 per 100 000) may be contrasted with those of 2044 – 4351 per 100 000 for gonorrhoea alone amongst those aged 20–24 years in the civilian populations of 14 American States during the same year (American Social Health Association 1974). Likewise in the Far East, in Thailand, Korea and Vietnam, where these rates are vastly exceeded, the venereal disease rates amongst the civilian population may also be vast. It was estimated at one time, for example, that 40 000 cases of gonorrhoea were occurring *each week* in Vietnam (Greenberg 1972).

However, it is more pertinent to attempt to establish who comprise the high-risk group within a high-risk group. The data of Siler (1943), quoted by Greenberg (1972), relating to servicemen leaving Korea showed that 72% contracted no venereal disease; of those who did threequarters had had only one attack and one-quarter (7% of the total) suffered 2–7 attacks. Does this 7% indicate the real high-risk group?

Migrant labourers: There are more than 6 million international migrant labourers of both sexes in Europe alone, the majority breaching an economic gap between developed and developing countries. Most are sexually active 18–35 year olds, the men tend to stay longer than the women (Radovanovic 1976), and 20–30% return to their homelands each year to be replaced by new recruits (WHO 1972).

There are also many internal migrant workers throughout the world such as lorry drivers, salesmen, &c., as well as seasonal workers engaged in agriculture or industry. These move from town to town and in many areas there may be a local male : female imbalance (Sowmini 1976). These persons have broken away from the traditional family and tribal circle and from racial, language and cultural barriers, and in consequence suffer from a sense of isolation and loneliness. With a lack of opportunity for a stable sexual relationship they consort either with prostitutes or with promiscuous young girls.

There is considerable evidence that migrant workers entering one country from another import very little venereal disease (Luger 1976, Fanta *et al.* 1976, Tardieu *et al.* 1976), and by contracting high rates in their host countries they are the victims rather than the cause (Tardieu *et al.* 1976). West Indian male immigrants in Britain, for example, have been shown to have gonorrhoea rates some 19 times higher than the same age groups of the home population (Willcox 1970).

Tourists: There are some 215 million tourists in the world today (Caletti 1975) who spend an average of two to five nights in one spot, which is shorter than the incubation period of many of the sexually transmitted diseases.

The group is a heterogenous one which includes students and young persons on holiday, families on vacation, business men and conference attenders. Students and young persons travelling alone are those at greatest risk.

Those not travelling with their families or girl friend frequently consort with other tourists on the same or kindred package tour ("The Dane in Spain consorts mainly with the Dane" – see WHO 1972; the same "like consorting with like" may be said of airline personnel). Indeed the prospect of a "conquest" with one or more persons is part of the anticipated "holiday". Hippy travellers are even more at risk being part of a closed group often involved with group sex. The businessman, on the other hand, frequently strays with the high-class prostitute or entertainer. Opportunity is related to the number of trips he may be required to undertake, as he may behave in this way only when removed from the restraining influences of his home environment and faced with the alternative of a lonely hotel or uncongenial lounge.

Some Behavioural Groups

Homosexuals: Since a more tolerant attitude towards homosexuality between consenting adults has been adopted in many countries a high proportion of male homosexuals has been found in patients with venereal disease, particularly primary and secondary syphilis in the larger cities – exceeding 50% in some areas (Guthe and Willcox 1971, Causse 1975). Such is by no means apparent in all areas but is so where homosexuals feel less inhibited in discussing their behaviour and cooperating in contact tracing. Data from the United Kingdom are shown in Table 6. The phenomenon at first sight appears less marked for gonorrhoea than for primary and secondary syphilis, but as gonorrhoea was 23.5 times more common than primary and secondary syphilis in the West End clinics and the proportion of syphilitic homosexuals only 2.7 times greater than those with gonorrhoea the numbers of known homosexuals with gonorrhoea were in fact nearly 8.9 times greater than those with primary and secondary syphilis (Willcox 1974).

Table 6

Percentage of homosexually acquired infections – UK 1971 (British Cooperative Clinical Group 1973)

Disease	*Total cases in study*	*Percentage homosexually acquired*				
		Wales	*Scotland*	*England*	*London*	*London West End*
Primary and secondary syphilis	924	9.5	13.5	45.9	62.1	73.3
Gonorrhoea	36 242	4.0	4.1	10.5	19.9	27.6

The reasons for high venereal disease rates amongst homosexuals compared with heterosexuals are many and complex and include the tendency of homosexuals to aggregate in large urban areas to preserve anonymity with consequent greater difficulties in contact tracing, considerable promiscuity amongst some and a tendency towards group exchange instead of mating in pairs. In addition there is a frequent unawareness of the disease among both patients and physicians and there are greater difficulties in diagnosis.

Prostitutes

Pattern of prostitution: Although prostitution in the classical sense was outlawed by the United Nations in 1959 it has in fact only altered its pattern. In many countries changing attitudes and behaviour have rendered the prostitute largely redundant, and in consequence she is now responsible only for the minority of infections. In others, especially in Africa, the Far East and South America, prostitutes are still the major source.

In such areas the economic framework, lack of employment for women and economic gain are all important. Almost universally, however, they will exist to fill the demand created largely by travellers and mobile groups.

Sociopsychiatric studies of prostitutes have frequently shown that they suffer from inadequate family and educational background, immaturity, low intelligence – sometimes with a history of alcohol and/or drug addiction – and psychopathological traits (Guthe and Willcox 1971), but the fact remains that women can earn more by this means than is otherwise possible in a manner they do not necessarily consider uncongenial

Society accepts prostitution – in Great Britain it can be said to be permitted if not causing a public nuisance – and in some areas of a number of countries (e.g. Germany, parts of the USA) there has even been a return to officially tolerated "houses".

Venereal infections in prostitutes: The prostitute comprises the greatest (and oldest) high-risk group for venereal disease. High rates of infection in prostitutes reaching 90–100% have in the past been reported in numerous countries, including for example, Austria, Egypt, France, Greece, India, Iraq, Malaysia, Philippines, Portugal and Turkey (Willcox 1958).

The possibility of infection depends on the number of partners per week, the infection rate in the clientele (which may or may not be open to selection), the precautions taken and the degree of voluntary or compulsory medical control.

The number of partners is dictated by the economics of the situation in relation to available clientele (Table 7). The equivalent of the prices indicated in sterling cover the wide range admitted as currently being paid by patients attending venereal disease clinics in many parts of the world. The richer the clientele the fewer the number of exposures likely.

With regard to anticipated infections in prostitutes it is the number of exposures per unit of time which is all-important. The anticipated number of infections likely to arise in prostitutes according to the number of exposures are shown in Table 8. It is apparent that if no precautions are taken all prostitutes with a clientele exceeding 1000 a year (20 a week) serving a population with one in 20 (5%) or more infected will acquire an infection at least once

Table 7

The economics of the prostitute, showing the price charged in relation to number of contacts and annual income

Annual no. of contacts	*Annual income*			
	£1000	*£2000*	*£4000*	*£8000*
10 000 (200 per week)	10p	20p	40p	80p
5000 (100 per week)	20p	40p	80p	£1.60
2000 (40 per week)	50p	£1.00	£2.00	£4.00
1000 (20 per week)	£1.00	£2.00	£4.00	£8.00
500 (10 per week)	£2.00	£4.00	£8.00	£16.00
100 (2 per week)	£10.00	£20.00	£40.00	£80.00

weekly and will be found, at weekly checks, to be continually infected. Such checks therefore serve little useful purpose in this situation. Even if only one in 100 of the clients is infected the same applies to women having 100 or more contacts in a week – which may be a female pattern in the poorer areas of a number of countries.

Even those charging £20–£80, and performing only twice weekly with clients of whom only one in 100 or one is 40 is infected will

Table 8

Anticipated infections per year in prostitutes (assuming 100% infected if exposed)

Annual no. of contacts	*No. of infections per year*	
	5–10% infection in partners	*1–2.5% infection in partners*
10 000 (200 per week)	500–1000	100–250
5000 (100 per week)	250–500	50–125
2000 (40 per week)	100–200	25–50
1000 (20 per week)	50–100	10–25
500 (10 per week)	25–50	5–12.5
100 (2 per week)	5–10	1–2.5

have 1–2½ infections per year. Unless they have regular voluntary medical checks a significant proportion can still be expected to be infected at any given moment, owing to the long spells of asymptomatic infection. But, as in many other aspects of life, the rich will fare better than the poor.

By the use of prophylaxis the numbers of infections can be modified, but precautionary methods are less satisfactory in the female than in the male.

Repeaters: If by definition a "repeater" is a person who obtains more than one infection of disease in a year it is not great sexual prowess that is implied, but considerable variety.

A female with 100% chance of being infected if exposed will be infected on an average once after 20 exposures if 5% of her consorts are infected and the second time only after 40 exposures. A male consorting with women 20% infected has a like record. Both imply a change of consort on an average of every nine days, little discrimination, and no precautions. A moderately active male homosexual has been stated to have 100 or more different contacts per year (Gebhard 1971) and therefore can be expected to be infected several times a year.

The psychologically inadequate or abnormal, the ignorant, the uneducable, the irresponsible and the careless belong in this group, in addition to those highly sexually charged. Behavioural studies (e.g. Boese 1953, Lentz *et al.* 1953, Bunderson *et al.* 1949) have shown them, although obviously physically mature, to be psychologically immature. They are irresponsible in the maintenance of their attendance and usually slow to benefit from past experience.

Conclusions

(1) Illustrations of high-risk groups indicate that age, domicile and occupation all contribute to the possibility of venereal infection in an overall climate of greater tolerance regarding heterosexual and homosexual behaviour in present-day society.
(2) Behavioural factors which have been foremost in the past are now even more important with the present-day vastly increased opportunities for sex encounter.
(3) Multiplicity of contacts associated with indiscriminate choice of partner and lack of precautions are the basic reasons why persons become infected. Many so indulge more moderately with some selection and use of precautions and escape classification as a high-risk group. Extremely high rates of infection exist in prostitutes,

and there are limitations in the control of venereal disease in these persons.

(4) It is probably true to say that virtually all society is now at risk of at least one sexually transmitted disease at some time. In order to be able to achieve the ideal of the integrity of personal health some return to a philosophy involving only one sexual partner at one time is required if a significant impact is to be made on the vast problem presented by these disorders to modern society.

References

American Social Health Association (1973, 1974, 1975). "Today's VD Control Problem". New York

Arya, O. P. and Bennett, F. J. (1967). *British Journal of Venereal Diseases* **43**, 275–279

Boese, R. (1953). *Journal of the Kansas Medical Society* **54**, 10

British Cooperative Clinical Group (1973). *British Journal of Venereal Diseases* **49**, 329–334

Bunderson, H. N., Plotke, F. and Eisenberg, H. (1949). *American Journal of Public Health and the Nation's Health* **39**, 1535

Caletti, G. (1975). *World Health* (May) 12–15

Causse, G. (1975). *World Health* (May) 3–5

Cross, A. and Harris, J. R. W. (1976). *see* IUVDT (1976)

Department of Health and Social Security (1973). "Annual Report of the Chief Medical Officer of the State of the Public Health for the Year 1972". HMSO, London

Eng, J. and Jensen, R. H. (1960). *Nordisk Medicin* **61**, 1285–1288

Fanta, D., Kokoschka, E. M. and Mescher, P. (1976). *see* IUVDT (1976)

Fiscina, B., Oster, G. K., Oster, G. and Swanson, J. (1973). *American Journal of Obstetrics and Gynecology* **116**, 86

Gebhard, P. H. (1971). *In* "The VD Crisis". American Social Health Association and Pfizer Laboratories, New York: pp 61–64

Greenberg, J. H. (1972). *Medical Clinics of North America* **56**, 1087–1100

Guthe, T. and Idsøe, O. (1964). *Tidsskrift for den norske Laegeforening* **84**, 1262–1268

Guthe, T. and Willcox, R. R. (1971). *Royal Society of Health Journal* **91**, 122–133

Hollander, X. (1973). "Xaviera!" Warner Communications Co, New York

Holmes, K. K., Johnson, D. W. and Throstle, H. J. (1970). *American Journal of Epidemiology* **91**, 170

IUVDT (International Union against the Venereal Diseases and the Treponematoses) (1976). Twenty-eighth General Assembly, Malta, 13–16 April 1975: *see British Journal of Venereal Diseases* (selected papers, in press)

Juhlin, L. (1968). *Acta Dermato-Venereologica* **48**, 82–84

Lee, T. Y., Utidjian, M. D., Singh, B., Carpenter, U. and Cutler, J. C. (1972). *British Journal of Venereal Diseases* **48**, 376–380

Lentz, J. W., Morton, H. E., Garrison, M. and Leberman, P. R. (1953). *American Journal of Syphilis, Gonorrhea and Venereal Diseases* **37**, 577

Luger, A. (1976). *see* IUVDT (1976)

McKenzie Pollack, J. S. (1970). *British Journal of Venereal Diseases* **46**, 114

Mid-West Association for Study of Human Sexuality (1975) (brochure), Chicago

Morton, R. S. (1973). *British Journal of Venereal Diseases* 49, 155–156
Radovanovic, M. F. (1976). *see* IUVDT (1976)
Siboulet, A. (1976). *see* IUVDT (1976)
Siler, J. F. (1943). *Army Medical Bulletin* 67, 238
Sowmini, C. N. (1976). *see* IUVDT (1976)
Tardieu, J. V., Wurtz, A. and Basset, A. (1976). *see* IUVDT (1976)
Willcox, R. R. (1958). *International Review of Criminal Policy* 13, 67–97; (1967*a*). *British Journal of Venereal Diseases* 43, 1–9; (1967*b*). Communication to the World Health Organization; (1970). *British Journal of Venereal Diseases* 46, 412–422; (1974). *British Journal of Venereal Diseases* 50, 169–178
World Health Organization (1972). The Intercountry Spread of Venereal Diseases. Report of a working group. WHO Regional Office for Europe, Copenhagen

Discussion

Dr Harold Auslander (*Jacksonville, Florida*) wondered what the situation was in regard to Chlamydia. He had noticed that no mention was ever made of that condition in the statistics.

Dr King (*Chairman*) said that the problem of Chlamydia as a cause of urethritis or genital infection was still under investigation. The matter had not been proven beyond question and there were few laboratories in which the Chlamydia could be isolated. It was a matter for further investigation and additional facilities. It might be shown in the future that there was more than one cause of "nonspecific" genital infection. It was premature to try to produce statistics of the kind mentioned by Dr Auslander.

Dr R S Morton (*Sheffield*) said Dr Wiesner had hinted that in the United States there were now sufficient basic data to permit some forecasting of the future incidence of gonorrhoea. He asked if Dr Wiesner had considered economic changes and forecasts and using these as guides to future trends of gonorrhoea, because in both the USA and the UK there had been, in the first phase of anti-inflationary measures (1971–1972), a slight fall or a slight deceleration in the rising rate of gonorrhoea. In fact, gonorrhoea was a most important index for venereologists and the quarterly returns in the UK had proved an excellent guide to the Stock Exchange — much more useful than the Dow-Jones Index. He wondered how Dr Weisner saw the future, not only in terms of economics but in terms of gonorrhoea incidence.

Dr Morton said his studies showed that the third quarter of the year was regularly the peak period for sexually transmitted infections in the UK. This peak became less obvious as the years went by. He suggested that economic prosperity might be reflected in the more widespread use of central heating and that this had made a contribution to the change.

Dr Morton asked Dr Antal if WHO now felt that STD rates had become so high that the Organization would revert to their original policy of having a regional adviser in STD for each and every region again.

Dr Willcox had mentioned prostitutes only to dismiss their impact in many developed countries. A study of prostitutes as vectors of gonorrhoea, just completed at Sheffield, suggested that the part they played in the spread of gonorrhoea was more marked than it had been in the late 1960s.

Dr Wiesner said that his attempt to depict a five-week moving average of gonorrhoea rates in the USA (Fig. 4, p 11), and its variations above or below the accepted deviation, was really an attempt to see whether in fact trends were moving in a different fashion from those of previous years; it did not attempt to explain that occurrence. He found it difficult to correlate the gonorrhoea rates with trends in other phenomena, though the Institute of Cycles in Cincinnati, Ohio, had done an interesting correlation between the gonorrhoea rates in the United States and pig-iron production in West Germany.

He thought that seasonality was important and should not be ignored by people interested in control; an epidemiologist looking at the seasonality indicating increased transmission during the summer months would have to conclude that control efforts should be intensified prior to those months and that some attempt to interrupt transmission during that time should be made. He had no knowledge of such an attempt being made. He agreed that seasonality was probably behaviourally related and would like to see if data on other sexually transmitted conditions with transmission rates similar to that of gonorrhoea showed the same seasonal variation. He thought the behavioural determinant of the seasonal transmission would be supported by the finding of seasonal variation in other diseases. That type of seasonal variation, with the same third-quarter peak, had been noticed for Chlamydia infections associated with ophthalmia neonatorum in Atlanta.

Dr Antal agreed with Dr Morton that it would be desirable to have an adviser on venereal diseases and treponematoses attached to each WHO Regional Office, but this was a question of finance and the decision would rest with the respective Regional Director. However, a start had been made by the Pan American Health Organization some years back with the appointment of Dr M L Brubaker as Regional Adviser on Leprosy and VD.

Dr Willcox was interested in what Dr Morton had said about the situation in Sheffield. He had certainly not been trying to minimize the role of the prostitute. In many parts of the world, particularly the Far East, 90–100% of these infections were still caught from prostitutes, but he thought the proportion in the UK was now below 20%.

Control Through Health Care Systems

Prevention and Control of the Sexually Transmitted Diseases in the United States

Richard B Roberts
Cornell University Medical College, New York

Introduction

The prevention and control of sexually transmitted diseases (STD) in the United States are dependent on medical services, both clinical and laboratory, education, and epidemiology. All three areas play an important role and the impact of each is difficult to assess. One of the unique characteristics which separates the STD from other common diseases is that they can be distributed widely and rapidly over significant distances. This fact demands a rapid response capability as well as a collaborative approach between federal, state, and local officials. This presentation will be limited to a brief review of the epidemiologic programs and health care systems employed in the United States for the control of these diseases.

A detailed reporting system exists in the United States for many communicable diseases. The information gained from this system is used for the planning, initiation, and reorganization of projects for the control of these diseases. In regard to the STD, syphilis, gonorrhea, lymphogranuloma venereum, granuloma inguinale, and chancroid are, by law, reported to the local public health authorities. The information reported includes, in addition to other data, the patient's name and, if applicable, that of the private physician. Other STD, such as nonspecific urethritis, genital herpesvirus and trichomoniasis are not reportable diseases. One exception at the present time is in the state of Massachusetts where nonspecific urethritis and genital herpesvirus infections are reported. Currently, control programs exist only for syphilis and gonorrhea. Less than 2000 cases of lymphogranuloma venereum, granuloma inguinale, and chancroid were reported in 1973, an incidence too low to warrant a national control program for these infections.

National Syphilis Control Program

The control of syphilis in the United States is primarily the responsibility of individual states. The functions of the federal government are (1) to provide financial support and personnel through grant or project programs, (2) to provide funds for basic and applied research studies, and (3) to investigate interstate spread. In 1974, 12% of 114 736 (or approximately 15 000) reports of sexual contacts lived in states other than those in which the index case received treatment.

The national control program for syphilis has been well established over a long period of time and has effectively reduced the incidence of infectious syphilis as well as the late complications of this disease. Historically, the federal government first established a Venereal Disease Division in the United States Public Health Service in 1918. This Division was established because venereal disease constituted a major cause of military service rejections in World War I. In 1938, the National Venereal Disease Control Act was enacted which provided annual grants-in-aid to individual states. This act subsequently served as the basic model for federal, state, and local cooperation in venereal disease control efforts which continues to the present time.

Therapeutic advances became evident in the 1940s. Rapid Treatment Centers were established in 1942 as a wartime emergency measure. Of the 12 million men inducted into the armed services, over 170 000 required treatment for syphilis before being placed on active duty. The purpose of these centers was to administer arsenical therapy over a period of 5–10 days instead of the period of weeks necessary on an outpatient basis. However, penicillin soon became available and from 1945 was the antimicrobial agent of choice for all stages of syphilis. Dramatic reductions in the late manifestations of syphilis were realized over the succeeding twenty years.

The present control system for syphilis is based on two programs, routine serology and contact investigation. In 1946 the VDRL was developed. This serologic test provided a standardized, reproducible, rapidly performed, sensitive test which could be used in routine screening programs. By 1960 most states had enacted laws requiring that a serologic test for syphilis (VDRL) be performed as part of every premarital and prenatal examination. Presently, serologic tests are also performed on blood donors and applicants for posts in industry and government. Many, but not all, private physicians and admitting physicians in hospitals also include serology as part of the initial evaluation of patients regardless of the presenting illness. In 1974 approximately 38 million serologic tests were performed of which one million were reactive. States require that all laboratories report patients with reactive serologic tests to the local public health department. As noted previously, the institution of penicillin therapy and effective serologic screening had a profound effect on the incidence of many complications of syphilis such as deaths (reduction by 85%), congenital syphilis (90% reduction) and hospital admissions for luetic psychosis (97% reduction).

An increase in the incidence of primary and secondary syphilis, however, was again noted in the late 1950s, and in 1961, a Surgeon General's Task Force recommended a "ten year eradication program". Additional federal funding was allocated and efforts were initiated to develop methods for the interruption in the transmission of syphilis. Case finding, which had been used in previous years, was replaced by case prevention. Infected patients were interviewed, given educational material, and contacts traced. All contacts, if seen within ninety days of exposure, were treated as if they had infectious syphilis. This has been termed epidemiologic treatment and is the second major program now employed in syphilis control. In 1974, contact investigation was used in 24 318 of the 25 141 reported cases (97%) of primary and secondary syphilis: 64 425 contacts were followed up of which 6940 new cases were diagnosed and treated and 22 225 individuals received epidemiologic treatment. This method of control has been questioned by foreign experts because it may promote lower standards of diagnosis, treatment and follow up; it may not always be in the best interest of the patient; and it may encourage antibiotic resistance particularly if examinations for gonorrhea are not performed. On the other hand, many epidemiologists in the United States feel that because of the mobility of our society and the difficulty in delivering comprehensive care to contacts because of the lack of patient cooperation, few alternatives to epidemiologic treatment exist at the present time.

National Gonorrhea Control Program

The control program for gonorrhea, when compared to that for syphilis, is not well established and must still be considered as in the developmental stages. From 1952 to 1955, the federal government sponsored the first gonorrhea control program which was termed "speed zone epidemiology". The goal of this program was to treat female contacts of infected male partners within 72 hours of exposure. Fifteen cities participated in the program. No obvious impact on the incidence of gonorrhea was observed and the program was terminated three years later. In retrospect, the fact that asymptomatic but infectious women were not taken into consideration could in part explain the negative results observed.

A marked increase in the incidence of gonorrhea occurred in 1968 and continued in subsequent years. Several city-sponsored programs were initiated which had four major elements that were incoporated into the 1972 Control Act. These included: (1) Routine screening of women employing the Thayer-Martin culture medium which was developed in 1964. (2) Epidemiologic treatment of asymptomatic female partners of infected males. (3) Expansion of diagnostic and treatment facilities. (4) Reemphasis of educational programs. Unfortunately, funds were restricted and most programs were on a city or local level. Thus, the national incidence of gonorrhea continued to rise by 10–15% annually. In 1972, under the National Venereal Disease Prevention and Control Act, federal appropriation of an additional \$16 000 000 in project grants to states and large cities was enacted by Congress. These funds were in addition to the \$6 300 000 allocated for syphilis control. The total federal appropriation for 1974–1975 was \$24 800 000. The monies have been designated for the following programs: (1) Venereal disease surveillance activities which include reporting, screening, and follow up of diagnostic tests. (2) Case finding, follow-up activities and contact-tracing. (3) Interstate epidemiologic referral and follow-up activities. (4) Professional and public education activities. (5) Special studies or demonstrations to evaluate or test venereal disease control.

The principal efforts for the prevention and control of gonorrhea since 1973 have been mass screening of asymptomatic women and case prevention. Recent estimates suggest that 800 000 women are asymptomatic but infectious. Attempts have been made to decrease this reservoir by mass screening using Thayer-Martin medium. Cervical cultures have been used routinely for female patients visiting venereal disease clinics, family planning clinics, prenatal clinics, outpatient and inpatient hospital facilities, neighborhood health centers, student and group health centers, free clinics, and private physician offices. In 1974, 8 016 879 cervical cultures were obtained; 345 090 (4.3%) were positive (Fig. 1). The estimated cost was \$15–\$20 per test. This expense and the low yield of positive cultures in facilities other than venereal disease clinics raises the question whether this method of control is practical on a long-term basis.

Because of the high incidence of gonorrhea and the short incubation period of the disease, the feasibility and practicality of case prevention has also been questioned. New approaches such as short interview techniques (15 minutes) with infected male patients and contact-tracing by the patient have been advantageous. In 1974, 151 798 and 36 024 contacts of infected male and female partners respectively were followed up at public clinics. Approximately 80%

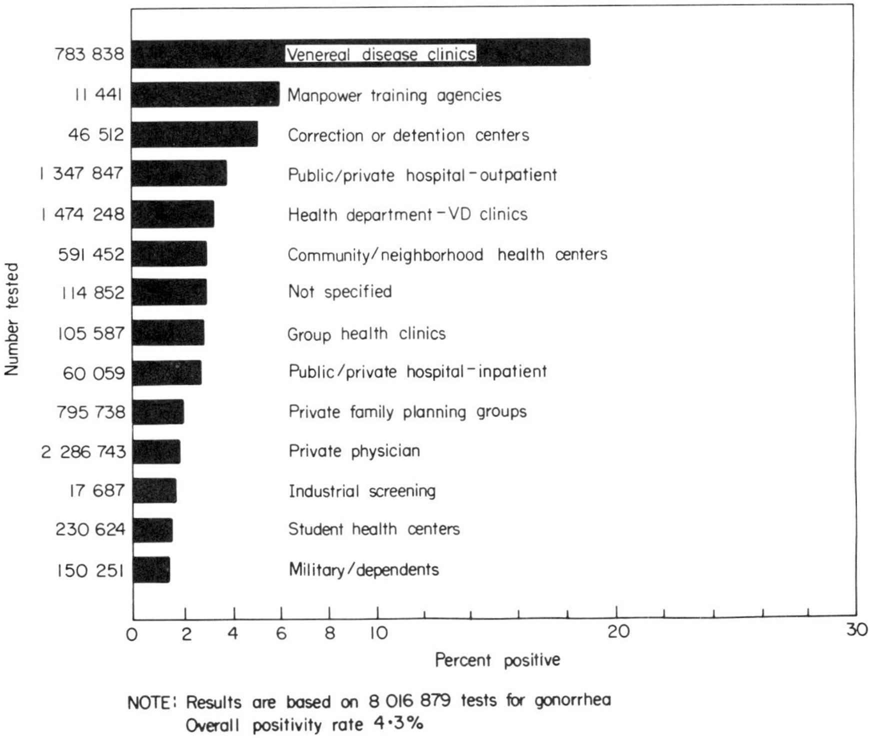

Fig. 1 *The gonorrhea screening program for women in 1973–1974: number and percent positive by facility*

of contacts in each group received epidemiologic treatment. Since the program has been in effect only for a short time, the impact is difficult to assess. However, certain factors suggest that case prevention will not be as effective as in the case of syphilis control: these include short incubation period; asymptomatic infections in both men and women; frequency of reinfection; and the relative resistance of the gonococcus to penicillin in certain geographical areas. New directions in gonorrhea control are needed, one of the most important being a sensitive and specific serologic test.

Health Care Systems for STD

As stated previously, the prevention and control of STD is a coordinated effort between federal, state, and municipal governments. At the federal level, the responsibility lies with the Venereal Disease Control Division (VDCD) at the Center for Disease Control (one of six agencies in the Department of Health, Education and

Welfare). Other divisions within the Bureau of State Services at CDC include Tuberculosis, Immunization, and Environment. The specific responsibilities of the VDCD are: (1) To provide grants-in-aid to states and localities for venereal disease control efforts. (2) To develop guidelines and standards and to coordinate, evaluate, and implement uniform control programs. (3) To provide training and technical assistance. (4) To conduct and foster research. The Director of the VDCD is Dr Ralph Henderson; Dr Paul Wiesner is Director of the Operational Research Branch.

The principal health care systems for STD with which the Venereal Disease Control Division collaborate are the public clinics and private physicians. The similarities and differences between the two systems with regard to patient management, case reporting, contact-tracing, patient education, quality of health care, the use of laboratory aids, and cost to the patient are listed in Table 1. What is

Table 1

Principal health care systems for the sexually transmitted diseases

	Public clinics	*Private physicians*
Patient management	20–30%	70–80%
Case reporting	100%	15–20%
Contact-tracing	Yes	Variable
Patient education	Variable	Variable
Quality of care	Variable	Variable
Laboratory aids	Used	Underutilized
Patient fee	No	Yes

immediately striking is that only 20–30% of patients with the STD, i.e. syphilis and gonorrhea, receive their health care in public clinics, whereas 70–80% of patients are treated by private physicians. Furthermore, it is estimated that private physicians report to the local health departments only 15–20% of patients treated (*see below*).

Public Clinics

The public clinic, supported by state and local taxes, is the major health department system for the care of patients with STD. Other types of clinics are available but are used less frequently by patients. These include model city and family clinics which are supported by federal funds; youth clinics, used also for other health needs such as pregnancy, drugs, and alcoholism, and financially supported by voluntary subscription; walk-in clinics staffed by voluntary physicians; and hospital clinics, which may be associated with state, city, or county hospitals, or with university teaching institutions. The advantages and disadvantages of university-based clinics are discussed in the section New Developments (*below*).

Public clinics are the reponsibility of the state and local health departments. They number over 2000 and work closely but independently with the public health laboratories. Many public clinics are staffed by public health advisors (*see below*). Since these clinics are supported and administrated locally, their capabilities for health care vary greatly. These will not be discussed in detail in this review but are presented in the Pan American Health Organization publication "Report of the International Travelling Seminar in the United States of America, 1974". This study, conducted over a three-week period in late 1971, concluded: "There are too few clinics for the case load of patients, and many clinics are inconveniently situated. Facilities vary considerably. The standard of doctors in many clinics is a serious drawback in the control of venereal diseases."

Private Physicians

Private physicians who manage patients with STD are in various medical specialties, including general practice, internal medicine, obstetrics and gynecology, urology, and dermatology. This diversity of medical disciplines is one of the principal reasons for the variability in the quality of patient care. As stated previously, private physicians treat 70–80% of patients with STD but report only 15–20% of them. Many physicians consider the medical significance and control of syphilis quite different from that of gonorrhea, which may in part explain their hesitancy in reporting patients with gonorrhea to the health department.

In the management of syphilis the VDRL is used not only as a screening test but also to confirm a clinical diagnosis. Private and public health laboratories in most states are required by law to report reactive serologic tests to the health authorities. This reporting system includes amongst other data the patient's name and, when applicable, the name of the private physician. The public health advisor in that locale contacts the physician for obtaining permission for contact-tracing and field investigation. Thus, a reporting system for syphilis exists which does not rely on the cooperation of the private physician. Such a system is critical since over the past decade intensive efforts have been made at state and local levels to encourage physicians to report, yet the percentage of cases reported has remained the same or decreased. Previous surveys asking physicians about their reluctance to report patients with syphilis gave the following reasons: (1) Physician-patient confidentiality. (2) Patient objection.

The prevention and control of gonorrhea in private practice is even more a concern to public health authorities. Serology is not available. The mass screening by cervical cultures of asymptomatic women recommended by the United States Public Health Service over the past few years is not universally performed by private physicians. Expense to the patient (approximately $15-$20), sensitivity of the patient, especially if married, and the small chance of isolation because of inadequate media or transport service have been given as reasons for the lack of cooperation by private physicians. Indeed, many patients with gonorrhea are treated without laboratory confirmation. Thus, case-reporting of patients with gonorrhea depends on the cooperation of the private physician. Confidentiality between the patient and physician is again given as a major reason for the low percentage of case-reporting. Other explanations reflect the belief by many private physicians that gonorrhea cannot be controlled by public health contact-tracing.

The alternative solutions for the control of STD in private medicine appear limited. Enforcing already existing laws is unrealistic and intensifying present methods for eliciting physician cooperation has been unsuccessful. Furthermore, these methods do not take into consideration physician-patient confidentiality. The reporting of reactive serologic tests for syphilis and contact-tracing by public health advisors working in collaboration with the private physician should be continued. Feedback to the physician from the health department should be ensured. In the case of gonorrhea, reporting should be separated from contact-tracing. Reporting should be encouraged for statistical purposes, thus conserving patient confidentiality. Contact-tracing should be conducted by the private physician or, more importantly, by the infected patient. For this process to be effective, public education must be intensified, a subject which is discussed in a subsequent section.

Public Health Advisers

The public health adviser (PHA) is responsible for the day-to-day activities related to the control program. This individual has also been referred to as the venereal disease program representative, field representative or field investigator. The PHA usually has a college degree and receives three months of training in interviewing techniques before being assigned to a public clinic. Career opportunities for federal PHA are available and many administrators in the United States Public Health Service are former public health advisers of the

Venereal Disease Control Branch. There are currently 500 PHA supported by federal funds and over 1000 by state and local funds that staff the 2000 clinics in the United States. The number of PHA assigned to public clinics varies as to population, funding, needs, &c. For example, in New York City in 1973–74, there were 175 PHAs, one-third of whom were either federal, city, or project employees.

In general, the public health adviser has four major responsibilities: epidemiology, professional relations, public education, and administration. The most important and time-consuming responsibility is epidemiology or case management. The adviser interviews, reinterviews and counsels the infected patient, conducts follow-up field studies of case contacts and cluster suspects (contact investigation), and maintains records of incidence, trends, and ensures reporting. Other public clinic personnel, such as physicians, nurses, and physician assistants may also conduct similar investigations. Professional relations include ensuring case-reporting and securing permission for field studies from private physicians, hospitals, and laboratories. Educational opportunities are encompassed in these activities. Public education and administration are activities which are dictated by the needs of the local public clinics.

New Developments

Future developments in the prevention and control of STD will depend on continued collaboration between federal, state, and local governments. Developments should be directed toward the health care systems and the public. They should include improvement of medical services, continued epidemiologic methods and education. To improve medical services, federal funding must be increased. Laboratory aids must be upgraded and maintained. Efforts to prevent and control STD other than syphilis and gonorrhea should be considered. Training of physicians at all levels of their education should be strengthened and competent physicians recruited for public clinics.

At present, medical services in public clinics may have to be provided by physician assistants. It is well recognized that it is difficult to attract full-time competent physicians. Many physicians in public clinics are either young or near retirement and thus mobile. Similarly, overcrowding in unattractive environs and performing a categorical service, not comprehensive care, make it difficult to attract physicians. On the other hand, physician assistants perform well in clinical settings similar to those in public clinics; that is, diseases of high frequency, diseases with relatively low clinical variability, efficient diagnostic procedures, effective therapy by protocol and few emergencies. A three-month training program is now available through the VDCD for physician assistants interested in staffing public clinics.

University hospital-based clinics will also improve medical services for patients with STD. These clinics have been strongly recommended by the International Travelling Seminar and the National Committee on Venereal Diseases. The advantages of such an affiliation are readily apparent: (1) Quality patient care with the problem-oriented approach, and ancillary diagnostic and therapeutic aids. (2) Training of medical students, post-graduate physicians and physician assistants. (3) Counselling patients including education and psychological assistance. (4) Promoting excellence in clinical research. However, there also are disadvantages to university hospital-based clinics. These include: (1) Cost to the patient depending on the patient's ability to pay. (2) The location of many university hospitals in areas of low risk for STD. (3) The difficulty in performing field studies. Despite these drawbacks, a university hospital clinic in each urban area or major city would help in meeting many of the current problems outlined above.

Epidemiologic methods such as case-reporting and contact-tracing should be continued. Case-reporting should be limited to surveillance, so that the confidentiality of the private patient be maintained. The responsibility for contact-tracing should be continued by the PHA, the physician assistant, or the infected patient. Epidemiologic treatment for syphilis which effectively interrupts transmission should be continued. Screening of women with repeated gonorrhea is currently being evaluated at the Venereal Disease Control Division. Finally, education of the public, especially students, parents and homosexuals, should be intensified and more effort should be made to inform legislators.

Summary

The prevention and control of the STD in the United States is a collaborative effort between federal, state, and local agencies. The control program for syphilis has been in effect for many years and is well established. The program consists of the mandatory reporting of reactive serologic tests, subsequent contact-tracing, and epidemiologic treatment. The control program for gonorrhea is still in its infancy. Mass screening of asymptomatic women may be replaced by screening of women with repeated infections. The success of contact-tracing by infected individuals will depend on the effectiveness of public education.

The major health care systems for STD are the public clinics and private physicians. Each has its limitations in the control of syphilis and gonorrhea and new developments will have to be individualized to take into consideration medical services (clinics) and patient confidentiality (private physicians). It must be realized, however, that in the past the incidence of syphilis in the United States has paralleled federal appropriations for control efforts. Unfortunately, the STD have always had a low priority in federal funding which explains in part why appropriations are usually crisis related. Furthermore, unlike narcotics, mental retardation and alcoholism, the STD are the only group of social diseases without a non-governmental constituency. Future control efforts will depend on adequate federal and state appropriations and the effective education of the public and Congress.

Acknowledgments

I am grateful to Dr Ralph Henderson and Dr Paul Wiesner from the Venereal Disease Control Division of the Center for Disease Control for their cooperation and advice in the preparation of this review and to Mr Norman Scherzer, Division of Prevention, New York, New York.

References

American Social Health Association (1975). "Today's VD Control Problem". New York

Dans, P. E. (1974). *Journal of the American Venereal Disease Association* 1, 70

Henderson, R. (1975). *Clinical Obstetrics and Gynecology* 18, 223

Pan American Health Organization

(1974*a*) Venereal Diseases. Report of the International Traveling Seminar in the United States of America. Washington, DC

(1974*b*) Section Reports of the International Traveling Seminar in the United States. *Journal of the American Venereal Disease Association* 1, 63

US Department of Health, Education and Welfare (1974). VD Facts Sheet 1974. Publication No. (CDC) 75-8195

The System in Britain

R D Catterall
James Pringle House,
The Middlesex Hospital, London W1

The failure to control the incidence of the sexually transmitted diseases during the past 25 years has been one of the most disappointing trends in medicine. Since the introduction of penicillin towards the end of the Second World War great hopes have been placed on antibiotics and chemotherapeutic agents. Although they have helped us to achieve substantial gains in some diseases, it has become increasingly clear that they are not in themselves the ultimate solution to the problem. Intensive contact-tracing and other epidemiological techniques were at one time believed to offer a possible solution to the problem and eradication campaigns were started in some countries, but proved to be both costly and disappointing. Health education and the wider dissemination of factual information to the public has recently been favoured by many health authorities and modern techniques of education have been used for these ends. Unfortunately the available evidence suggests that knowledge of the facts does not necessarily influence human behaviour, as has been shown in the cases of cigarette smoking and lung cancer, seat belts and motor car accidents, obesity and its medical consequences, alcoholism, drug taking and many other health matters.

Another method of control is through a well-developed health care system in which high quality facilities for investigation, diagnosis, treatment and contact-tracing are widely available to the public. There is general agreement that the ideal service should be free, easily accessible to patients, available for long hours each day, situated in the outpatient departments of general hospitals and staffed by doctors and nurses with special training in the subject. It should be supported by efficient laboratory services and properly trained social workers to carry out contact-tracing and help with the social problems of the patients. At university teaching hospitals time and facilities should be available for teaching both undergraduate and postgraduate students, as well as nurses and social workers. In the larger departments research should form an important part of the programme and ideally there should be one or more academic chairs in the subject.

For well over 50 years the principle policy for the control of sexually transmitted diseases in the United Kingdom has been directed towards the establishment of a high quality service of this type. The initial legislation was passed by Parliament in 1916 and was known as the Venereal Diseases Regulations. Under these regulations free and confidential consultations were provided by the local health authorities at regional hospitals and in special clinics. A second Bill, known as the Venereal Diseases Act of 1916, provided legislation to protect the public from quacks and charlatans. Heavy fines or imprisonment may be imposed on any unqualified individual who offers advice or gives treatment to patients with veneral diseases. Under this act the venereal diseases are defined as syphilis, gonorrhoea and chancroid.

When the National Health Service was introduced in 1948 the clinics became the responsibility of the Regional Hospital Boards and the Boards of Governors of Teaching Hospitals. This was an important development as the specialty of venereology became established on an equal status with the other medical specialties, such as general internal medicine, cardiology, neurology and gastroenterology. During the past 25 years the service has expanded and developed, until there is now a comprehensive and sophisticated service throughout the whole country.

The estimated population of the United Kingdom in 1974 was just over 56 000 000 people. To serve this population there are 230 special clinics for sexually transmitted diseases of which 187 are in England, 18 in Scotland, 14 in Wales and 11 in Northern Ireland. Of the 187 clinics in England, 30 are in Greater London and 157 in the provinces. There are clinics at all of the 25 university teaching hospitals.

There is a physician in charge of each clinic who is reponsible for the organization of the service and the management of the patients. In the majority of the larger clinics there are two consultants. The Department of Health and Social Security consider that one consultant in sexually transmitted diseases is required for every half million population. This means that in the United Kingdom there should be 110–120 consultants.

The consultants are supported by a staff of medical assistants, clinical assistants and junior staff in training at senior house officer, registrar and senior registrar level. Some general practitioners are attached to the clinics on a sessional basis. In addition each clinic has a staff of trained nurses of both sexes, a laboratory staff, health workers who carry out contact-tracing, medical social workers who are available for counselling patients, as well as receptionists and secretarial staff. Some clinics have a psychiatrist who attends for one or two sessions a week.

The larger clinics are open for medical consultations for 9 or 10 hours daily each week day. Many of the smaller clinics are open only part-time. All patients have free access to the clinics and can attend of their own accord without a letter of introduction from their general practitioner. A few clinics have an appointment system but at the majority the patients attend at a time of their own choosing without an appointment. Many are referred by their general practitioner and a substantial number attend because of contact-tracing. Others are referred by consultants in other medical and surgical specialties.

Responsibility for the service of sexually transmitted diseases in the United Kingdom rests with the Secretary of State for Health and Social Security, who is a member of the Cabinet. She works through the Department of Health and Social Security which administers the National Health Service. An adviser in sexually transmitted diseases is appointed from among the more senior specialists to advise about England. There is a separate adviser for the Scottish Home and Health Department, for the Welsh Office and for the Northern Ireland Department of Health and Social Security. The advisers play an important role in helping to plan policy on all matters related to sexually transmitted diseases.

The administration of the National Health Service was completely reorganized in 1974 and there are now Regional, Area and District Health Authorities between the physicians in charge of clinics and the Department of Health and Social Security. However, the clinics are organized on a regional basis and the clinic directors have direct access to the adviser for discussion and advice.

Undergraduate medical students receive teaching about the sexually transmitted diseases at all the 25 medical schools in the United Kingdom. The arrangements vary from school to school but usually take the form of lectures, seminars, demonstrations and clinical teaching in outpatients and on the wards. The number of hours devoted to the sexually transmitted diseases depends upon the policy of the school and the enthusiasm of the venereologist and ranges from 10 to 24 hours. Students are encouraged to spend their elective period in the clinics and questions about sexually transmitted diseases are included in the final examinations from time to time.

Recently a postgraduate course in sexually transmitted diseases has been established in London and is administered by the British Postgraduate Medical Federation. The course is of three months' duration and includes lectures, seminars, demonstrations and periods of clinical attachment to some of the larger clinics at London teaching hospitals. It is designed for overseas students but a number of trainees in venereology from the United Kingdom may attend it on a day-release basis. There are two courses each year.

Those who have completed the course and others with suitable training and experience may take the examination for the Diploma in Venereology. This diploma is awarded to successful candidates after a written, multiple choice question, clinical and oral examination held by the Society of Apothecaries of London twice a year. This society is the oldest non-university organization granting medical diplomas in Britain, having been founded by James I in 1617.

A small number of postgraduate students are able to obtain clinical attachments to the larger departments at teaching hospitals and are usually sponsored by their own government or university, the World Health Organization, the British Council or the British Postgraduate Medical Federation. General practitioners and consultants in other specialties are kept up to date with developments in the field by lectures at postgraduate centres throughout the country and by suitable patients being presented at clinical meetings in hospitals.

The programme of training for a specialist in sexually transmitted diseases has been laid down by the Royal Colleges of Physicians. After five years of undergraduate training the newly qualified doctor has to perform a compulsory year as a resident house physician or surgeon. This is followed by three years of general professional training in internal medicine or in some of the medical specialties. During this period the trainee specialist would normally be expected to pass an examination for membership of one of the Royal Colleges of Physicians. The period of general professional training is followed by a further period of approximately four years of specialist training, during which time the trainee will usually work at a large department for sexually transmitted diseases and gradually take increasing responsibility for patient care, teaching, administration and research, all under the direct supervision of the physician in charge of the clinic. Some trainees may spend up to one year abroad at a large centre and some will undertake studies leading to a higher university degree such as the MD, PhD or MSc. Trainees may be attracted from other specialties and in such cases the training programmes are interpreted in a very flexible manner.

Specialist training in the United Kingdom is supervised by a Joint Committee on High Medical Training established by the Royal Colleges of Physicians and each medical specialty has a Specialist Advisory Committee. The Joint Committee arranges for training posts to be investigated and maintains a list of hospital posts suitable for specialist training.

Once the trainee has completed his training he may apply for a consultant post in the specialty. These posts are advertised in the medical press as they become available and the application of the trainee will be considered in competition with other applicants by a committee of representatives of the Royal Colleges of Physicians, the university, the hospital concerned and the Regional and Area Health Authorities. When he is finally appointed to a consultant post he can choose whether he will be full-time or part-time in the National Health Service. If he is part-time he may undertake private practice. Trainee consultants are not allowed private practice.

Post-registration training for nurses takes the form of courses of six months' duration held at some teaching hospitals at which advanced training in up-to-date methods is given. The Health Workers who are responsible for contact-tracing have their own professional organization and hold an annual conference.

Health education in the United Kingdom is the responsibility of the Health Education Council, a government-sponsored organization.

It is responsible for keeping the public informed about important health matters and for developing improved methods of health education.

There are a number of organizations in the United Kingdom devoted wholly or partially to the sexually transmitted diseases. The Medical Society for the Study of Venereal Diseases is a professional organization of doctors which holds regular scientific meetings in London and elsewhere. It publishes the *British Journal of Venereal Diseases* in conjunction with the *British Medical Journal* and organizes the British Cooperative Clinical Group, a collaborative research organization.

The Venereologists Group of the British Medical Association is an elected body concerned with conditions of service, pay and other political matters. The British Federation against the Venereal Diseases is an organization of medical and non-medical bodies concerned with the social and educational aspects of the subject. It is a member organization of the International Union against the Venereal Diseases and Treponematoses.

The evolution of the service for sexually transmitted diseases in the United Kingdom has led to the establishment of a high standard clinical service to patients, substantial undergraduate and post-graduate medical teaching and expanding research programmes. Health education and the preventive aspects of the subject are as yet less well developed. Nevertheless, the rates of infection per hundred thousand of population are only 3.26 for early infectious syphilis and 126.10 for gonorrhoea and are appreciably lower than in many comparable industrial countries, suggesting that a comprehensive service does produce some measure of control of the diseases.

In many countries without a National Health Service the majority of patients with sexually transmitted diseases are treated in the private sector of medicine. Thus, in the United States of America it is estimated that over 80% of the cases of gonorrhoea are treated by private physicians and only minimal efforts are made to notify the diseases diagnosed or trace the contacts of the infected patients. In the United Kingdom, with a free sexually transmitted diseases service widely distributed throughout the country, the majority of general practitioners and other doctors refer their patients to the clinics or the patients go directly to a clinic of their own accord. This enables an accurate diagnosis to be made and confirmed by microbiological methods, the correct treatment to be given, follow-up tests to be carried out to establish that the patient is cured and that the cure is permanent, contact-tracing to be efficiently performed and any social, personal or psychiatric problems to be dealt with. Equally important is the fact that undergraduate medical students and postgraduate doctors can be given proper clinical teaching about the sexually transmitted diseases.

References

American Social Health Association (1974). "Today's VD Control Problem". New York

Catterall, R. D. (1972). *Lancet* **ii**, 321

Department of Health and Social Security (1974). Annual Report of the Chief Medical Officer on the State of the Public Health. HMSO, London

Department of Health and Social Security (Medical Staffing Division) (1974). *Health Trends* **6**, 30

Pan American Health Organization (1974). Venereal Diseases. Report of the International Traveling Seminar in the United States of America. Washington, DC

Discussion

Dr A G Lawrence (*St Stephen's Hospital, Chelsea, London*) asked Dr Roberts for his views on the failure of potential patients to attend at public health clinics in America. The number of clinics – about 2000 – appeared to be adequate. The UK had 200 for a population one-third that of America. He thought clinics in all countries tended to have very poor facilities but felt that could not be a reason for non-attendance in America.

Dr Roberts said that in the USA many such clinics were in urban areas where there was a high risk for sexually transmitted diseases and therefore, geographically, they had a service role and many young people living in urban areas attended them. Many were not affilitated with university teaching hospitals and it had been difficult to recruit physicians of good calibre.

In the USA many patients had private physicians and preferred to have their medical care by private physicians in their offices. This was also true in ward patients in university teaching hospitals. What would happen when there was some form of national health insurance whereby everyone would be able to pay for private physicians would be another matter.

Dr Wiesner said that in the USA they were limited by legislation which was related specifically to the support of public health advisers and had been extended, expanded and interpreted in different fashions in as many situations as possible to provide increased support for clinical services. He thought, however, that at the national level they were committed to increasing the quality of clinical services for sexually transmitted diseases. The real issue was the mechanism by which it should be done. Support from both state and local governments would be needed to assure continuity of care.

Dr Wiesner thought that, while there were pitfalls in comparing rates of various venereal diseases between countries, it would be interesting to compare the rates of increase of various sexually transmitted diseases in that way. He doubted whether there would be any evidence that comprehensive health care had limited the rate of increase of sexually transmitted diseases in England. He wondered if Dr Catterall would comment on this.

Dr Catterall said no one was more aware of the pitfalls of statistics than himself and did not claim that his figures proved anything other than that the UK rate was fairly low.

He thought Dr Wiesner's suggestion of comparing rates of increase was important. He had actually done this as far as he could with the statistics available and had obtained a result which showed that the rate of increase in the UK was slower than that in the USA and in Sweden and in other countries where data were available. He thought the weakness in the UK was that health education had not been developed to anything like the same extent as it had been in the USA; prevention had not been examined at all.

Miss Elspeth Robertson (*Devon Area Health Aurhority, Exeter*) said that health education was the responsibility of Area Health Authorities in the UK, who employed Health Education Officers. The Health Education Council had a responsibility in proposing measures which might be utilized by Health Education Officers. She personally found publicity material less effective than the spoken word and was currently running a school campaign in Exeter and East Devon, speaking to school children from 12–13 years old or older. These talks were proving very popular and were well received. She was now being asked to address parent–teacher associations, and talks concerning STD would now be a permanent feature of Health Education Programmes in her district. She worked in close cooperation with the area venereologist and the committees concerned.

Dr Catterall said that health education would be discussed in a later session.

Mr Alan Hilton (*Lancashire Area Health Authority, Preston*), while not wishing to deprecate the value of clinical knowledge on the subject, suggested that there was some lack of agreement by venereologists on what they wished to communicate in the field of health education. He also thought that present campaigns were too general and needed more specificity, and wondered whether the authorities were trying to moralize and prevent people involving themselves in risk behaviour, or trying to get them into the clinics for treatment. He thought there was a need for clinicians and health educators to share their information, expertise and respective skills to produce planned programmes.

Mr R Irtizaali (*Barking and Havering Health Education Officer, Romford, Essex*) endorsed Mr Hilton's remarks.

Dr Catterall had suggested that although health education was not very well developed, there had been a considerable change. The Barking and Havering area had a VD Answer-Phone service running; so had London, Sheffield, Bristol and many other areas. Dr Catterall had also suggested that knowledge of facts did not necessarily alter behaviour, but it did influence behaviour to some extent. In Barking and Havering the number of calls increased just before the summer months, in May and early June, and started falling about September. In June and July the number dropped again. He was trying to suggest an explanation for the third-quarter peak of the new cases.

The point Dr Catterall had made was that educational models were used. This was so, but behavioural models were also used for altering or influencing the behaviour of the individual. In fact health educators probably had much more armoury in primary and secondary prevention than did clinicians.

Mr Irtizaali thought it would be helpful to travellers abroad, at least in Europe, if there were available some form of guide as to where treatment might be sought.

Mr J D Bloom (*Cambridge Area Health Authority* (*Teaching*)) asked what system for control of STD was used amongst troops who were abroad, such as the American troops in the UK or British troops in Europe.

Dr Antal said that his knowledge was limited to Korea where the Preventive Medicine Officer was responsible for health education in venereal infections among the US troops stationed there. The approach and intensity of these activities changed with the interest of the incumbent officer and was relative to the large number of troops. Health education in VD was stepped up during the periods of elevated risk of infection in the course of the 12-month tour of duty of the soldier. Unfortunately, a fearsome picture of venereal diseases and their sequelae was drawn. It was recommended to abstain from frequently changing partnership.

In principle, no repressive measures were applied to soldiers reporting with venereal infections. Local commanders and their medical officers being responsible for venereal disease control among their troop frequently assisted local health authorities with supplies for the screening and treatment of high-risk groups.

Dr Willcox noted that Dr Antal had indicated that research of the WHO would be orientated towards techniques which would help with future prevention and asked if, as he hoped, this would be taken in the broadest sense. In the past few years the WHO and other bodies had fostered much wider, more fundamental research, particularly in relation to the gonococcus; this had paid off to a remarkable degree, as would be learned at the next session.

Dr Antal in reply to Dr Willcox, explained that the Venereal Diseases and Treponematoses Unit of WHO would continue to support basic research aiming at the development of techniques which would be beneficial in public health programmes directed towards the control of sexually transmitted diseases and the problems arising in developing countries.

Dr E M C Dunlop (*London Hospital*) put forward statistics on the relative incidence of venereal infection in the USA and in England and Wales.

The ASHA had estimated that only some 11% of cases were being reported in the USA; therefore their estimates should be used for comparing the relative incidences of fresh venereal infection in the two countries. There were some 1600 cases of infectious syphilis in England and Wales per annum. Assuming the true figure to be 2000, to allow for 25% of cases being treated outside the clinics, then the USA, if the rate of infection was the same, would have 8000 cases per annum because their population is four times greater than that of England and Wales. In fact the USA had some 24 000 reported cases (of primary and secondary syphilis) and an estimated rate of 85 000. That, and the estimated gonorrhoea rate of 2 500 000 cases per annum, suggested that the USA had some ten times the infection rate found in England and Wales. That was the difference that must be used in assessing the relative effectiveness of the STD control systems in the two countries.

Dr Morton was interested in the idea of a guide book produced by the WHO, but wondered if that was the best way to tackle the problem, since different types of guide book would be required for undeveloped countries, for more developed countries, and for the most advanced countries. He felt that the reports of WHO regional seminars provided a better method of dealing with the matter; that on the West Pacific region by Dr Guthe and Dr Willcox (WHO 1969, Report on Second Symposium on VD Control in Western Pacific Region. Document WHO/WPRO/VDT/69, 0144) was a classic and should be read by every venereologist.

In trying to improve technological means the WHO had been instrumental in establishing reference laboratories in various places which, numerically, had concerned syphilis much more than gonorrhoea which was the real public health problem of today. There was still only one GC reference laboratory and he thought it was time the WHO took further action.

Dr Antal was not convinced that reports (and their annexes) of WHO seminars on VDT control contained the detailed information on techniques which would be expected of a guide-book on STD control. Ideally, the book should be designed in such a way that it could be of service to the majority of health administrators and health care institutions.

He agreed that there was an urgent need for more regional reference laboratories for gonococci, assisting national laboratories in surveillance and training. Proposals were awaited from the WHO regional offices. At present, the WHO Collaborating Centre for Reference and Research in Gonococci in Copenhagen rendered a word-wide service.

Dr John M Knox (*Houston, Texas*) thought it was probably accurate to say that the rate of VD in the USA was about 10 times that in the UK.

He personally believed that the British system of VD control was better than that of the USA; however, there could be additional reasons why the VD rate was higher in the USA. The population in the USA was very heterogenous, with many minority groups; much of the VD was in the black population, which continued to be more numerous than in the UK, and there were other minority groups, such as Latin Americans, in poverty areas. In addition, the population was constantly mobile and it was recognized that when people left home they were more promiscuous. He was not happy with the current system in the USA, but felt the problem could not be simply explained away by the system.

The Changing Clinical Picture in Gonorrhoea and Non-gonococcal Infections

Chairman
Dr Richard Krause
Rockefeller University, New York

Dr Krause (*Chairman*), in introducing the session, commented that it was a remarkable one. Had it been held five years earlier there would not have been nearly so much of substance to report in the bacterial, immunological and genetic side of gonococci or Chlamydia. The picture had changed in the interval; there had been substantial progress in each of these areas for both organisms. In the USA this new research effort had been a collaboration among the Centre for Disease Control, the National Institute for Allergy and Infectious Diseases and, most especially, a new generation of physicians and scientists at these institutions, and also in the universities and research institutes, who had been trained in the rigorous disciplines of cell biology, molecular biology, immunology and genetics. It was this new generation of scientists who were posing fundamental questions about immunology and immunity, and from this work might flow reliable serological tests for the detection of gonorrhoea and serological classification, an important advance for fundamental epidemiological investigations on transmission. Mechanisms of pathogenesis and drug resistance were being examined at the cellular and molecular level and similar research was under way for the Chlamydia. It should be borne in mind that all this, which rested on the fundamental biological principles learnt by the study of bacteria, was of theoretical interest but was of little practical importance from a medical point of view.

Dr Krause felt that the speakers in this session would be the first to recognize their debt to those who had elucidated fundamental biological principles. It was also his conviction that mastery over gonococci and Chlamydia would lead to the development of new insights into the basic processes of infection, and that this work would be the basis in the future for the study of other bacterial diseases yet to be controlled and conquered.

Clinical Epidemiology and Change in Clinical Manifestations of Gonococcal Infection

King K Holmes, David A Eschenbach and Joan S Knapp
Departments of Medicine and Obstetrics and Gynecology, University of Washington, and the US Public Health Service Hospital, Seattle

The emergence during the past few years of new knowledge concerning the epidemiology and clinical manifestations of gonococcal infection has resulted partly from the development and application of new laboratory techniques, and partly from the increasing use of formal methods of epidemiologic study. Clinical venereologists have long been active in both clinical and epidemiologic research, but the bias inherent in the patient populations available to clinical venereologists for study has at times led to erroneous conclusions concerning the clinical epidemiology of venereal lesions. These have been passed on as misleading paradigms which even today serve to impede control measures and to obfuscate the actual manifestations of these lesions. It is only during the past few years that formal methods of epidemiologic investigation, employing cohort, case-control, and sampling techniques, have been used to study gonococcal infection. The apparent "changes" in the manifestation of gonorrhea thus probably represent changes in perception more than actual changes in the manifestations. On the other hand, the relationship of the host-gonococcus interaction to contraceptive and sexual practices, which are changing, and the apparent existence of geographic differences in clinical manifestations, suggest that real temporal changes in the manifestations of gonococcal infection have probably occurred.

This paper presents a general overview of the clinical epidemiology of gonorrhea, as elucidated by epidemiologic studies and by application of a method for typing gonorrhea, called auxotyping.

Usual Clinical Manifestations

A concept has emerged, based primarily upon observations made in venereal disease clinic patients, that gonococcal infection produces no symptoms in the great majority of infected women (Brown 1971, Fiumara 1972) and nearly always produces symptoms in men (Brown 1971, Fiumara 1972, Pedersen and Harrah 1970). In the United States this led to a major emphasis upon detection of nonsymptomatic female carriers by routine "screening" endocervical cultures and by contact-tracing. Recent studies of the clinical epidemiology of gonorrhea in men have given interesting results which on the surface appear contradictory. A US Navy Cohort Study (Harrison *et al.* 1973) observed that only about 3% of men who became newly infected in Southeast Asia remained nonsymptomatic longer than two weeks. On the other hand, a study of the point prevalence of gonorrhea in a sample of US Army men (Handsfield *et al.* 1974) showed that approximately a third of men found to have gonorrhea had symptoms and signs of urethritis, a third had signs but no symptoms, and a third had neither symptoms nor signs. These two studies are not contradictory if one assumes that most men who develop symptoms eventually seek treatment. Those who never develop symptoms, together with those whose symptoms subside after an initial "wait and see" period, and those who develop symptoms or signs which they ignore ("noniatrotrophic" symptoms and signs), comprise the population of males who have gonorrhea at any point in time.

Although these observations bear on military personnel only, evidence that about half to two-thirds of men who carry infection at any point in time are nonsymptomatic is also provided by recent studies of the male sex contacts of women who present as self-referred patients. When women, because of symptoms of gonococcal pelvic inflammatory disease or disseminated gonococcal infection have been interviewed, it has been found that over half of their male sex partners brought to examination as a result of contact-tracing, have untreated gonococcal infection, and about half of those with infection have no symptoms while the other half have noniatrotrophic, or ignored, symptoms (Handsfield *et al.* 1974, Eschenbach *et al.* 1975). Examination of male sex partners of women whose gonorrhea was detected by routine screening culture examination gives similar results (Blount 1972). It is only when women who attend venereal disease clinics are interviewed that a high proportion of the men named as sex contacts are found to have symptomatic gonorrhea – often already treated (Pedersen and Harrah 1970). This is because the woman who comes to a venereal disease clinic typically does not have recently acquired acute symptomatic disease. She has come because she herself has been identified by a male sex partner who has developed symptomatic gonorrhea. Interviewing such a woman will usually yield only the names of the same symptomatic men who originally identified her as being infected, and perhaps other men she has recently infected, most of whom will also have developed symptoms by the time they are found by the contact-investigator.

It is less clear how commonly symptoms occur in women with gonorrhea. Certainly the notion that 80% of infected women never develop symptoms seems inaccurate. It does seem that the prevalence of specific symptoms among all women with gonorrhea at any point in time is low since the prevalence of such symptoms is low among infected women identified as sex partners of men with acute, recently acquired gonococcal urethritis. On the other hand, the prevalence of symptoms is much higher among female patients who attend hospital emergency room, walk-in, or gynecology clinics and who are found to have gonorrhea. For example, a recent survey of women who attended clinics at the University of Washington Hospital and who were found to have gonorrhea, disclosed that 81% sought help because of symptoms attributable to gonorrhea (Handsfield *et al.* 1974). Curran *et al.* (1975) demonstrated that endocervical gonococcal infection was correlated with dysuria, unexplained abnormal menstrual bleeding, bartholinitis, and pelvic inflammatory disease among women examined at the City of Memphis Hospital Emergency Room.

Thus, it should be acknowledged that an unknown proportion of women who acquire gonorrhea develop transient or progressive symptoms such as low abdominal pain or abnormal menstrual bleeding (due to endometritis and salpingitis); purulent vaginal discharge (due to cervicitis); dysuria (due to urethritis); anal discomfort, discharge or bleeding; painful labial swelling (due to acute bartholinitis); sore throat (due to pharyngeal infection) or arthralgias and skin lesions (due to disseminated gonococcal infection – DGI). The proportion who develop symptoms could best be determined by a prospective cohort study. It is possible that the manifestions of gonorrhea differ in initial and recurrent infections, and, as discussed below, the risk of certain complications appears to be influenced by certain definable host factors, as well as by recognizable strain-to-strain variation in gonococcal virulence. Before considering the two principal complications of gonorrhea, however, we should like to discuss two manifestations of gonococcal infections which have only recently been recognized. These are pharyngeal gonococcal infections and the perinatal manifestations of gonococcal infection.

Pharyngeal Gonococcal Infection

Pharyngeal gonococcal infection has been recognized with increasing frequency in the US and in Scandinavian countries since the report of Fiumara *et al.* (1967). Pharyngeal infection is acquired by fellatio, and to a lesser extent by cunnilingus, and is found in 20–30% of women and male homosexuals with gonorrhea who have performed fellatio with their sex partner, and in perhaps 5–10% of heterosexual men who have performed cunnilingus with their current sex partner (Wiesner, Tronca *et al.* 1973, Bro-Jorgensen and Jensen 1973). Infection appears to be limited to the pharynx in a large proportion of pregnant women found to have gonococcal infection (Corman *et al.* 1974). Anecdotal experience suggests pharyngeal gonococcal infection probably causes transient or chronic pharyngitis, although it has not yet been possible to prove this point. We have encountered rare instances of apparent transmission of gonococcal infection from the pharynx by kissing or fellatio. However, the major threat of pharyngeal gonococcal infection appears to be to the infected individual himself, since disseminated gonococcal infection can arise from a pharyngeal focus. In fact, pharyngeal gonococcal infection has been significantly more common among heterosexual men with disseminated gonococcal infection than among those with uncomplicated anterior urethritis (Handsfield 1975), suggesting that pharyngeal infection may carry a particular risk of causing DGI in men, perhaps partly because it is more likely than urethral infection to escape detection and go untreated.

The diagnosis of pharyngeal gonococcal infection requires recovery of *N. gonorrhoeae* from the posterior pharynx on selective medium, and identification of the isolate by sugar fermentation tests. Treatment of pharyngeal infection with 4.8 million units of aqueous procaine penicillin G plus 1.0 g of probenecid is usually successful (Wiesner, Tronca *et al.* 1973, Adams *et al.* 1976) but spectinomycin (Pedersen *et al.* 1975), oral ampicillin (Karney *et al.* 1974) or 5.0 million units of sodium penicillin G in lidocaine given with probenecid (Bro-Jorgensen and Jensen 1973, Adams *et al.* 1976) have been considerably less effective for pharyngeal infection than for genital or anal infection, particularly in male patients.

Perinatal Gonococcal Infection

The effects of gonococcal infection upon early pregnancy have not been well studied. Disseminated gonococcal infection has been observed during the second and third trimester (Holmes, Counts *et al.* 1971). Other complications occur rarely during the second and early third trimester, suggesting that pregnancy confers protection against these complications. However, retrospective study suggests that gonococcal infection near term is associated with premature rupture of membranes with prolonged labor, premature delivery, maternal post-partum fever, chorioamnionitis and funisitis, and orogastric gonococcal contamination of the newborn (Handsfield *et al.* 1973). Recovery of *N. gonorrhoeae* from the orogastric aspirate of the newborn is frequently associated with nonspecific signs compatable with sepsis, and occasionally with pneumonitis or meningitis. This constellation of findings has been termed the "gonococcal amniotic infection syndrome", which has become more common than gonococcal conjunctivitis during the neonatal period. Institution of routine endocervical culturing for *N. gonorrhoeae* at the initial prenatal visit and at the 36th week of pregnancy appears to have largely prevented further occurrence of this syndrome at the University of Washington Hospital in Seattle.

Complications of Gonorrhea

Disseminated Gonococcal Infection

The onset of disseminated gonococcal infection is usually characterized by polyarthralgias and/or inflammation of the extensor tendon(s), particularly involving the wrists, ankles, knees, and small joints of the hands and feet. This is associated with skin lesions which commonly are petechial or papular, but which more distinctively are pustular, hemorrhagic or necrotic, and are usually distributed over the extremities rather than the trunk. Fever and chills may be, but are not necessarily, present. *N. gonorrhoeae* can often be recovered from the blood and demonstrated by fluorescent antibody staining in the skin lesions of patients who present early after the onset of symptoms (Tronca *et al.* 1974). Other patients who do not seek treatment during the bacteremic stage may present with monoarticular arthritis. At this stage blood cultures are usually negative, but *N. gonorrhoeae* can often be recovered from the synovial fluid. The probability of recovering the gonococcus from the synovial fluid is directly related to the duration of the monoarticular arthritis and to the number of polymorphonuclear leukocytes present in the synovial effusion at the time the fluid is aspirated (Handsfield 1975).

In Seattle, an estimated 3% of persons with gonococcal infection develop DGI (Holmes, Wiesner *et al.* 1971). This complication has been observed less commonly in other areas. It is important to stress that genital gonococcal infection is usually nonsymptomatic in men and women with DGI, and nonsymptomatic pharyngeal infection may also give rise to DGI. In many cases the bacteriologic diagnosis depends upon routine performance of genital, pharyngeal, and blood cultures when clinical evidence suggests DGI. None the less, it appears likely that regional differences do exist in the ratio of DGI incidence to total incidence of gonococcal infection. This may be due to regional differences in the prevalence of gonococcal strains which are capable of causing DGI. In Seattle, the majority of gonococci which are isolated from patients with DGI are susceptible to $\leqslant 0.015$ μg/ml of penicillin G (Wiesner, Handsfield *et al.* 1973). Recent application of the auxotyping method described by Catlin (1973) has disclosed that all penicillin-hypersensitive gonococci recovered from patients with DGI are classifiable as auxotype 11 or 14, because they have auxotrophic requirements for arginine, hypoxanthine, and uracil (AHU) (Knapp and Holmes 1975). It is not yet clear whether penicillin-hypersensitivity and/or the requirements for AHU are genetically linked to virulence; or whether these are coincidental markers which, although not linked to virulence, permit recognition of strains capable of producing DGI.

It is of interest to note that in Seattle during 1973, approximately 40% of gonococci recovered from patients with uncomplicated gonorrhea were susceptible to ⩽0.015 μg/ml of penicillin G, and required AHU. All isolates which were susceptible to ⩽0.015 μg penicillin/ml required AHU.

Table 1

Auxotrophic requirements of *N. gonorrhoea* recovered from patients with DGI or with uncomplicated gonorrhea in Seattle and from males with urethritis in London

Minimal inhibitory concentration of Penicillin G	*Seattle patients with DGI*		*Seattle uncomplicated gonorrhea*		*London uncomplicated gonorrhea*	
	AHU •	*Other* ■	*AHU*	*Other*	*AHU*	*Other*
⩽0.008	33	0	15	0	3	0
0.015	8	0	11	0	8	19
0.03	0	0	2	8	1	1
0.06	0	0	0	4	1	3
0.125	0	0	0	7	0	3
0.25	0	2	0	10	0	1
0.50	0	2	0	15	0	3
1.0	0	1	0	4	0	1

• AHU indicates number of isolates which require arginine, hypoxanthine, and uracil. Only one isolate per patient is included in this table

■ Other indicates number of isolates which are prototrophic or require arginine, proline, or arginine plus proline, but do not require hypoxanthine or uracil. Only one isolate per patient is included

Examination of 44 strains of *N. gonorrhoeae* isolated from consecutive uncomplicated cases of gonorrhea at St Thomas's Hospital in London, and kindly provided by Dr Ian Philips, showed somewhat different results (Table 1). Thirty percent of 44 isolates required AHU, and although all of these were susceptible to ⩽0.015 μg/ml of penicillin G, only about half of the London strains which were susceptible to 0.015 μg/ml actually required AHU.

A more interesting finding is that penicillin-hypersensitive, AHU-requiring strains of *N. gonorrhoeae* recovered from patients with DGI are resistant to the complement-mediated bactericidal activity of normal human serum, whereas a large percentage of AHU-non-requiring strains recovered from patients with uncomplicated infection are rapidly killed by normal human serum in the presence of complement (Schoolnik *et al.* 1975). Individuals who lack certain precursors required for the terminal sequence of complement activation may be uniquely susceptible to DGI (Petersen *et al.* 1975). The relationship of penicillin hypersensitivity, serum resistance, AHU requirement, and virulence of *N. gonorrhoeae* remains to be defined.

Pelvic Inflammatory Disease

Dr Wiesner has presented data suggesting that for every 100 cases of gonorrhea in women there are approximately 20 cases of PID. Studies of 204 women with PID examined consecutively during 1973 and 1974 in Seattle have shown that gonococcal infection was directly responsible for approximately half these cases (Eschenbach *et al.* 1975). Gonococci recovered from women with PID have not yet been found to have distinguishing characteristics.

An attempt was therefore made to elucidate factors which predispose women with gonorrhea to develop PID, and also to determine the cause(s) of nongonococcal PID. For this purpose, a case-control study design was employed, in which women with acute PID were matched with female controls who did not have PID. Matching was accomplished for age, race, marital status, parity, socioeconomic status, number of recent sex partners, and presence or absence of gonorrhea. It was found that IUD usage was significantly more common among PID patients than among controls (Eschenbach 1975). Three previous studies have also shown that the risk of PID is increased among IUD users (Wright and Laemmle 1968, Noonan and Adams 1974, Targum and Wright 1974). Because the Seattle study involved PID patients who were studied prospectively, it was possible to show that IUD usage was predominately associated with nongonococcal PID. Several types of IUD were found to be associated with PID. An unexpected finding was that oral contraceptive use was less common among women with gonococcal PID than among their matched controls who had uncomplicated gonorrhea. This suggests that, whatever the influence of oral contraceptives upon the risk of acquisition of gonoccal infection, their use may somehow decrease the risk of PID once gonococcal infection occurs.

A large proportion of cases of nongonococcal PID were found to be associated with pelvic peritoneal infection by vaginal commensal bacteria – particularly by *Bacteroides fragilis*, peptostreptococci and peptococci (Eschenbach 1975). As has previously been noted (Falk 1965), the onset of gonococcal PID and, to a lesser extent, of nongonococcal PID, coincides with menstruation. A history of mild PID occurring with previous attacks of gonorrhea (analogous to the clinical syndrome described by Rees and Annels (1969)) was often elicited from women presenting with nongonococcal PID. Prospective follow up of the cohort of Seattle women treated for gonococcal PID then confirmed the fact that an initial episode of gonococcal PID is often followed by subsequent attacks of nongonococcal PID.

Conclusions

The natural history and usual manifestations of gonorrhea in men have been studied by a number of methods, most extensively in military populations. It remains to be determined whether exceptions exist to the general concepts emerging from these studies. For example, it is not known whether the incubation period and usual manifestations of infection caused by penicillin-hypersensitive, AHU-requiring, serum-resistant gonococci are different from those of infection caused by other types of gonococci. None the less, increased awareness of the importance of interviewing self-referred women, to identify their nonsymptomatic male sex partners, has emerged during the past few years. The clinical epidemiology of gonorrhea in women has not been subjected to a cohort study, and the frequency of occurrence of the various clinical manifestations of gonorrhea has not been determined. In fact, one might point out that the absence of data concerning the prevalence, manifestations, and diagnosis of gonorrhea in women seen in casualty departments and non-STD clinics in Great Britain has been almost as conspicuous as the absence of the word service from the various descriptive titles used at this meeting to characterize the venereal disease program in the United States. The present incidence of gonorrhea in Great Britain appears to be much lower than in the US, perhaps as a result of the well-organized venereal disease service in Britain. It seems appropriate to point out at this Anglo-American Conference that the reported case rate of gonorrhea among persons 20–24 years of age – the peak incidence group – was over three times higher during 1973 in the United States than in the United Kingdom. Since reporting is considered more complete in the UK, the true difference was probably much greater. If these differences are indeed due to the venereal disease service success in the UK, it might be that further progress could be made by directing attention to the diagnosis of gonorrhea in symptomatic women seen outside the STD clinic.

Pharyngeal gonococcal infection and the perinatal gonococcal amniotic infection syndrome represent manifestations of gonorrhea which undoubtedly have been with us for a long time, but which have been recognized only relatively recently. The effect of gonococcal infection upon pregnancy requires more careful study. The observed incidence of DGI may vary from one region to another, in relation to the regional prevalence of unique strains of *N. gonorrhoeae* which appear to cause DGI. Host factors such as menstruation and contraceptive practices are particularly important determinants of the risk of PID in women with gonorrhea. A major unanswered question concerns the nature of host factors which determine susceptibility to gonococcal infection, particularly the nature and extent of acquired immunity.

Acknowledgments

We are grateful to the Center for Disease Control, Department of Health, Education and Welfare, for support by Contract HSM 21-73-535, and to the National Institutes of Health for research grant AI-12192.

References

Adams, H. G., Turck, M. and Holmes, K. K. (1976). *In* "Genital Infections and Their Complications". Proceedings of the Symposium held in Stockholm, October 9–11, 1974. Ed. D. Danielsson *et al.* Almquist and Wiksell, Stockholm; p 1925

Blount, J. H. (1972). *American Journal of Public Health and the Nation's Health* **62**, 710–712

Bro-Jorgensen, A. and Jensen, T. (1973). *British Journal of Venereal Diseases* **49**, 491–499.

Brown, W. J. (1971). *Journal of Infectious Diseases* **123**, 682–688

Catlin, B. W. (1973). *Journal of Infectious Diseases* **128**,178–194

Corman, L. C., Levison, M. E., Knight, R., Carrington, E. R. and Kay, D. (1974). *Journal of the American Medical Association* **230**, 568–570

Curran, J. W., Rendtorff, R. C., Chandler, R. W., Wiser, W. L. and Robinson. H. (1975). *Obstetrics and Gynecology* **45** 195–198

Eschenbach, D. A. (1975). Paper presented at the 15th Interscience Conference on Antimicrobial Agents and Chemotherapy, Washington DC

Eschenbach, D. A., Buchanan, T. M., Pollock, H. M., Forsyth, P. S., Alexander, E. R., Lin, J. S., Wang, S. P., Wentworth, B. B., McCormack, W. M. and Holmes, K. K. (1975). *New England Journal of Medicine* **293**, 166–171

Falk, V. (1965). *Acta obstetrica et gynecological Scandinavica* **44**, 65–118

Fiumàra, N. J. (1972). *Medical Clinics of North America* **56**, 1105–1114

Fiumàra, N. J., Wise, H. M. Jr and Many, M. (1967). *New England Journal of Medicine* **276**, 1248–1250

Handsfield, H. H. (1974). Paper presented at the 14th Interscience Conference on Antimicrobial Agents and Chemotherapy, Washington DC

Handsfield, H. H., Hodson, W. A. and Holmes, K. K. (1973). *Journal of the American Medical Association* **225**, 697–701

Handsfield, H. H., Lipman, T. O., Harnisch, J. P., Tronca, E. and Holmes, K. K. (1974). *New England Journal of Medicine* **290**, 117–123

Harrison, W. O., Hooper, R., Wiesner, P. J. and Holmes, K. K. (1973). Paper presented at the 13th Interscience Conference on Antimicrobial Agents and Chemotherapy, Washington DC

Holmes, K. K., Counts, G. W. and Beaty, H. N. (1971). *Annals of Internal Medicine* **74**, 979–993

Holmes, K. K., Wiesner, P. J. and Pedersen, A. H. B. (1971). *Annals of Internal Medicine* **75**, 470-471

Karney, W. W., Turck, M. and Holmes, K. K. (1974). *Journal of Infectious Diseases* **129**, 5250-5253

Knapp, J. S. and Holmes, K. K. (1975). *Journal of Infectious Diseases* **132**, 204-208

Noonan, A. S. and Adams, J. B. (1974). *American Journal of Public Health and the Nation's Health* **64**, 700

Pedersen, A. H. B. and Harrah, W. D. (1970). *Public Health Reports* **85**, 997-1000

Pedersen, A. H. B, Wiesner, P. J., Holmes, K. K., Johnson, C. J. and Turck, M. (1972). *Journal of the American Medical Association* **220**, 205-208

Petersen, B. H., Graham, J. A. and Brooks, G. F. (1975). *Clinical Research* **23**, 259a

Rees, E. and Annels, E. H. (1969). *British Journal of Venereal Diseases* **45**, 205-215

Schoolnik, G. A., Buchanan, T. M. and Holmes, K. K. (1975). Paper presented at the 15th Interscience Conference on Antimicrobial Agents and Chemotherapy, Washington DC

Targum, S. D. and Wright, N. H. (1974). *American Journal of Epidemiology* **100**, 262-271

Tronca, E., Handsfield, H. H., Wiesner, P. J. and Holmes, K. K. (1974). *Journal of Infectious Diseases* **129**, 582-586

Wiesner, P. J., Handsfield, H. H. and Holmes, K. K. (1973). *New England Journal of Medicine* **288**, 181-185

Wiesner, P. J., Tronca, E., Bonin, P., Pedersen, A. H. B. and Holmes, K. K. (1973). *New England Journal of Medicine* **288**, 181-185

Wright, N. H. and Laemmle, P. (1968). *American Journal of Obstetrics and Gynecology* **101**, 979-990

Chlamydial Infection of the Genital Tract in the Mothers and Fathers of Babies Suffering from Ophthalmia Neonatorum due to TRIC Agent

E M C Dunlop and David Goldmeier
Diagnostic Clinic, Moorfields Eye Hospital, and
Whitechapel Clinic, The London Hospital,
S Darougar and Barrie R Jones
The Virus Laboratory, Department of Clinical Opthalmology,
Institute of Ophthalmology, London

The mothers of babies who develop ophthalmia neonatorum due to TRIC agent must have transmitted the infection from the genital tract to their babies at the time of delivery. If the fathers of such babies have urethritis it is likely to be due to the same cause. Hence material from such mothers and fathers was used to test the sensitivity of cell culture as a diagnostic method for chlamydial infection of the cervix, urethra and rectum, in women, and of the urethra in men.

Methods and Patients

Twenty-five mothers and 19 fathers of babies who had developed ophthalmia neonatorum due to TRIC agent were studied, using the methods for collection of specimens that have been outlined (Dunlop *et al.* 1964, Dunlop *et al.* 1965, Dunlop *et al.* 1969, Dunlop *et al.* 1971, Dunlop *et al.* 1972). The simplified cell-culture techniques that were used have been outlined (Darougar *et al.* 1971, Darougar, Kinnison and Jones 1971, Darougar *et al.* 1972).

An additional 9 mothers were excluded from this assessment. In 3 cases the mother had already received treatment, for pelvic inflammatory disease (one case), dysuria (one case) and fever (one case), sufficient to make isolation of Chlamydia unsuccessful. In 3 cases the baby had been treated prior to diagnosis, so that tests of conjunctival material for Chlamydia gave negative results and ocular infection by TRIC agent could not be proved. In one case, that of a baby clinically suffering from partly treated ophthalmia neonatorum due to TRIC agent, tests of baby and mother did not show that agent, although it was found in urethral material from the father, who had urethritis. In 2 cases the results of genital tests of the mother and father are not yet available.

Table 1

Genital findings in 25 mothers of babies suffering from TRIC-positive ophthalmia neonatorum

	No. of cases	
Symptoms (discharge, abdominal pain, dysuria)	24	
Cervix: mucosal change:		
"Follicles", lumps	22	23
"Follicles" and "splash" scarring	1	
Pus	21	
Pelvic inflammatory disease:		
Salpingitis	6	8 •
Endometritis	1	
Salpingitis and endometritis	1	
Rectum:		
Mucosal change	9	
Pus	6	
Cell culture Chlamydia-positive:		
Cervix	19/25	23
Urethra	10/20	
Rectum	5/25	
Fixation in LGVCFT:		
Any	11	
>1 in 16	6 ■	

•Excluded: 1 R_X already for PID

■ All Chlamydia-positive

Results

Twenty-five mothers were studied. Two mothers had previously been treated for sexually transmitted disease: one for gonorrhoea twice, trichomoniasis twice, genital warts and early latent syphilis; the other for trichomoniasis and candidiasis. There were symptoms of infection (vaginal discharge, dysuria, lower abdominal pain) in 24 cases (Table 1), mucosal changes in the marginal area of the cervix in 23, pus on microscopy of the endocervical mucus (maximal count 25 or more polymorphonuclear leukocytes per high-power field (HPF)) in 21 and evidence of pelvic inflammatory disease (PID) in 8. There were mucosal changes in the anorectum in 9, there was pus on the anorectal mucosa (maximal count 10 or more polymorphonuclear leukocytes per HPF) in 6. TRIC agent was grown from cervical material in cell culture in 19 of the 25, from urethral material in 10 of 20, raising the number of Chlamydia-positive cases to 23 of 25 (because in 4 cases the agent was grown from urethral material alone), and from anorectal material in 5 of 25; in each of these 5 the agent was also grown from cervical material.

A complement-fixation test (LGVCFT) for antibody to group anti-chlamydial antibody gave some fixation in 11 cases; in 6 (2 with PID) the titre was greater than 1 in 16.

Two mothers had candidiasis initially, 2 developed it during follow-up. Two mothers had trichomoniasis, and one of these developed gonorrhoea during follow-up, after her husband had been found to have gonococcal urethritis following extramarital intercourse.

Table 2

Genital findings in 19 fathers of 25 babies suffering from TRIC-positive ophthalmia neonatorum

	No. of cases	
History of urethritis	6	
Urethritis:		
"Non-specific" urethritis	13	14
Trichomonas vaginalis positive	1	
Cell culture Chlamydia-positive:		
Urethral meatus swab	5/18	8
Endourethral swab	6/18	
Urethral scrape	8/19	
Fixation in LGVCFT:		
Any	4	
>1 in 16	0	

Nineteen fathers of the 25 babies were studied. Five had previously been treated for sexually transmitted disease: one for non-specific urethritis (NSU) and for latent syphilis or yaws; one for gonorrhoea twice and NSU once, 2 for NSU, and one for gonorrhoea. Two developed gonorrhoea during follow-up. Six gave a history of urethral discharge (Table 2), with or without dysuria. On examination, including tests of the overnight urethral secretion in those without obvious discharge, 14 had urethritis. Trichomonads were present in the urethral secretion of one of these, the remainder had "non-specific" urethritis. Chlamydia was isolated from 8 of the 14 men with urethritis. No isolate was obtained from those without urethritis.

The LGVCFT showed some fixation in 4 cases; in no case was the titre greater than 1 in 16.

Discussion

In 1966 Dunlop *et al.* (1967) reported the detection of TRIC agent in cervical material from 8 of 28 mothers similar to those in the present series. In 4 cases agent was grown in yolk sac, in 3 cases it was grown and inclusions detected in smears, in one case an inclusion was found. Dr Francis Gordon was present at the meetings in San Francisco and Asilomar at which these findings were presented. He then came to the Institute of Ophthalmology, London, and set up his cell-culture system, using irradiated McCoy cells (Gordon *et al.* 1969), which has been continued with modifications.

Some of you will know that, after Francis Gordon retired as Director of the Department of Microbiology of the US Naval Medical Research Institute, he was awarded a Medical Research Council fellowship. This was to study cellular immunity in chlamydial infection at the Institute of Ophthalmology. He and his wife Mary set sail from New York in a container ship on 19 October 1973 to take up this fellowship. Two days out of New York the ship caught fire; when their lifeboat was being launched Francis and Mary Gordon were swept out and drowned. This tragedy was a major loss, not only for all of us who knew them, but also for the study of chlamydial infection.

The increase in the positive findings in the present series using cell culture, compared with the earlier series (Dunlop *et al.* 1967) which used culture in yolk sac and the examination of smears, was due to a number of factors. Pre-eminent among these was the greater sensitivity of cell culture. Others were the selection of patients in the present series, and the changes in the technique for collecting speciments from women, so that urethral material was collected and multiple specimens were obtained.

In the selection of patients 3 women were excluded because they had received or were receiving treatment with antibiotics, sufficient to affect the result of tests for Chlamydia. Two such cases were included in the previous series. Deducting these, the positive findings in that series would become 8 of 26 compared with 23 of 25 in the cell-culture series.

In the present series urethral tests yielded an additional 4 positive cases, 2 in routine tests, 2 in multiple tests. Deducting these results the remaining 19 positive cases of the 25 in the cell culture series can be compared with the 8 positive cases of the 26 in the early series. One of the urethral isolates was obtained from a mother (Mrs Y H) with marked "burning" dysuria but no increase in frequency of micturition. An addition endourethral swab (Dunlop *et al.* 1972) was used to obtain urethral material. An isolate was obtained from this specimen. All others gave negative results.

The taking of multiple specimens was another factor in the cell-culture series. They were taken from 13 women. In these cases 18 of 34 swabs of cervical material were positive, as were 14 of 32 cervical scrapings, 9 of 30 swabs of urethral material, and 7 of 32 swabs of anorectal material. Thus, in these 13 cases 48 isolates were obtained from 128 specimens.

The taking of multiple specimens yielded 2 additional positive cases which were missed by culture of the first specimen in each series of tests. One of these 2 cases has already been deducted because the only positive finding was in urethral material. Deduction of the remaining one leaves 18 positive cases of 25 tested, compared with 8 of 26 in the earlier yolk-sac series.

Of 19 fathers studied using cell culture 14 had urethritis; isolates were obtained from urethral material from 8 of the 14. This compares with 19 fathers (Dunlop *et al.* 1967) in the series studied by means of culture in yolk sac and by smear. Seventeen had urethritis, and 8 of this number had positive tests. It is possible that some of these isolations in yolk sac were pseudo-isolations as none was first pass. In contrast no control specimen has given a positive result during work in this laboratory on cell culture.

Summary

Twenty-five mothers of babies suffering from ophthalmia neonatorum due to TRIC agent were studied. There were symptoms of infection in 24 cases, mucosal changes in the marginal area of the cervix in 23, excess of pus in the endocervical mucus in 21, PID in 8, mucosal changes in the anorectum in 9 and pus on the anorectal mucosa in 6.

Results of culture for Chlamydia in cell culture of cervical, urethral and rectal material were positive in 23 cases. In 4 cases isolates were obtained from urethral material only. This compares with positive results from only 8 of 26 similar mothers previously studied by culture of material in yolk sac, and by the examination of smears. The difference is because culture in cell culture is a more sensitive method of testing for Chlamydia; and because tests of urethral material, and of multiple specimens, were carried out in the present study.

Urethral material from 19 fathers of these 25 babies was cultured for Chlamydia in cell culture. Fourteen fathers had urethritis, isolates were obtained from 8 of these men. Positive findings were earlier obtained from 8 of 19 such fathers by means of culture in yolk sac and the examination of smears. Some of these isolates in yolk sac may have been due to cross-contamination in the laboratory. Control studies show that culture in cell culture is free from the risk of such cross-contamination.

Acknowledgments

We are grateful to our colleagues for referring patients for investigation, and to Dr A E Wilkinson, Director of the VD Reference Laboratory, The London Hospital, for carrying out serological tests for syphilis and cultures for bacteria, for Candida and for *Trichomonas vaginalis.* Dr David Goldmeier's work at The London Hospital was supported by a grant from the Medical Research Council.

References

Darougar, S., Dwyer, R. St. C., Treharne, J. D., Harper, I. A., Garland, J. A. and Jones, B. R. (1971). *In* "Trachoma and Related Disorders". Ed. R. L. Nichols. Excerpta Medica, Amsterdam; p 445

Darougar, S., Jones, B. R., Kinnison, J. R., Vaughan-Jackson, J. D. and Dunlop, E. M. C. (1972). *British Journal of Venereal Diseases* **48**, 416

Darougar, S., Kinnison, J. R. and Jones, B. R. (1971). *In* "Trachoma and Related Disorders". Ed. R. L. Nichols. Excerpta Medica, Amsterdam; p 63

Dunlop, E. M. C., Al-Hussaini, M. K., Garland, J. A., Treharne, J. D., Harper, I. A. and Jones, B. R. (1965). *Lancet* **i**, 1125, 1286

Dunlop, E. M. C., Freedman, A., Garland, J. A., Harper, I. A., Jones, B. R., Race, J. W., Du Toit, M. S. and Treharne, J. D. (1967). *American Journal of Ophthalmology* **63**, 1073

Dunlop, E. M. C., Hare, M. J., Darougar, S. and Jones, B. R. (1971). *In* "Trachoma and Related Disorders". Ed. R. L. Nichols. Excerpta Medica, Amsterdam; p 494

Dunlop, E. M. C., Hare, M. J., Darougar, S., Jones, B. R. and Rice, N. S. C. (1969). *Journal of Infectious Diseases* **120**, 463

Dunlop, E. M. C., Jones, B. R. and Al-Hassaini, M. K. (1964). *British Journal of Venereal Diseases* **40**, 33

Dunlop, E. M. C., Vaughan-Jackson, J. D. and Darougar, S. (1972). *British Journal of Venereal Diseases* **48**, 421

Gordon, F. B., Harper, I. A., Quan, A. L., Treharne, J. D., Dwyer, R. St. C. and Garland, J. A. (1969). *Journal of Infectious Diseases* **120**, 451

Interaction of Gonococci with Host Cells

Professor Peter J Watt, M E Ward and Janet N Robertson
Microbiology, Faculty of Medicine,
University of Southampton
Medical and Biological Sciences Building,
Bassett Crescent East, Southampton SO9 3TU

Inflammatory Response in Gonorrhoea

A profuse, purulent discharge is so typical of acute gonorrhoea that the diagnosis can be made with a 95% certainty by simple examination of the patient (Jacobs and Kraus 1975). A visual impression of

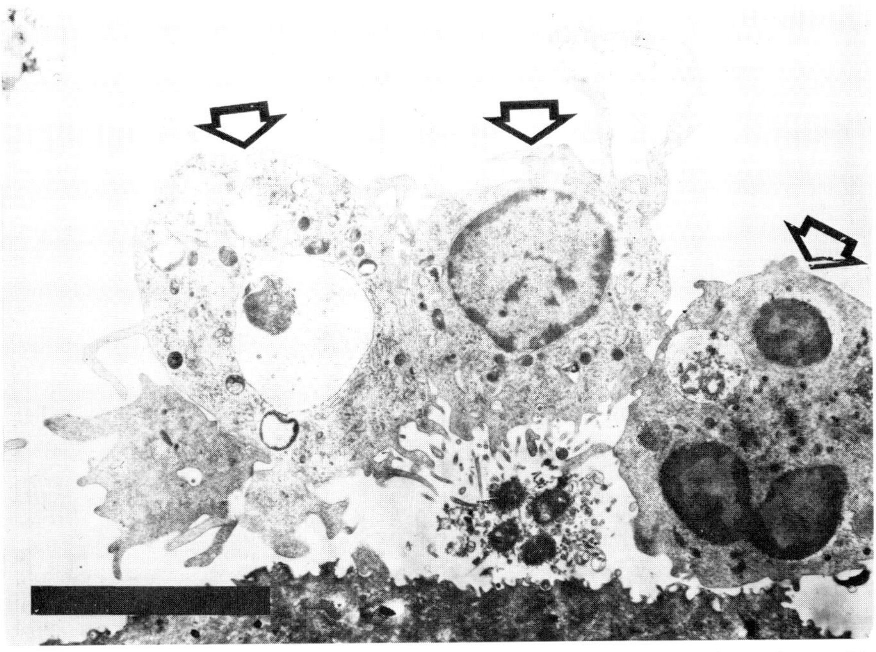

Fig. 1 *Electron micrograph of urethral material taken from a male patient with symptomatic gonorrhoea of less than one day's duration. Polymorphs (arrows) are clearly readily attracted towards the invading gonococci. The bar represents 10 μm*

this marked propensity of gonococci to attract polymorphonuclear leukocytes (PMN) is shown in Fig. 1. In this electron micrograph of urethral pus from a male with acute gonorrhoea, 3 PMN can be seen converging on a cluster of gonococci associated with the surface of an epithelial cell.

In order to identify the stimulus which attracts these enormous numbers of PMN we have used the Boyden chamber. In this system the chemotactic stimulus is separated from human PMN by a membrane with 3 μm pores. After incubation at 37°C for 90 min, the distance the polymorphs have migrated towards the stimulus is assessed by measuring the depth of penetration of PMN into the membrane. The first proposition to be excluded is that during growth gonococci generate chemotactic factors, for example metabolic products or budded-off cell-wall vesicles (Stead *et al.* 1975). When pilated gonococci were suspended at a concentration of 5×10^9 organisms/ml, only one of 3 strains tested was weakly chemotactic. On testing purified fractions of the gonococcus for chemotactic activity, we found a solubilized fraction of the cell wall enhanced chemotaxis fourfold over the media blank while high concentrations of gonococcal lipids were found to inhibit PMN migration.

If we are to assess the biological significance of these findings, we should ask the critical question: "Are chemotactic factors liberated from invading gonococci or damaged human cells when virulent gonococci invade a mucosal surface isolated from host defence systems?" We have looked for chemotaxins liberated from human fallopian tube organ cultures infected with pilated gonococci and maintained 48 hours after challenge. Both the culture supernatant and homogenized tissue were found to be weakly chemotactic but we had identical results in our noninfected organ culture controls. If, then, the potent chemotaxins of acute gonorrhoea are not generated by the organism nor result from damage of mucosal cells, we must examine the interaction of gonococci with antibodies and complement. The difficulty of studying this in the laboratory is that normal serum and plasma are potent chemotaxins (Frei *et al.* 1974); perhaps the factors concerned are normally cleared from the circulation *in vivo*. Accepting the high plasma control migration, we find that when serum from a single individual was reacted with 3 different strains of gonococci there was a marked difference in the chemotaxins generated. The likely reason is variation in the specificity of natural antibodies for different gonococcal strains. One might further postulate that the phagocytosis of gonococci by PMN would produce new chemotaxins, thus enhancing the inflammatory response. This appears likely, as we have demonstrated chemotaxins released when PMN phagocytose washed opsonized gonococci in the absence of complement. The obvious next step will be to determine if the serum of asymptomatic carriers fails to generate chemotaxins on reaction with the infecting strain of gonococcus. Failure to generate chemotaxins and thus inflammation might be an easy explanation for the lack of symptoms.

Phagocytosis of Gonococci by Human PMN

In an earlier study (Ward *et al.* 1972), we investigated the fate of gonococci in PMN from men with acute gonorrhoea using the electron microscope to look for ultrastructural damage in the bacteria. We demonstrated that PMN degranulate normally into vacuoles containing gonococci and that obviously degenerate forms were present in older vacuoles. More recently there has been a

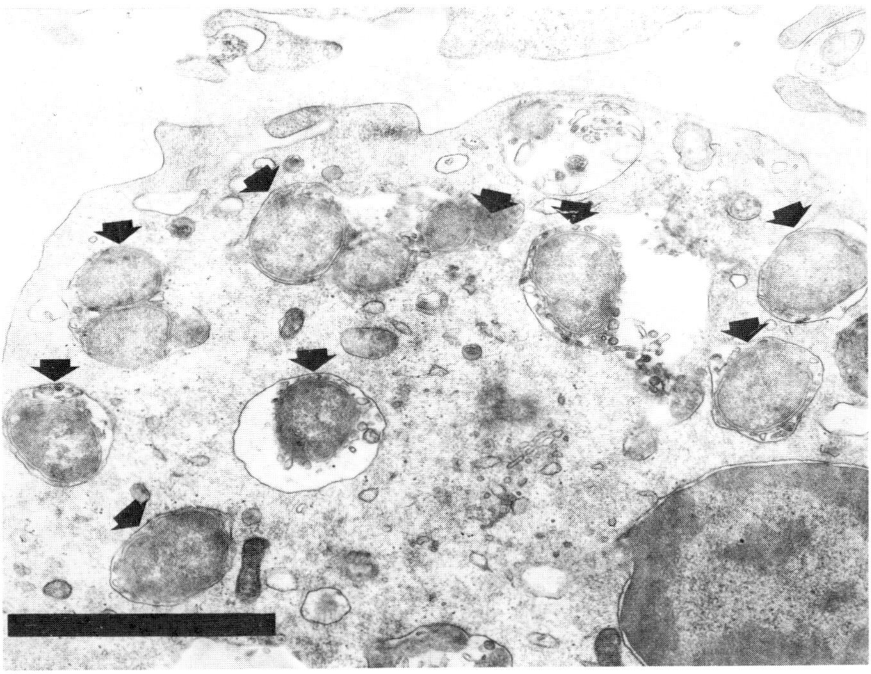

Fig. 2 *Electron micrograph of a portion of a polymorphonuclear leukocyte from a male patient with early symptomatic gonorrhoea. Numerous gonococci (arrows) may commonly be seen within polymorph phagosomal vacuoles, demonstrating, in contrast to some reports in the literature, that virulent gonococci are readily phagocytosed. The bar represents 2 μm*

considerable outflow of laboratory studies on the interaction of gonococci and PMN. Thongthai and Sawyer (1973), using gonococci from agar plates, suggest that gonococcal pili act as an antiphagocytic virulence factor inhibiting phagocytosis by PMN. Gibbs and Roberts (1975), using gonococci grown in the chick embryo, suggest that pilated gonococci grown into the log phase attach to but are not phagocytosed by PMN. This property was lost in log-phase organisms. In contradistinction, the results of Swanson *et al.* (1974) showed that pilation was of minor importance in the attachment-ingestion of gonococci by human PMN. It seems to us pertinent to question the relevance of these laboratory studies to human disease. Surely we all recognize gonococcal pus by the numerous gonococci associated with the PMN. Having examined scores of urethral exudates using the electron microscope, we know that these gonococci lie inside phagocytic vacuoles. Fig. 2 shows such a PMN from urethral pus; a

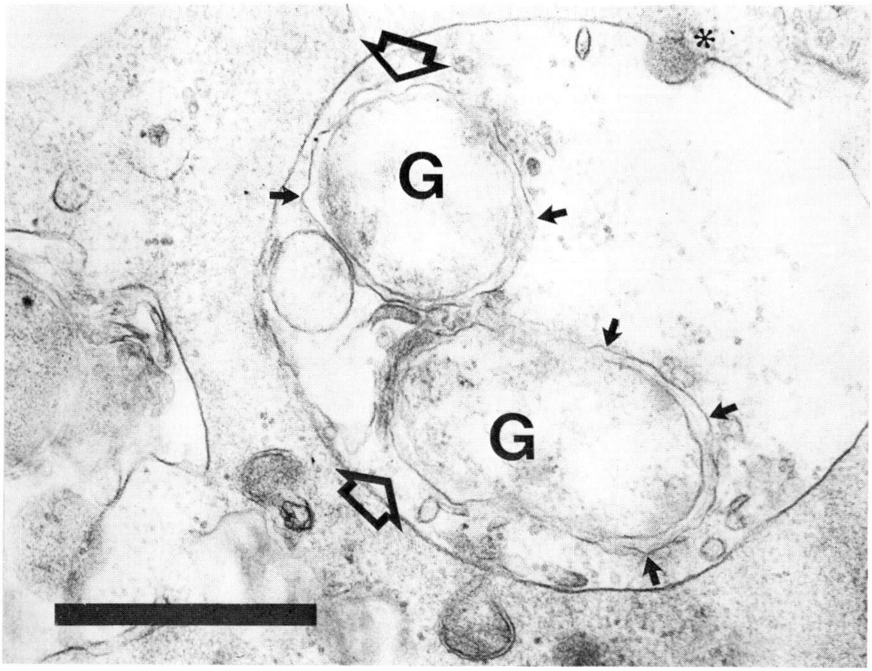

Fig. 3 *Ultrathin section of the phagolysosomal vacuole of a polymorph from a patient with early acute gonorrhoea. A lysosome (asterisk) is in the process of being released into the vacuole demonstrating that gonococci* (G) *do not inhibit degranulation. The gonococci are clearly being destroyed: note the absence of ribosomes, the detaching outer envelope (arrow heads) and the presence of breaks in the cell wall (hollow arrows). The bar represents 1 μm*

dozen gonococci can be seen lying in phagocytic vacuoles inside the cell.

Laboratory studies of the fate of gonococci within PMN have produced conflicting results. Gibbs and Roberts (1975) accept that after ingestion gonococci do not survive or multiply intracellularly but are rapidly killed by human PMN. Certainly there can be no doubt that in the natural disease many of the gonococci ingested by PMN are dead, as evidenced by disintegration of the cell wall and loss of ribosomes (Fig. 3). However, Veale *et al.* (1975) have made the interesting suggestion that "a significant aspect of the pathogenicity of gonococci appears to be that, while some are killed within human phagocytes, others survive and possibly multiply". The data presented by these workers indicate that some 88% of phagocyte-associated gonococci are killed after 2 hours' incubation. Veale *et al.* believe that the persisting 12% of PMN-associated gonococci lie within host cells and the fact that they were destroyed by incubation with 2 μg/ml penicillin in the presence of fresh serum indicates that the antibiotic penetrates phagocytes infected with gonococci. They go on to state that at a lower concentration, 0.2 μg/ml, penicillin fails to enter PMN but will destroy extracellular gonococci. Examining their data, we see that in the presence of 0.2 μg of penicillin the numbers of intracellular gonococci increase from 500 to 9675 in 2 hours; this indicates a division time of 28 min. Thus we are faced with deciding between the possibilities that every gonococcus within these PMN was dividing three times faster than the best growth rates we have achieved using enriched media in the laboratory, or that the experimental method was subject to an eighteenfold error. Mandell (1973), using radio-labelled penicillin and a marker to determine extracellular water, clearly demonstrated that PMN which had phagocytosed staphylococci remained impermeable to penicillin. Until such sophisticated technology is applied to laboratory studies on the phagocytosis of gonococci, we see no reason to modify our earlier claim that in acute gonorrhoea the gonococci are readily phagocytosed and destroyed by PMN.

Growth of Gonococci on Mucosal Surfaces

The undoubted attachment of gonococci to the mucosal cells lining the urethra and cervix (Ward and Watt 1972, Ward *et al.* 1975) permits the organism to multiply at these sites despite the flows of urine and mucous secretions. Multiplication on the mucosal cell surface presumably precedes invasion of the submucosa; thus it is to be expected that factors affecting the growth rate of gonococci would modify the outcome of the infection. Undoubtedly biological factors other than immunity influence the clinical features of gonococcal infections. Thus gonococcal salpingitis rarely presents in the luteal phase of the menstrual cycle and it is more difficult to isolate gonococci from the cervix at this time. Morse and Fitzgerald (1974) have sought an explanation in an inhibitory action of progesterone on the multiplication of gonococci. The system used was to add varying amounts of progesterone to cultures of 10 million gonococci in broth. At concentrations of progesterone less than 20 μg/ml considerable variation was found in the degree of growth inhibition, but all gonococcal strains were markedly inhibited at progesterone concentrations of 40 μg/ml. A concentration of 40 μg/ml progesterone is 4000 times the plasma level in the luteal phase of the cycle, moreover all but 1.3% of plasma progesterone is avidly bound to protein. Given that the concentration of progesterone in the fallopian tube fluid is comparable to the plasma level (Hoskins and Casillas 1975), it is difficult to accept the relevance of this type of work. We have been interested in gonococcal infection of the human fallopian tube maintained in organ culture. Because the fallopian tube is susceptible to changes in the concentration of oestrogen and progesterone, it is a valid model for investigating the

Table 1

Effect of progesterone on the growth of gonococci on human fallopian tube organ cultures

Inoculum counts		*Growth after 8 hours' incubation*	
		Control	*Progesterone* 10^{-5} g/ml
	1×10^2	1.6×10^3	5.6×10^2
	2×10^1	4.2×10^3	2.8×10^2
	5×10^2	1.4×10^2	6.2×10^2
	6×10^1	5.6×10^2	2.6×10^2
	6×10^1	1.9×10^3	4.4×10^2
	5.6×10^2	6.8×10^3	3.4×10^3
	1.8×10^2	3×10^2	1.4×10^3
	1.6×10^2	4×10^1	7.2×10^2
	1.1×10^2	3.8×10^2	8×10^1
	1.6×10^2	3.4×10^2	2.6×10^2
Mean	1.07×10^2	5.01×10^2	4.8×10^2

Mean generation time no progesterone	3.59 h
Mean generation time 10^{-5} g/ml progesterone	3.70 h

effect of sex hormones on gonococcal infection: in our experiments we have infected the mucosal surface of fallopian tube organ cultures with a challenge dose of 100 pilated gonococci. Groups of 10 organ cultures were incubated without hormone, in the presence of the peak physiological level of hormone and in a concentration a thousandfold higher. The multiplication of gonococci was determined by viable counts after 8 hours' incubation. Table 1 shows the results of one such experiment; the mean generation time of gonococci growing on the mucosal surface in the absence of progesterone was 3.59 hours. Progesterone did not inhibit growth; at a concentration of 10^{-5} g/ml, 4, Pregnen-3,20 dione (a thousandfold higher than physiological), the mean generation time was 3.70 hours. Most certainly in our system, physiological concentrations of progesterone do not impair the growth of gonococci. In other experiments we found a mean division time of 4.01 hours in controls without oestradiol 17β and 3.88 hours in physiological concentrations of 10^{-9} g/ml oestrogen. These small differences are nowhere near to being statistically significant. Thus, our experimental results fail to support the concept that changes in the seriousness of gonococcal infections at different phases of the menstrual cycle are due to the direct action of hormones on gonococci. Surely, it is more likely that the effect of hormones on the infection is secondary to changes in host physiology. One simple suggestion has been that progesterone increases the acidity of vaginal mucus thus inhibiting gonococcal growth. A more sophisticated hypothesis would be that oestrogens and progesterones act by altering the concentrations of the secondary cell messengers, cAMP and cGMP. Thus, oestradiol 17β stimulates adenyl cyclase increasing cellular concentrations of cAMP (Singhal and Sutherland 1975). Drugs that increase intracellular levels of cAMP in phagocytes inhibit the rate of ingestion (Stossel 1974) and we know that the mucosal cells lining the genital tract phagocytose gonococci (Ward *et al.* 1975). Perhaps, then, the reduced incidence of gonococcal salpingitis during the phase of the menstrual cycle when oestrogen levels are high is explained by a relative inhibition of the uptake of gonococci into mucosal cells. Clearly more work is needed in this area.

Interaction of Gonococci and Mucosal Cells

In order to grow on a mucosal surface, gonococci must not only anchor to the cell membranes but each daughter organism must be capable of holding on to its partner. There is now abundant evidence that pili facilitate attachment of gonococci to each other (Swanson *et al.* 1971), to human cells in tissue culture (Swanson 1973) and to human sperm (James-Holmquest *et al.* 1974). As yet we know little of the molecular mechanisms involved in this attachment.

Using electrofocusing, we have demonstrated that gonococci have a pI of 5.6, that is, they have a net negative charge due to an excess of ionized acidic groups on their surfaces. Mammalian cells have a comparable negative surface charge so that one might expect forces of electrostatic repulsion to interfere with the attachment of gonococci to the host cell membrane. In order to investigate this problem, we have looked at the effect of modifying the gonococcal surface charge on the attachment of gonococci to Wish cells grown on coverslips. We use differential centrifugation to remove aggregated gonococci and standardize the numbers of diplococci using a Coulter counter. We have deposited standard numbers of 10, 50 and 100 gonococci on to the upper surface of each cell using minimal centrifugal force. After 30 min incubation, we wash off nonadherent gonococci, stain the coverslip and count the attached bacteria. In this test system, we find the pili confer a threefold advantage in attachment to Wish cells. The importance of surface charge is confirmed by the fact that when we modify carboxyl groups giving the gonococcus a positive surface charge (pI 8.17), the numbers of gonococci attaching to cells doubles. Conversely, when we increase the negative charge by modifying amino groups (pI 3.97), fewer gonococci attach. We have postulated (Ward and Watt 1974) that a function of pili is to circumvent the problem of electrostatic forces of repulsion between the gonococcus and the host cell. The fact that when the surface charge of the gonococcus is reversed pili confer no advantages in attachment is consistent with this theory. If pili indeed function in this way, one can anticipate that they should have a low charge density. Using cationised ferritin (Danon *et al.* 1972), an electron dense positively charged protein prepared by coupling ferritin with dimethylpropane diamine, we have confirmed, by electron microscopy, that the pili have a much lower charge density than the surrounding outer envelope.

The other point emerges from these studies that when both carboxyl and amino groups of proteins were blocked, gonococci still attached to cell membranes. The possible implication is that the critical groups on the gonococcal surface involved in attachment are sugars. One way of determining if a sugar is involved is to treat the gonococcus with sodium periodate, as this destroys sugars with two adjacent free hydroxyl groups. We find periodate treatment enormously enhances the attachment of gonococci to glass but impairs attachment to cell membranes. This nonspecific effect suggests that major changes occur in the outer surface of the gonococcus when sugar groups are oxidized. Undoubtedly, attempts to modify cell surfaces, for example with plant lectins, lead to unwanted changes in the membrane. Such data require careful interpretation.

Invasion of Mucosal Surfaces

We know from the classical studies of Harkness (1948) that in patients with acute gonococcal urethritis by the third day of infection gonococci have penetrated the mucosal lining and have become established in the subepithelial connective tissue. We have suggested (Ward *et al.* 1975) that gonococci penetrate the intact mucosal surface by invasion through the cells rather than passsing between cell junctions. We demonstrated the intracellular penetration of gonococci into mucosal cells desquamated from the cervix and urethra of patients with acute gonorrhoea. Further, in infected fallopian tube organ cultures we observed cells laden with gonococci rupturing into the submucosa (Ward *et al.* 1974).

Pathogenic micro-organisms are known to invade mucosal cells by phagocytosis or by erosion of the host cell membrane and sub-

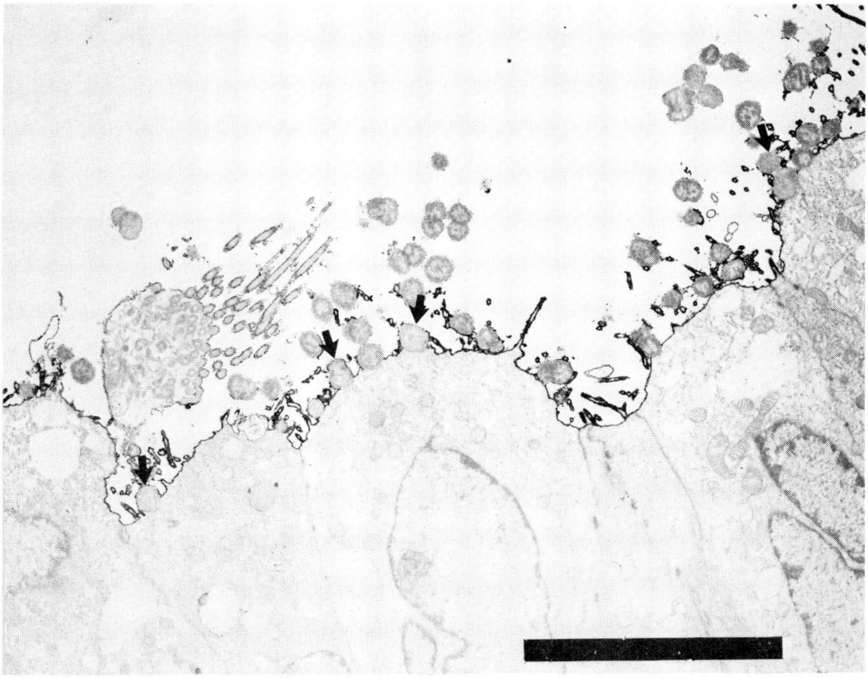

Fig. 4 *Electron micrograph of the mucosal surface of a fallopian tube organ culture 8 hours after infection with a pilated gonococcus strain P9. The fixed tissue has been stained* en bloc *with 1% colloidal thorium hydroxide (Taab Laboratories) in 3% acetic acid pH 2.6 for 24 h and the section examined without counterstaining. Positively charged colloidal thorium particles can be seen bound to the negatively charged cell coat. The attached gonococci (arrows) have not damaged the adjacent cell membrane, as shown by the failure of the 10–30 nm colloidal thorium particles to penetrate the cell. The bar represents 10 μm*

sequent penetration. This latter mechanism has been demonstrated in Salmonella infections (Takeuchi 1967). Fig. 4 shows an electron micrograph of an infected fallopian tube organ culture 8 hours after challenge. Although numerous gonococci are seen attached to the mucosal surface, the host cell membrane adjacent to the organism remains intact, as shown by the complete exclusion of the 10–30 nm particles of colloidal thorium. This excludes the possibility that gonococci penetrate cells by destruction of their outer membrane.

In an attempt to assess the numbers of gonococci which have invaded the mucosal surface of an infected fallopian tube organ culture 8 hours after challenge, we have used spectinomycin to destroy attached but nonpenetrated gonococci (Ward *et al.* 1975). The method presents difficulties in that we are limited as to the number of organ cultures we can prepare from each fallopian tube, and the ratio of mucous cells to ciliated cells is determined by the

Table 2

The use of spectinomycin to assess the penetration of the pilated gonococcus P9 into human fallopian tube maintained in organ culture

	Control		*+ Cytochalasin B 4 μg/ml*	
	Log_{10} viable gonococci		*Log_{10} viable gonococci*	
	Pre-treatment	*Post spectinomycin*	*Pre-treatment*	*Post spectinomycin*
	6.43	4.04	6.18	2.93
	6.45	2.71	6.18	2.95
	6.57	4.61	6.61	4.11
	6.74	3.89	6.73	4.08
	6.80	5.18	6.86	3.72
	6.83	5.11	6.93	3.18
	6.86	3.82	7.00	3.00
	6.91	5.63	7.00	3.86
	7.04	3.38	7.08	3.83
Log_{10} mean	6.73	4.26	6.73	3.52
% persisting	0.34		0.06	

Gonococci were centrifuged on to the mucosal surface of the fallopian tube. After washing to remove unattached bacteria organ culture blocks were cut and incubated in organ culture medium (OCM) at 37°C for 8 hours. Viable counts were determined after washing the organ culture blocks and pulping in OCM. The number of gonococci surviving exposure to 300 μg/ml spectinomycin for 30 min is expressed as a percentage of the log_{10} mean count before treatment

hormonal state of the patient at operation. Nevertheless we can test the validity of the system by demonstrating that treatment of infected organ cultures with cytochalasin B reduces the number of gonococci persisting after spectinomycin treatment. Cytochalasin B would block the phagocytic uptake of gonococci by disrupting the microfilament system of the mucosal cell. At a concentration of 4 μg/ml cytochalasin did not affect the multiplication of gonococci on the organ culture blocks but the numbers surviving spectinomycin treatment was reduced fivefold from 0.36% to 0.06% (Table 2). This is consistent with the concept that the initial step in invasion is phagocytosis by mucosal cells.

Because pili are involved in the attachment of gonococci to mucosal cell membranes, we must consider if they also function to stimulate phagocytosis. The real problem in testing this hypothesis is that nonpilated gonococci adhere less effectively to the mucosal surface than pilated organisms of the same strain. Table 3 shows that

Table 3

The use of spectinomycin to assess the penetration of the pilated gonococcus P9 into human fallopian tube maintained in organ culture

Pilated			*Non-pilated*	
	Log_{10} viable gonococci		*Log_{10} viable gonococci*	
	Pre-treatment	*Post spectinomycin*	*Pre-treatment*	*Post spectinomycin*
	6.6	4.9	5.9	3.6
	6.6	4.4	5.9	2.7
	6.4	4.4	5.8	3.2
	6.4	4.6	5.7	3.3
	6.3	3.7	5.7	3.3
	6.3	4.6	5.6	3.3
	6.2	4.0	5.5	4.0
	6.1	3.7	5.5	3.8
	6.0	3.4	5.5	3.8
	5.9	4.6	5.4	3.1
	5.9	3.6	5.3	3.6
	5.9	3.6	5.3	3.2
	5.6	3.6	5.3	3.2
	5.6	3.6	5.3	2.8
Log_{10} mean	6.12	4.05	5.55	3.35
% persisting	0.85		0.67	

Gonococci were centrifuged on to the mucosal surface of the fallopian tube. After washing to remove unattached bacteria organ culture blocks were cut and incubated in organ culture medium (OCM) at 37°C for 8 h. Viable counts were determined after washing the organ culture blocks and pulping in OCM. The number of gonococci surviving exposure to 300 μg/ml spectinomycin for 30 min is expressed as a percentage of the log_{10} mean count before treatment

after 8 hours' growth following challenge with comparable numbers, the log_{10} mean viable count per organ culture was 6.12 for pilated gonococci and 5.55 for the non-pilated mutant. However, when we look at the percentage of gonococci surviving exposure to spectinomycin, we find no significant difference between pilated and non-pilated gonococci. Thus it appears that pili, while important for attachment to mucosal cell membranes, are not a critical determinant in invasion of the cell.

Conclusions

For those interested in the pathogenesis of gonorrhoea many critical questions remain unanswered. Much more work will be needed before we can understand the molecular basis of such fundamental problems as why gonococci sitting on genital mucosal cells cause disease, whereas the commensal organisms on the same cells give no trouble. The recent increased interest in the gonococcus has taken us some way towards this understanding, but unfortunately some of the published data are contradictory or confusing.

Acknowledgments

We are grateful to the Medical Research Council for a Programme Grant in support of this work.

References

Danon, D., Goldstein, L., Marikovsky, Y. and Skutelsky, E. (1972). *Journal of Ultrastructural Research* **38**, 500–510

Frei, P. C., Baisero, M. H. and Ochsner, M. (1974). *Journal of Immunological Methods* **5**, 375–386

Gibbs, D. L. and Roberts, R. B. (1975). *Journal of Experimental Medicine* **141**, 155–171

Harkness, A. H. (1948). *British Journal of Venereal Diseases* **24**, 137–147

Hoskins, D. D. and Casillas, E. R. (1975). *In* "Molecular Mechanisms of Gonadal Hormone Action". Ed. J. A. Thomas and R. L. Singhal. HM and M, Aylesbury; p 283

Jacobs, N. F. and Kraus, S. J. (1975). *Annals of Internal Medicine* **82**, 7–12

James-Holmquest, A. N., Swanson, J., Buchanan, T. M., Wende, R. D. and Williams, R. P. (1974). *Infection and Immunity* **9**, 897–902

Mandell, G. L. (1973). *Journal of Clinical Investigation* **52**, 1673–1679

Morse, S. A. and Fitzgerald, J. J. (1974). *Infection and Immunity* **10**, 1370–1377

Singhal, R. L. and Sutherland, D. J. B. (1975). *In* "Molecular Mechanisms of Gonadal Hormone Action". Ed. J. A. Thomas and R. L. Singhal. HM and M, Aylesbury; p 225

Stead, A., Main, J. S., Ward, M. E. and Watt, P. J. (1975). *Journal of General Microbiology* **88**, 123–131

Stossel, T. P. (1974). *New England Journal of Medicine* **290**, 774–781

Swanson, J. (1973). *Journal of Experimental Medicine* **137**, 571–589

Swanson, J., Kraus, S. J. and Gotschlich, E. C. (1971). *Journal of Experimental Medicine* **134**, 886–906

Swanson, J., Sparks, E., Zeligs, B., Siam, M. A. and Parrott, C. (1974). *Infection and Immunity* **10**, 633–644

Takeuchi, A. (1967). *American Journal of Pathology* **50**, 109–136

Thongthai, C. and Sawyer, W. D. (1973). *Infection and Immunity* **7**, 373–379

Veale, D. R., Smith, H. and Witt, K. (1975). *Lancet* i, 306–308

Ward, M. E., Glynn, A. A. and Watt, P. J. (1972). *British Journal of Experimental Pathology* 53, 289–294
Ward, M. E., Robertson, J. N., Englefield, P. M. and Watt, P. J. (1975). *Microbiology* 2, 188–199
Ward, M. E. and Watt, P. J. (1972). *Journal of Infectious Diseases* 126, 601–605
(1974). International Conference on Genital Infections, Stockholm (in press)
Ward, M. E., Watt, P. J. and Robertson, J. N. (1974). *Journal of Infectious Diseases* 129, 650–659

Discussion

Professor L H Collier (*Lister Institute of Preventive Medicine, Elstree*) commented that Dr Dunlop had referred to the method of isolating Chlamydia in irradiated McCoy cells. That technique represented a great advance in methods for isolating these micro-organisms, but those concerned with laboratory techniques should know that the use of irradiated cells was not obligatory. Blyth and Taverne (1974, *Journal of Hygiene* 72, 121) had demonstrated that isolations could be made just as efficiently in non-irradiated BHK-21 cells.

Professor Collier said Dr Dunlop had referred to the efficacy of tetracycline for treating chlamydial infections and asked if he had any information about the long-term results of such treatment, and whether serotyping of isolates was of any value in distinguishing between relapses and reinfections.

Dr Dunlop said that cure of chlamydial genital infection was difficult to assess. Babies treated for eye infection with chlortetracycline eye ointment for six weeks were cured providing the ointment was put in properly. Mordhorst and Dawson (1971, *American Journal of Ophthalmology* 71, 861) had shown that the development of scarring and pannus was obviated if effective treatment had been started by the time the baby was 13 days old.

All Dr Dunlop's adult patients were now treated with oxytetracycline for genital infection due to Chlamydia for longer (three weeks) than was formerly the case. They were re-tested at three and six weeks and at three months. The isolation of Chlamydia following such treatment was exceptional. Clinical resolution resulted. The serotyping of isolates and the measurement of the serological response to chlamydial infection was being carried out.

All Dr Dunlop's patients were tested at three weeks, six weeks and three months. Positive isolation following treatment was exceptional. There was certainly clinical resolution following treatment.

Dr J D J Parker (*London*) asked Dr Dunlop if anyone had ever demonstrated Koch's postulate in chlamydial urethritis by inoculating material from a positive McCoy cell culture into the normal male urethra. He appreciated that there were ethical considerations in such experiments.

Dr Dunlop said that for genital infection the answer was "No".

Dr M A Waugh (*Leeds*) asked Dr Holmes if there was any evidence in regard to the incidence of virus isolation rates in pelvic inflammatory disease (PID) in women.

Dr Holmes said that cytomegalovirus and herpes virus had been sought. The former had been recovered from 36% of women with PID and 23% of women who had come into the VD clinic with complaints unrelated to PID. The geometric mean titre of CMV antibody in the CF test was a little lower in the PID group than in the VD clinic group, but the percentage of patients who had antibody to CMV was 76% in the PID group and 56% in the female VD clinic population. There was no evidence of sero-conversion or titre rises.

Herpes virus was recovered from 7% of patients with PID; this did not differ from the prevalence of herpes virus in the VD clinic population, as determined by culture of the cervix.

Dr Denys K Ford (*Vancouver, Canada*) thought no one would dispute that Chlamydia caused urethritis. However, Shepard had demonstrated the very clear relationship between the number of T strain mycoplasmas in the urethra and the onset of symptoms.

It was unfortunate that tetracycline cured both conditions. He wondered if there were any antibiotics that would not eradicate Chlamydia but would eradicate T strain mycoplasma, or vice versa. He thought that was the only way to settle the argument. Some people believed that T strain mycoplasmas caused many cases of urethritis.

Dr David Taylor-Robinson (*Clinical Research Centre, Harrow*), in reply to Dr Ford, said that Shepard's experiments on the quantitative isolation of T strain mycoplasmas, in which he had treated patients suboptimally with tetracyclines, showed there was a parallel between the disappearance of the organisms and the disappearance of symptoms and then the reappearance of organisms when the symptoms returned; from this Shepard had suggested that the T strain mycoplasmas were responsible for the symptoms. Dr Taylor-Robinson thought, however, that this was not conclusive as the presence of Chlamydia was not investigated. He mentioned that rifampicin was a drug which inhibited Chlamydia but not T strain mycoplasmas.

Dr Elisabeth Rees (*Liverpool Royal Infirmary*) said that during the past 18 months, in Liverpool, Chlamydia had been isolated from the cervix of 130 of 440 women (29.5%) who had comprised a selected series containing a high proportion of NSU contacts. The method of culture, using non-irradiated McCoy cells, was that described by Hobson, Johnson, Rees and Tait (1974, *Lancet* **ii**, 555–556). Tests had been repeated before treatment in 94 positive cases and 88 had again been positive; in 48 negative cases 46 had again been negative. The original report had therefore been confirmed in 95% of cases, suggesting that the method was reasonably sensitive.

Isolates had been obtained from 15 babies in maternity units. The mothers of 6 of these babies had already been receiving antibiotics for post-partum infection; this was a very high incidence of post-partum infection. Isolates were obtained from 7 of 8 mothers examined who had not been receiving antibiotics. Dr Rees asked Dr Dunlop the age of the babies in his series and whether he had found a similar incidence of post-partum infection.

Dr Dunlop said that the average age of the babies was about five weeks at the time that the mother was examined. The oldest was about four months old, and the youngest nine days old. Many babies were now being treated for "sticky eye" by midwives to avoid the diagnosis of ophthalmia neonatorum. One baby with "sticky eye" was referred when he was nine weeks old when both gonococci and Chlamydia were isolated from the conjunctiva.

Of the 25 mothers in the present series 8 had pelvic inflammatory disease at the time of examination, which was a high proportion. A further 3 mothers were excluded from the study because they had already received large amounts of antibiotics because of post-partum infection. One had had high fever, another had had salpingitis, and the third had had severe dysuria.

Dr Holmes, referring to antibiotics that might be differentially effective, said he believed sulphonamides were active against Chlamydia but not against T strain mycoplasmas. He had found that Chlamydia-positive cases responded to sulphonamides and that Chlamydia-negative cases did not. That fact, together with the evidence that Chlamydia-negative cases did not show an antibody response to Chlamydia and their sex partners did not have Chlamydia infections, suggested there was a category which was not Chlamydial in origin.

Dr Emil C Gotschlich (*New York*) said the idea of the abolition of the negative charge by both the cell and the organism by the pili was interesting, but he thought Professor Watt did not emphasize that this was probably only an initial step. There still existed a specific mechanism at the terminal end of the pilus for its attachment to the epithelial cell which could be demonstrated in certain cases.

Professor Watt accepted Dr Gotschlich's comment, but said that for gonococci such attachment might be an artifact; certainly inhibitions by sugars cannot be demonstrated. The one thing gonococci did *par excellence* was to stick to each other, and undoubtedly the pili formed bundles all along their length, not just at their tips.

Dr Morton made a comment about progesterone and gonococci in the cervix. Bhattacharyya and Jephcott (in preparation) had done some clinical work on this to see if there was any difference in the incidence of positive smears and in cultures from the cervix in women on "the pill" and women not on "the pill".

Dr Morton was not clear on Dr Holmes's views about the intrauterine device and pelvic inflammatory disease and asked whether he recommended that the IUD be removed before a woman who had gonorrhoea was treated.

Dr Holmes said that the IUD should be removed from women with gonorrhoea since its presence increased susceptibility to non-gonococcal PID.

There was a problem in following up patients seen and treated for PID, whether gonococcal or non-gonococcal; the recurrence rate was extremely high, 30% in his series of 200 women. If the initial episode was gonococcal the next was usually non-gonococcal, so that the gonorrhoea was producing both the gonococcal PID and the subsequent episode of non-gonococcal PID. The IUD might be a risk factor here, but there was no proof.

Dr Wiesner asked Dr Holmes whether Chlamydia played a role in non-gonococcal PID.

Dr Holmes said that cultures from the cervix had been examined for Chlamydia and compared with a control group; the antibody response had also been considered, and cultures for Chlamydia had been taken from the cul-de-sac of some women with PID. Chlamydia had been recovered from 1 in 30 cul-de-sac fluids and from 20% of the cervices of women with non-gonococcal PID. The same rate was found in women with gonococcal PID and in women seen in the clinic without PID. A fourfold rise in micro IF antibody to *C. trachomatis* had been seen in about 15-20% of women with PID.

A speaker asked Dr Dunlop if he had done a prospective study of women with positive Chlamydia in the cervix to see if any of their babies developed ocular disease or infection.

Dr Dunlop said that he had not. In the UK research projects have to be approved by hospital ethical committees; in his view such a study would be unethical and should not be approved.

In reply to a further comment he said that, in addition to the morbidity in the mother and the father, since the papers by Jones *et al.* (1965, *Revue Internationale du Trachome* **42**, 27) and by Freedman *et al.* (1966. *Transactions of the Ophthalmological Society of the United Kingdom* **86**, 313) there was an increasing body of evidence, such as that of Mordhorst and Dawson, and Collier *et al.* (1969, *Lancet* **i**, 101), showing that trachomatous scarring and pannus could develop in infected babies. The diagnosis and treatment of chlamydial infection were important matters.

Immunology of Gonococcal Infections — Immunization Prospects

Emil C Gotschlich
The Rockefeller University,
New York, New York 10021

Bacterial antigens may be loosely divided into those which are defined operationally — that is to say, by the method used for their extraction — and those which are defined by physicochemical or immunochemical means. Operationally defined antigens in selected instances can be extremely useful, a notable example being the acid extraction method developed by Lancefield (1928) for the grouping and typing of streptococci. In general, however, such antigens are too complex and variable to give readily interpretable results. I shall, therefore, limit the present discussion to two gonococcal antigens where the materials have been physicochemically defined to a greater or lesser extent; these are gonococcal pili and the major outer membrane protein.

Gonococcal Pili

Jephcott *et al.* (1971) and Swanson *et al.* (1974) found independently that some gonococci carried pili on their surfaces. In addition, it was found that pilation correlated with the colonial typing system developed by Kellogg *et al.* (1968), suggesting strongly that pili had a role in gonococcal virulence. This line of investigation has been pursued in several laboratories, and it has been found that pilated gonococci are more virulent in a chick embryo system (Bumgarner and Finkelstein 1973, Buchanan and Gotschlich 1973) as well as in the subcutaneous chamber model developed by Arko (1974). The mechanism for such increased virulence is presumed to be that pili confer adhesiveness to gonococci. This has been shown to be the case in several systems, ranging from explanted epithelial cell monolayers in tissue culture (Swanson 1973) to the organ culture experiments with human fallopian tube segments carried out by Ward *et al.* (1974). The influence of pilation on the interaction of gonococci with white cells has also been studied extensively, but the interpretation of this line of investigation has proved more complex. Sawyer and his associates (Thongthai and Sawyer 1973, Punsalang and Sawyer 1973) and Ofek *et al.* (1974) have concluded that pili have antiphagocytic properties and that they interfere in the phagocytic process. Swanson and his associates (Swanson *et al.* 1974, Swanson 1975) on the other hand, feel that pili are not very relevant in the association between gonococci and polymorphonuclear leukocytes, but that other surface proteins as yet uncharacterized are far more important. Thomas *et al.* (1973) and Dilworth *et al.* (1975) have obtained evidence that pilated organisms become associated with polymorphonuclear leukocytes but remain attached to their surface and resist ingestion. Clearly, it is a complex issue which requires further work to be fully understood; nevertheless, the sum of the work indicates that pili are important in pathogenesis.

The immunochemistry of gonococcal pili has been studied in considerable detail by Buchanan *et al.* (1973) and by Brinton (1975) and his associates. Both groups have developed methods for the purification of gonococcal pili; the structures can be prepared in milligram quantities and in high purity. Buchanan (1975) has reported that gonococcal pili consist of a single kind of protein subunit with a molecular weight of 24 000, that the pili contain no detectable hexose, and that they have a density of 1.28 g/cm^3. Brinton(1975) has reported that pili consist of a subunit of 21 000 molecular weight with, possibly, a very small amount of another kind of protein with a larger subunit molecular weight associated with the pili. He has also found 1–2% hexose and 1–2 moles of phosphorus per subunit. He reports a buoyant density of 1.34 g/cm^3 on cesium chloride gradients. Thus, there are some differences in the physicochemical characteristics of the pili purified by the two investigators, and these will need to be resolved by further comparative studies. Both Brinton (1975) and Buchanan (1975) have reported antigenic variability between gonococcal pili. The work is still in the preliminary stages, and we lack solid information on the degree of homology between various kinds of pili as well as on the number of determinants that are subject to variation.

Buchanan *et al.* (1973) have carried out an extensive series of investigations on the human immune response to gonococcal pili, employing a quantitative radioimmunoassay. The results are summarized in Fig. 1. The immune response of individuals known not to have had gonorrhea ranges from undetectable to approximately 1.6

μg/ml of antibody, with a mean of 0.5 μg/ml. On the left are listed the immune responses of men with asymptomatic or symptomatic genitourinary gonococcal disease. While the average immune response is significantly different from that seen in the controls, there is extensive overlap between the two groups. On the right are depicted the responses observed in women with asymptomatic gonococcal infection. Their mean antibody response is considerably higher than that seen in men, and the overlap between this group and the controls is rather small. Interestingly, men with pharyngeal gonococcal infection have antibody responses similar to those seen in the

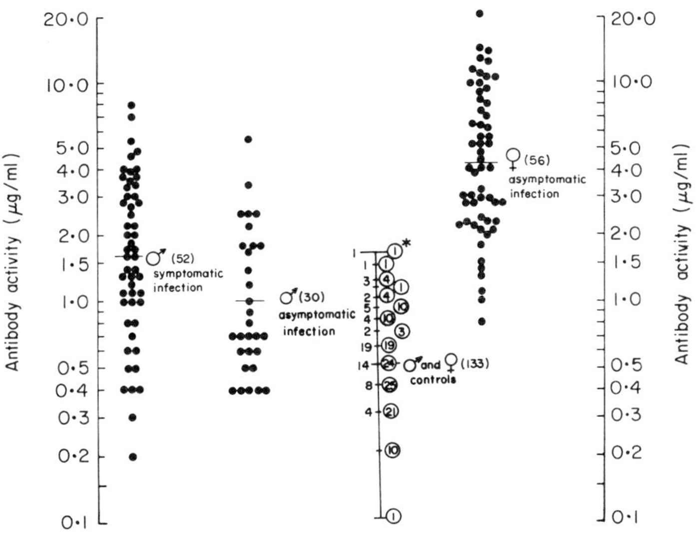

Fig. 1 *Radioactive antigen binding activity of human sera. For the 133 controls, the circled numbers (*) represent the total group and the uncircled numbers the adults within that group. The geometric mean for the latter was 0.6 μg/ml*

asymptomatic women. Work is in progress in several laboratories to determine the usefulness of the measurement of antibodies to gonococcal pili either by this radioimmunoassay or by other methods for the serodiagnosis of gonorrhea, particularly in the asymptomatic female.

The question of whether antibodies to gonococcal pili are protective has not yet been settled in a definitive manner. On the one hand lack of clear evidence for natural immunity to gonococcal infection conferred by a prior infection would tend to suggest that antibodies to these structures are not protective; on the other hand as we have already mentioned, there is antigenic variability among pili of different strains. Brinton (1975) has reported some increased resistance to reinfection in chimpanzees and humans following immunization with purified gonococcal pili. Before more definite plans for the use of pili for human vaccination can be made, however, we shall need to know a great deal more concerning their antigenic diversity and relatedness, their immunogenicity in experimental animals and man, and the level of protection that can be achieved by active immunization.

Serotype Antigens

Another family of antigens has been studied intensively by Johnston and Gotschlich (in preparation). These are located in the outer cell wall membrane and, unless the organism is encapsulated, they are a part of the layer which is in direct contact with the host. It has been shown for Gram-negative organisms in general and for the gonococcus in particular that the isolated outer cell wall membrane has a relatively simple protein composition when examined by SDS gel electrophoresis (Johnston and Gotschlich 1974). Usually, one protein markedly dominates the spectrum, and for the purposes of this discussion it is called the major outer membrane protein. This is illustrated in Fig. 2, which shows the SDS polyacrylamide gel electrophoretic pattern of a purified outer membrane of gonococcal strain 29 prepared by sucrose gradient centrifugation of membranes

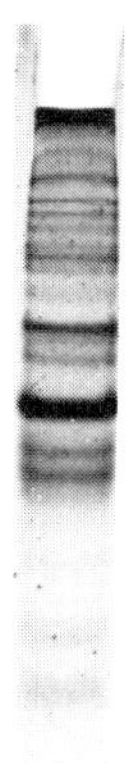

Fig. 2 *Pattern obtained with isolated gonococcal outer membrane upon sodium dodecyl sulfate polyacrylamide electrophoresis according to the methods of Weber and Osborn (1969). A slab gel electrophoretic system as described by Maizel (1971) was used. The outer membranes were purified by the method of Johnston and Gotschlich (1974).*

obtained from EDTA lysozyme induced spheroplasts according to the methods of Johnston and Gotschlich (1974). Extracts rich in the major outer membrane protein can be prepared much more readily by lithium chloride extraction of intact organisms according to the methods of Frasch and Gotschlich (1974). When extracts were prepared by this method from a number of gonococcal strains, it was found that the molecular weight of their major outer membrane protein was not identical in every instance, and that the strains segregated into several well-defined classes. This can be seen in Fig. 3,

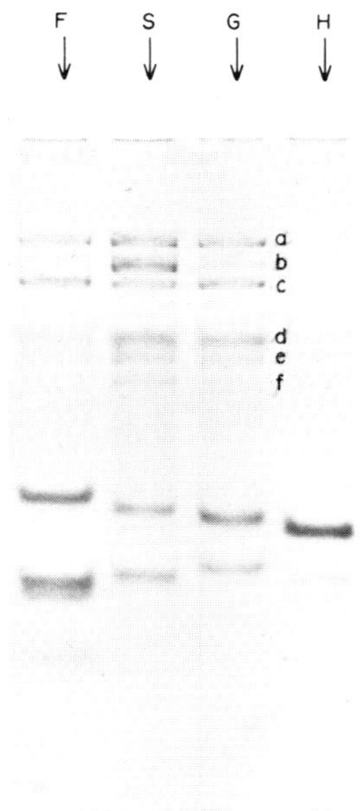

Fig. 3 *Slab gel electrophoretic pattern obtained with lithium chloride extracts of four different gonococcal strains (Frasch and Gotschlich 1974). SDS polyacrylamide electrophoresis was carried out according to the methods of Weber and Osborn (1969) in an apparatus described by Maizel (1971).*

which is a SDS gel electrophoresis of extracts obtained from four serotypes of gonococci, designated F, G, H and S. The molecular weight of the major outer membrane protein ranges from 37 000 to 32 000. When antiserum was prepared to such an extract, it was found that all extracts containing a major outer membrane protein of identical molecular weight reacted with the antiserum, whereas extracts containing major outer membrane proteins with different molecular weights failed to react with it. The results are shown in Table 1. On the left are the results obtained with 166 strains obtained in the New York City area: 95% of these could be typed with seven antisera, A–G. However, when 58 strains obtained from various places overseas (supplied by Dr King Holmes) were examined with these seven sera, only 50% of them could be typed. When an additional 5 antisera were developed to new major outer membrane proteins encountered in the collection, 96% of the foreign strains, and all of the New York strains, were typable.

This serotyping system appears to be stable in the sense that a large number of the strains were typed on more than one occasion and in more than one colonial form, and always gave identical results. In addition, all contact pairs were of the same serological type. To date, no association has been seen between this gonococcal typing system and virulence as defined by invasiveness. If immunity

Table 1

Distribution of serotypes among gonococcal strains

Serotype	*Strains from New York City (166)* %	*Strains from overseas (58)* %
A	24.7	0.0
B	10.8	10.3
C	16.3	1.7
D	19.3	15.5
E	7.2	5.2
F	8.4	1.7
G	10.2	17.2
H	1.8	6.9
N	1.2	19.0
R	0.0	3.4
S	0.0	8.6
T	0.0	6.9
Untypable	0.0	3.4

to gonococcal infection is type-specific, it is understandable that natural immunity is not readily observed. A great deal needs to be known about the epidemiology of gonococcal serotypes and their stability in the community before one can hazard a guess as to whether it would be worth while attempting to produce a vaccine based on the serotype antigens.

To sum up, I believe that an effective vaccine to prevent gonorrhea is not on the immediate horizon, but that the search for such an agent, which has already given us much fundamental information concerning the host-parasite relation in the disease, will, if pursued in a rational way, continue to do so and will eventually produce a solution to the problem.

References

Arko, R. J. (1974). *Journal of Infectious Diseases* **129**, 451
Brinton, C. C. jr. (1975). Presented at 75th Annual Meeting, American Society for Microbiology
Buchanan, T. M. (1975). Presented at 75th Annual Meeting, American Society for Microbiology
Buchanan, T. M. and Gotschlich, E. C. (1973). *Journal of Experimental Medicine* **137**, 196
Buchanan, T. M., Swanson, J., Holmes, K. K., Kraus, S. J. and Gotschlich, E. C. (1973). *Journal of Clinical Investigation* **52**, 2896
Bumgarner, L. R. and Finkelstein, R. A. (1973). *Infection and Immunity* **8**, 919
Dilworth, J. A., Hendley, J. O. and Mandell, G. L. (1975). *Infection and Immunity* **11**, 512
Frasch, C. E. and Gotschlich, E. C. (1974). *Journal of Experimental Medicine* **140**, 87
Jephcott, A. E., Reyn, A. and Birch-Andersen, A. (1971). *Acta pathologica et microbiologica Scandinavica* **Section B**, 79, 437
Johnston, K. H. and Gotschlich, E. C. (1974). *Journal of Bacteriology* **119**, 250
Kellogg, D. S. jr, Cohen, I. R., Norins, L. C., Schroeter, A. L. and Reising, G. (1968). *Journal of Bacteriology* **96**, 596
Lancefield, R. C. (1928). *Journal of Experimental Medicine* **47**, 91
Maizel, J. V. (1971). *Methods in Virology* **5**, 179
Ofek, I., Beachey, E. H. and Bisno, A. L. (1974). *Journal of Infectious Diseases* **129**, 310
Punsalang, A. P. Jr and Sawyer, W. D. (1973). *Infection and Immunity* **8**, 255
Swanson, J. (1973). *Journal of Experimental Medicine* **137**, 571
Swanson, J. (1975). Presented at 75th Annual Meeting, American Society for Microbiology
Swanson, J., Kraus, S. J. and Gotschlich, E. C. (1971). *Journal of Experimental Medicine* **134**, 886
Swanson, J., Sparks, E., Zeligs, B., Siam, M. A. and Parrott, C. (1974). *Infection and Immunity* **10**, 633
Thomas, D. S., Hill, J. C. and Tyeryar, S. J. jr (1973). *Infection and Immunity* **8**, 98
Thongthai, C. and Sawyer, W. D. (1973). *Infection and Immunity* **7**, 373
Ward, M. E., Watt, T. J. and Robertson, J. N. (1974). *Journal of Infectious Diseases* **129**, 650
Weber, K. and Osborn, M. (1969). *Journal of Biological Chemistry* **244**, 4406

Immunology of Chlamydia

S Darougar
Institute of Ophthalmology, London WC1H 9QS

Chlamydia is the causative agent of a variety of ocular, oculogenital, genital and systemic diseases in man (Table 1).

Hyperendemic trachoma, spread by eye-to-eye transmission, is the world's most common eye disease, affecting 500 million people and causing blindness in some 2 million of these (Tarizzo 1973). The sexually transmitted TRIC (trachoma-inclusion conjunctivitis) infection of the eye, i.e. inclusion conjunctivitis, TRIC punctate kerato-conjunctivitis, trachoma and TRIC agent ophthalmia neonatorum, are not uncommon in the developed countries.

Nongonoccocal urethritis (NGU), which is mainly caused by Chlamydia, is the commonest sexually transmitted disease. The number of cases of NGU attending venereal disease clinics in the United Kingdom in 1973 was over 70 000 (*see* Dunlop, p 83). Nonspecific cervicitis (NSC) due to Chlamydia is common amongst women attending VD clinics (up to 31%) (Hilton *et al.* 1974, Oriel *et al.* 1974, Burns *et al.* 1975). Chlamydial proctitis and urethritis are commonly detected in women suffering from chlamydial cervicitis (Dunlop *et al.* 1971, Vaughan-Jackson *et al.* 1972). The recent microbiological and serological findings in our laboratory indicate that Chlamydia may also be associated with Reiter's disease, cystitis, salpingitis and spontaneous abortion.

Table 1

Chlamydia infection of man

Subgroup A	Subgroup B
Ocular:	*Systemic disease:*
Trachoma	Psittacosis
	Ornithosis
Oculogenital:	Enzootic abortion of ewes
Inclusion conjunctivitis	Feline pneumonitis
TRIC punctate keratitits	
Ophthalmia neonatorum	*Ocular but uncommon:*
Urethritis (NSU)	Guinea-pig conjunctivitis
Cervicitis (NSU)	Cat kerato-conjunctivitis
Urethritis in women	
Proctitis	
LGV	
Reiter's disease?	
Cystitis?	
Salpingitis?	
Abortion?	

In recent years studies have been carried out in human and animal models to elucidate the nature of host-parasite relationships in chlamydial infections. The purpose of this paper is to present the results of some of these investigations regarding the nature and antigenicity of Chlamydia.

Chlamydia is an obligate intracellular parasite which produces inclusion bodies in cells. The chlamydial inclusions contain two types of particles: (1) Mature infectious elementary bodies, which measure approximately 0.3 μm in diameter. (2) Noninfectious reticulate or initial bodies, whose size varies between 0.5 and 10 μm.

The chlamydial particles, in common with bacteria, contain DNA and RNA, multiply by binary fission, possess enzymes and have some metabolic activity of their own, have cell walls and are sensitive to certain antibiotics.

The family Chlamydiaceae is divided into two main species: *Chlamydia trachomatis* and *Chlamydia psittaci*. These two species are related to each other because both are obligate intracellular parasites and contain a common group antigen. However, the presence of

Table 2

Distribution of serotyped TRIC and LGV isolates (total = 235)

Area	*Hyperendemic trachoma serotypes*				*Paratrachoma serotypes*						*LGV serotypes*		
	A	*B*	*Ba*	*C*	*D/E*	*F*	*G*	*H*	*I*	*K*	*L1*	*L2*	*L3*
Africa	26	6	1	1	1	1							
Asia	2	40		34	9	1	1	2					
Australasia		2		1									
America				1	5	2	1	1	1	1	2	12	1
Europe		2		1	63	9	12	5	2	3			1
Clinical site													
Ocular strains:													
Hyperendemic trachoma	28	48	1	36	2								
Paratrachoma		2			32	4	6	1					
Genital strains				2	44	9	8	7	3	4	2	12	2

glycogen in the inclusion of *C. trachomatis*, the presence of type-specific antigen, the sensitivity of *C. trachomatis* to sulfadiazine and D-cycloserine and the difference in DNA homology separate these two species from each other.

The two subspecies of *C. trachomatis*, i.e. lymphogranuloma venereum (LGV) and TRIC agent, are divided immunologically into a number of serotypes using the microimmunofluorescence test (micro-IF) (Wang and Grayston 1970, Treharne *et al.* 1972). To date there are 3 known serotypes of LGV, L_1, L_2, and L_3; 4 TRIC agents commonly associated with hyperendemic trachoma of eye-to-eye transmission in developing countries, A, B, Ba and C; and a further 7 (D, E, F, G, H, I and K) associated with the sexually transmitted oculogenital and genital infections in the developed countries (Table

2). The antigenic differences between these serotypes appear to play an important role in the immunity and pathogenesis of chlamydial infections.

C. trachomatis as well as *C. psittaci* organisms contain 7 distinct antigenic components. Of these antigens, 3 are heat stable and group-specific, 2 are soluble in deoxycholate and one is a cell wall antigen (Kuo, Kenny *et al.* 1971, Katzenelson and Bernkopf 1967, Barron and Collins 1967); finally, an acidic polysaccharide antigen has been isolated from both species. The antigenicity of the latter can be destroyed by periodate and mild acid hydrolysis. A group-specific haemagglutinin as well as a strain with species-specific antigenicity, has been obtained from *C. trachomatis* (Zakay-Rones *et al.* 1968, Mitsui *et al.* 1962).

Antichlamydial Antibodies in Sera

The type-specific antibody has been detected in the blood of patients suffering from ocular and genital chlamydial infections using a micro-IF test (Tables 3 and 4). (Dwyer *et al.* 1972 and Treharne *et al.* in preparation).

In NSU patients with positive culture of Chlamydia the antibody was detected in the blood of up to 51% of these patients, with a

Table 3

Chlamydial antibodies in sera of patients suffering from genital infection by micro-IF test

Syndrome	*Culture in irradiated McCoy cells*	*No. of patients*	*% positive*	*GMT*
NSU				
(Dwyer *et al.*	Positive	17	88	27
1972)	Negative	24	29	16
NSU				
(Treharne 1975)	Positive	35	51	35
	Negative	30	10	5
Cervicitis				
(Treharne 1975)				
	Positive	120	80	70
	Negative	90	10	<8
Parents of babies	Mothers			
with TRIC	positive	16	100	112
ophthalmia				
neonatorum	Fathers positive	10	63	16
Reiter's disease	Isolate negative	18	77	26
LGV	Positive	6	100	512
Psittacosis	Not done	17	100	580
Control	Not done	40	0	0

maximum geometric mean titre (GMT) of 1 in 35. In NSU patients with isolate-negative culture the antichlamydial antibody was present in 10–29%. The GMT of antibody in this group was markedly less than positive NSU cases (1 in 5 to 1 in 16). In women suffering from chlamydial cervicitis the prevalence of antibody in sera was similar to that of NSU positive cases (80%) but the GMT in this group was markedly higher than men with chlamydial urethritis.

Antichlamydial antibody (GMT 1 in 112) was detected in the blood of all mothers of babies with TRIC agent ophthalmia neonatorum. Chlamydia was isolated from the cervix of 90% of these mothers. A few sera obtained from patients suffering from LGV and psittacosis showed the presence of specific antibody in all the sera with a very high GMT of 1 in 512 and 580 respectively. The most interesting finding was the detection of antichlamydial antibody in the blood of patients suffering from Reiter's disease. The prevalence

Table 4

Chlamydial antibodies in sera of patients suffering from ocular infection detected in micro-IF test

Syndrome	*Isolation of Chlamydia*	*No. of patients*	*Percentage positive sera*	*GMT*
Oculogenital (London)	Positive	36	94	51
Trachoma	Positive	21	90	40
(Tunisia)	Negative	73	70	9
Trachoma (Iran)	Not done	147	66	48

and GMT of antibody in these patients were similar to that of NSU patients with positive chlamydial culture. Patients suffering from proven adenovirus or herpes virus keratoconjunctivitis without a history of urethritis were selected as control serum group in this study and no antichlamydial antibody was detected in any of these patients.

Antichlamydial antibody was detected in up to 94% of the sera of patients suffering from ocular TRIC infection in London or from hyperendemic trachoma in Tunisia and Iran. The GMT of antibody in the patients with positive culture for Chlamydia was markedly higher (1 in 48 to 1 in 51) in comparison to that in patients with negative culture (1 in 9). The analysis of species of antibody has shown the presence of IgG (7S) IgM (19S) and IgA (7S) in the sera of patients suffering from hyperendemic trachoma and chlamydial oculogenital and genital infections (Jawetz *et al.* 1971, Reeve *et al.* 1974, Treharne, in preparation).

Characterization of Antichlamydial Antibody

Complement-fixing antibody: In rabbits the group-specific complement-fixing antibody developed 5–7 days following the injection of chlamydial antigen. The maximum amount of antibody developed within 30 days, then the titre declined over a period of several months. In humans the complement-fixing antibody was detected in patients suffering from ocular and genital diseases as well as in Reiter's disease (Barwell *et al.* 1967, Schachter 1970).

Neutralizing antibody against homologous strains has been detected in the serum of immunized rabbits. Mogg *et al.* (1971) reported a low titre of neutralizing antibody in IgG and IgM fractions of antichlamydial antibody.

Antibody to cell-wall antigen: A strain-specific antibody was obtained following the inoculation of cell-wall antigen. This antibody has been used for the study of relationships between LGV and TRIC strains (Phillips *et al.* 1967).

Agglutinating antibody: The group-specific agglutinating antibody develops in early stages of infection but rapidly declines before the appearance of complement-fixing antibody. It appears that there is a close association between the titre of agglutinating antibody and the activity of the disease.

Local antibodies: Antichlamydial antibody has been shown to be present in the eye secretions (tears) of patients suffering from trachoma (Bernkopf *et al.* 1966, McComb and Nichols 1969 and 1970, Jawetz *et al.* 1971, Jones 1974). Studies in our laboratory have shown that the presence and titre of antibody in tears are directly related to the severity of the disease and the presence of infectious agents (Table 5) (Treharne *et al.* in preparation).

The analysis of antichlamydial antibody in tears indicated the presence of IgG, IgA and IgM in trachomatous patients (Jawetz 1971, Collier *et al.* 1972).

Preliminary work in our laboratory has demonstrated the presence of local antibody in the genital tract and rectum (Table 6) (Darougar *et al.* 1971).

Cell-mediated responses have been demonstrated in patients suffering from chlamydial infection of the eye and genital tract. The results of skin tests in patients with NSU, the sexual consorts of patients with NSU and patients suffering from Reiter's disease are shown in Table

Table 5

Comparison of reciprocal geometric mean antibody titres and positivity in sera and tears, correlated with the activity of clinical disease (Jones 1974)

Clinical activity	*Sera*			*Tears*		
	GMT positive sera ●	*All sera*	*Percentage positive sera*	*GMT positive tears* ●	*All tears*	*Percentage positive tears*
Severe	51	25	82	43	14	70
Moderate	37	14	88	12	2.5	31
Mild	25	14	81	4	1.7	17

● Positive = 1 in 8 or more

7. Using an acid extract antigen from the LGV agent the skin tests were positive in 9 out of 50 cases of NSU and in 2 out of 26 consorts of NSU. In patients with Reiter's disease the skin test showed the highest rate of positivity: 8 out of 13 and 9 out of 13 using acid extract antigens obtained from LGV and TRIC agent respectively.

Table 6

Antichlamydial antibody in body fluids (Darougar *et al.* 1971)

Specimen	*No. of patients*	*No. of positives*	*Antibody titres* neat	*1 : 5*	*1 : 10*	*1 : 20*
Synovial fluid	9	2		1	1	
Prostatic fluid	4	3	3			
Urine	17	1	1			
Lymph node extract	1	1	1			
Vaginal fluid	61	2		2		
Cervical fluid	61	4	1	2	0	1
Rectal fluid	61	2	2			

In guinea-pigs infected with guinea-pig inclusion conjunctivitis agent (Gpic) the skin test using different antigens, i.e. intact elementary bodies, delipidized particles or acid extract compound, was positive in the early stage of infection and remained positive for a long period (Kuo, Wang *et al.* 1971).

Table 7

Skin test in genital infection (Dunlop 1975)

Disease	*LGV-acid extract*		*TRIC-acid extract*	
	No. of patients	*Positive*	*No. of patients*	*Positive*
NSU	50	9	–	–
Contact of NSU	26	2	26	1
Reiter's disease	13	8	13	9

In guinea-pigs sensitized subcutaneously with *C. trachomatis* the lymphocyte transformation test was positive when an antigen prepared from *C. trachomatis* was used.

Immunity: No natural immunity against chlamydial infections of the eye or genital tract has been reported. The acquired immunity which may develop following an infection of the eye or genital tract, or vaccination, is only relative; thus relapses and reinfection are common amongst patients suffering from trachoma and chlamydial infection of the genital tract.

Studies in our laboratory have shown that baboons injected with TRIC agent in the eye and genital tract, and guinea-pigs injected with Gpic in the eye, were relatively sensitive to reinfection.

Recent studies by Murray and Charbonnet (1971), and Murray *et al.* (1973), using the guinea-pig model, have shown that circulating antibody plays little or no role in the development of resistance to infection. The role of secretory IgA and cell-mediated reponses in resistance to infection is not yet fully understood. It has been suggested that secretory IgA may interact with Chlamydia either by agglutinating the free particles or by inhibiting the adherence of elementary bodies to epithelial cells. Also the coating of elementary bodies by such antibody may direct phagocytes against these particles.

Delayed hypersensitivity: Studies carried out in monkeys infected with Chlamydia indicate that delayed hypersensitivity may play an important role in the pathogenesis of blinding trachoma (Kuo, Wang *et al.* 1971, Grayston *et al.* 1971).

Vaccination: Several attempts have been made to provide a vaccine against trachoma. Studies in Taiwan (Grayston *et al.* 1962), India (Dhir *et al.* 1967), Saudi Arabia (Nichols *et al.* 1969), Gambia (Sowa *et al.* 1969) and Iran (Jones 1975), have shown that vaccination with a live or dead antigen may provide relative protection for one to three years against trachoma.

References

Barron, A. L. and Collins, A. R. (1967). *American Journal of Ophthalmology* 63, 1487–1491

Barwell, C. F., Dunlop, E. M. C. and Race, J. W. (1967). *American Journal of Ophthalmology* 63, 1527–1534

Bernkopf, H., Orfila, J. and Maythar, B. (1966). *Nature (London)* **209**, 725–726

Burns, D. C. M., Darougar, S., Thin, R. N., Lothian, L. and Nicol, C. S. (1975). *British Journal of Venereal Diseases* 51, 314–318

Collier, L. H., Sowa, J. and Sowa, S. (1972). *Journal of Hygiene* **70**, 727–740
Darougar, S., Dwyer, R. St. C., Treharne, J. D., Harper, I. A., Garland, J. A. and Jones, B. R. (1971). *In* Nichols (1971). pp 445–460
Dhir, S. P., Agarwal, L. P., Detels, R., Wang, S. P. and Grayston, J. T. (1967). *American Journal of Ophthalmology* **63**, 1639–1644
Dhir, S. P., Hakomori, S., Kenny, G. E. and Grayston, J. T. (1972). *Journal of Immunology* **109**, 116–122
Dunlop, E. M. C. (1975). *In* "Recent Advances in Sexually Transmitted Diseases". Ed. R. S. Morton and J. R. Harris. Churchill-Livingstone, Edinburgh and London; p 267
Dunlop, E. M. C., Hare, M. J., Darougar, S. and Jones, B. R. (1971). *In* Nichols (1971). pp 507–512
Dunlop, E. M. C., Vaughan-Jackson, J. D., Darougar, S. and Jones, B. R. (1972). *British Journal of Venereal Diseases* **48**, 425–428
Dwyer, R. St. C., Treharne, J. D., Jones, B. R. and Herring, J. (1972). *British Journal of Venereal Diseases* **48**, 452–459
Grayston, J. T., Kim, K. S. W., Alexander, E. R. and Wang, S. P. (1971). *In* Nichols (1971). pp 377–385
Grayston, J. T., Woolridge, R. L. and Wang, S. P. (1962). *Annals of the New York Academy of Sciences* **98**, 352–367
Hilton, A. L., Richmond, S. J., Milne, J. D., Hindley, F. and Clarke, S. K. R. (1974). *British Journal of Venereal Diseases* **50**, 1–10
Jawetz, E., Dawson, C. R., Schachter, J., Juchau, V., Nabli, B. and Hanna, L. (1971). *In* Nichols (1971). pp 233–242
Jones, B. R. (1974). *British Journal of Ophthalmology* **58**, 438–454
Jones, B. R. (1975). *Transactions of the Ophthalmological Societies of the United Kingdom* **95**, 16–33
Katzenelson, E. and Bernkopf, H. (1967). *American Journal of Ophthalmology* **63**, 1483–1487
Kuo, C. C., Kenny, G. E. and Wang, S. P. (1971). *In* Nichols (1971). pp 113–123
Kuo, C. C., Wang, S. P. and Grayston, J. T. (1971). *In* Nichols (1971). pp 158–176
McComb, D. E. and Nichols, R. L. (1969). *American Journal of Ophthalmology* **90**, 278–284
McComb, D. E. and Nichols, R. L. (1970). *Infection and Immunity* **2**, 65–68
Mitsui, Y., Higai, H. and Kitamuro, T. (1962). *Archives of Ophthalmology* **68**, 651–652
Mogg, A. E., Collier, L. H. and Harris, R. G. (1971). *In* Nichols (1971). pp 185–195
Murray, E. S. and Charbonnet, L. T. (1971). *In* Nichols (1971). pp 369–376
Murray, E. S., Charbonnet, L. T. and MacDonald, A. B. (1973). *Journal of Immunology* **110**, 1518–1525
Nichols, R. L. (ed.) (1971). "Trachoma and Related Disorders Caused by Chlamydial Agents". Exerpta Medica, Amsterdam
Nichols, R. L., Bell, S. D., Haddad, N. A. and Bobb, A. A. (1969). *American Journal of Tropical Medicine and Hygiene* **18**, 723–730
Oriel, J. D., Powis, P. A., Reeve, P., Miller, A. and Nicol, C. S. (1974). *British Journal of Venereal Diseases* **50**, 11–16
Phillip, R. N., Lackman, D. B., Frank, F. W., Morrison, J. D., Casper, E. A. and Greaves, A. B. (1967). *American Journal of Ophthalmology* **63**, 1499–1505
Reeve, P., Gerloff, R. K., Casper, E., Phillip, R. N., Oriel, J. D. and Powis, P. A. (1974). *British Journal of Venereal Diseases* **50**, 136
Schachter, J. (1971). *American Journal of Ophthalmology* **71**, 857–860

Sowa, S., Sowa, J., Collier, L. H. and Blyth, W. A. (1969). *Journal of Hygiene* 67, 699–717

Tarizzo, M. (1973). "Field Methods for the Control of Trachoma". World Health Organization, Geneva; p 9

Treharne, J. D., Davey, S. J., Gray, S. J. and Jones, B. R. (1972). *British Journal of Venereal Diseases* **48**, 18–25

Vaughan-Jackson, J. D., Dunlop, E. M. C., Darougar, S., Dwyer, R. St. C. and Jones, B. R. (1972). *British Journal of Venereal Diseases* **48**, 445–451

Wang, S. P. and Grayston, J. T. (1970). *American Journal of Ophthalmology* **70**, 367–374

Zakay-Rones, Z., Katzenelson, E. and Levy, R. (1968). *Israel Journal of Medical Sciences* **4**, 305–306

A Possible Model for the Development of Plasmid-mediated Penicillin Resistance in the Gonococcus

Stanley Falkow, Lynn P Elwell, Johannes de Graaff,
Fred Heffron & Leonard Mayer
Department of Microbiology, School of Medicine,
University of Washington, Seattle, Washington 98195

Current Status of Resistance and its Genetic Basis

Antibiotic resistance among gonococci has been gradually increasing in many areas of the world. For example, it has been shown (Martin and Price 1970) that gonococci resistant to 0.06–0.3 μg/ml of penicillin comprised only 1% of randomly isolated strains in the USA in 1955 but that this proportion had increased to 51% of the strains by 1969. Strains resistant to 1 μg or more of penicillin per ml are still relatively rare, but there is little doubt that this increasing resistance to penicillin (and to other drugs) has made therapy more difficult. Nevertheless, although the extensive use of penicillin has produced ample selective pressure to ensure the survival and spread of resistant strains, penicillin is still the antibiotic most commonly used in the treatment of gonorrhea and it is still usually an effective regimen.

Resistance to chemotherapeutic agents may result from mutation or plasmid transfer followed by selection during therapy. The genetic basis of gonococcal resistance has been the subject of several recent investigations, particularly by Sparling and his associates. Resistance of gonococci to antibiotics falls into two general categories (Sparling 1972): low-level resistance (2–8 μg/ml at most) to penicillin (Pen), erythromycin (Ery), tetracycline (Tet) and chloramphenicol (Chl), and high-level resistance (usually 1 mg/ml or greater) to streptomycin (Str) and spectinomycin (Spc). Two laboratories (Sarrubi *et al.* 1974, Maier *et al.* 1975) have recently mapped the loci for resistance to several antibiotics in laboratory-derived strains and clinical isolates by genetic transformation. The data clearly show that independent genes for resistance occur in a linked cluster in the apparent order Str, Tet, Chl, Spc, Ery. The locus for resistance to penicillin was transferred independently of the Str cluster.

The biochemical basis for resistance to streptomycin and spectinomycin has been examined by Maness *et al.* (1974). Resistance to these two aminoglycoside antibiotics in both laboratory-derived mutants and clinical isolates is associated with 30S ribosomal resistance to the respective antibiotics. The genetic clustering of Str, Tet, Chl and Ery is similar to that seen in *Escherichia coli* and *Bacillus subtilis*, as is the mechanism of resistance to the aminoglycosides. It seems likely, therefore, that in the gonococcus all the genes in the Str cluster are loci for structural ribosomal proteins. Resistance of gonococci to penicillin is not known to be associated with a β-lactamase. This fact, together with the epidemiological observations on the appearance of gonococcal strains with decreased sensitivity to penicillin, is consistent with the step-by-step selection of chromosomal mutations affecting the phenotypic response of the cell to the antibiotic.

Multiple antibiotic resistance due to a single or limited number of genes has also been observed in both laboratory strains and clinical isolates of the gonococcus. Maness and Sparling (1973) showed that the simultaneous loss of low level resistance to a group of drugs (Pen, Ery, Tet, Chl as well as amino-acridine dyes) could be restored by a single back mutation to any one. Although several plausible explanations for multiple resistance were presented, including the unlikely possibility of plasmid-mediated multiple resistance, it now appears that this phenomenon is due to a single-step chromosomal mutation which occurs at a locus (Env) affecting cell envelope permeability (Sarrubi *et al.* 1974).

The genetic analysis of antibiotic resistance in the gonococcus indicates that resistance is, for the present at least, mediated solely by chromosomal genes. This is a far cry from the experience with enteric micro-organisms and staphylococci where high-level multiple drug resistance is common and is mediated by plasmids which are directly or indirectly transmissible. The gonococci do not stand alone as bacterial species which have shown relatively small changes in antibiotic resistance despite widespread selective pressure. No group A β-hemolytic streptococcus resistant to penicillin has been isolated from man. Pneumococci significantly resistant to penicillin are rare and, like the gonococcus, resistance is of chromosomal origin and of a relatively low magnitude. Similarly, *Haemophilus influenzae* was considered to be uniformly susceptible to ampicillin since its availability in 1964, and in no case was the failure of ampicillin treatment attributed to resistance of the *H. influenzae* isolates.

A few years ago the situation changed dramatically; indeed, meningitis due to ampicillin-resistant strains has been increasing in frequency during the past year (Clymo and Harper 1974, Kahn *et al.* 1974, Tomeh *et al.* 1974). The resistant strains of *H. influenzae* showed several characteristics which were not consistent with simple mutation to resistance, in that cells were resistant to relatively high levels of ampicillin (25 μg/ml or greater) due to the presence of a β-lactamase similar to that found in Gram-negative bacilli harboring R plasmids (Kahn *et al.* 1974, Farrar and O'Dell 1974).

The implication that ampicillin resistance in *H. influenzae* might be plasmid-mediated led us to examine this question directly. The results, coupled with other studies in our laboratory on the origin of plasmid-mediated ampicillin resistance and the plasmid pool of *N. gonorrhoeae*, are presented in the following sections. These data seem to be worth considering as a possible model showing that the gonococcus may eventually acquire antibiotic resistance by other than a mutational mechanism.

The Origin of β-lactamase Genes in the R Plasmids of Enteric Bacteria

Plasmid-mediated resistance to penicillins and cephalosporins in enteric bacteria is almost universally associated with the elaboration of a β-lactamase. Two broad classes of drug resistant (R) plasmid-mediated β-lactamase are now recognized (Hedges *et al.* 1974, Dale and Smith 1974). TEM-type β-lactamase (TEM) has a high absolute activity against benzyl penicillin, ampicillin and cephaloridine substrates but low activity against isoazolyl penicillin such as oxacillin. The other type of R-factor-mediated β-lactamase (0) can be differentiated from TEM by its lower absolute activity against benzyl penicillin and its ability to hydrolyze oxacillin at an appreciable rate. TEM is by far the most common R-factor-mediated β-lactamase and is found on a wide variety of naturally occurring plasmids. While the R plasmids of enteric bacteria come in a variety of sizes and guanine + cytosine (G + C) contents, and are isolated from many different bacterial species around the world, it has been consistently observed that the TEM β-lactamase protein is essentially identical in its molecular properties, substrate profile, &c.

About a year ago we had cause to examine a rather small, 5.5×10^6 dalton (5.5 MDal) plasmid which encoded for a TEM β-lactamase. This plasmid, which we called RSF1030 (referred to hereafter as R-Amp), possessed several unique replicative properties (Crosa *et al.* 1975) which led us to examine its molecular fine structure by DNA-DNA hybridization studies. At the time we were looking for a clue to the replication properties of R-AMP; instead we found the rather striking correlation summarized in Table 1. Much to our surprise we found that R-Amp shared 30–40% of its DNA sequences with a variety of R plasmids that coded for a TEM β-lactamase, but showed no DNA sequence homology with plasmids that did not specify ampicillin resistance or that coded for an O β-lactamase (Heffron, Sublett *et al.* 1975). The implication of this observation was that R-Amp and any other plasmid which specified the TEM β-lactamase shared a common DNA segment of about 3 MDal. Such a DNA segment was of sufficient size to encode not only for the TEM β-lactamase, a 22 000 dalton protein, but for several additional proteins as well.

Table 1

Demonstration of a common DNA sequence between plasmids which specify the TEM β-lactamase

R plasmids	*Percentage guanine plus cytosine*	*Size (MDal)*	*Type β-lactamase*	*DNA homology with RSF1030*
RSF1030	49	5.5	TEM	100
R388	62	21.0	None	1
R7K	62	22.0	TEM	30
R1	52	62.0	TEM	44
R222	52	68.0	None	1
R16	50	48.0	O	1
R684	50	60	TEM	36
R64	50	72	None	1
R55	?	?	O	1
R746	?	?	TEM	32
N3	49	32	None	3
R390	?	?	TEM	46

Since it appeared that the DNA segment encoding for TEM was of a common origin, we were led to examine the possible genetic mechanism which would explain the widespread dissemination of this DNA segment. Several laboratories (Richmond and Sykes 1972, Hedges and Jacob 1974) had previously reported that some R plasmid genes, including those specifying ampicillin resistance, could be transposed or translocated from plasmid to plasmid, or from a plasmid to the bacterial chromosome. Consequently, in collaboration with R W Hedges and Alan Jacob of the Royal Postgraduate Medical School, London, we obtained a series of plasmid pairs that differed only in whether or not they contained the genetic information for ampicillin resistance (Heffron, Sublett *et al.* 1975). Such plasmid derivatives are quite simple to prepare in the laboratory. For example, if one has a bacterial cell carrying a 5.5 MDal plasmid encoding for resistance to sulphonamide and streptomycin, it is a simple matter to introduce a much larger (say 60 MDal) unrelated plasmid which encodes for the TEM β-lactamase. It is then possible to isolate the total plasmid DNA from this strain, separate the larger plasmid from the smaller by sedimentation in a sucrose gradient, and use the sucrose gradient fractions containing only the smaller plasmid DNA molecules to transform $CaCl_2$-treated *E. coli* with selection for linked streptomycin and ampicillin resistance. If the smaller plasmid has in fact received the genes encoding for ampicillin resistance from the larger plasmid, then one can examine the recombinant plasmid to gain some view of the genetic mechanism involved.

Table 2

DNA-DNA hybridizations between plasmids differing only in the TEM β-lactamase sequence

R plasmid	*TEM β-lactamase*	*Homology with RSF1030*
RSF1010	—	<1
RSF1010-1 •	+	39
Sa	—	<1
Sa-1	+	37
R483	—	<1
R483-1	+	30
R66a	—	<1
R66a-1	+	30
R64	—	<1
R64-1	+	36

• Each of the plasmids designated-1 has received the TEM β-lactamase gene and has increased in size by an average of 3.2 MDal

Table 2 illustrates the results obtained when paired plasmids differing only by the acquisition of ampicillin resistance were hybridized against R-Amp. The results confirm the impression that there is a common 3 MDal DNA segment which is associated with ampicillin resistance. Figure 1 provides a rather clear insight into the genetic mechanism that is operating in the acquisition of the ampicillin genes from one plasmid by another. This Fig. is an electron micrograph of a DNA heteroduplex molecule formed between the single strand of a plasmid before the acquisition of the genes determining ampicillin resistance, and a single strand of the same plasmid species after the acquisition of ampicillin resistance genes. The molecules are prepared and mounted for inspection in the electron microscope so that regions of DNA homology appear as relatively smooth darkly staining regions, while nonhomologous

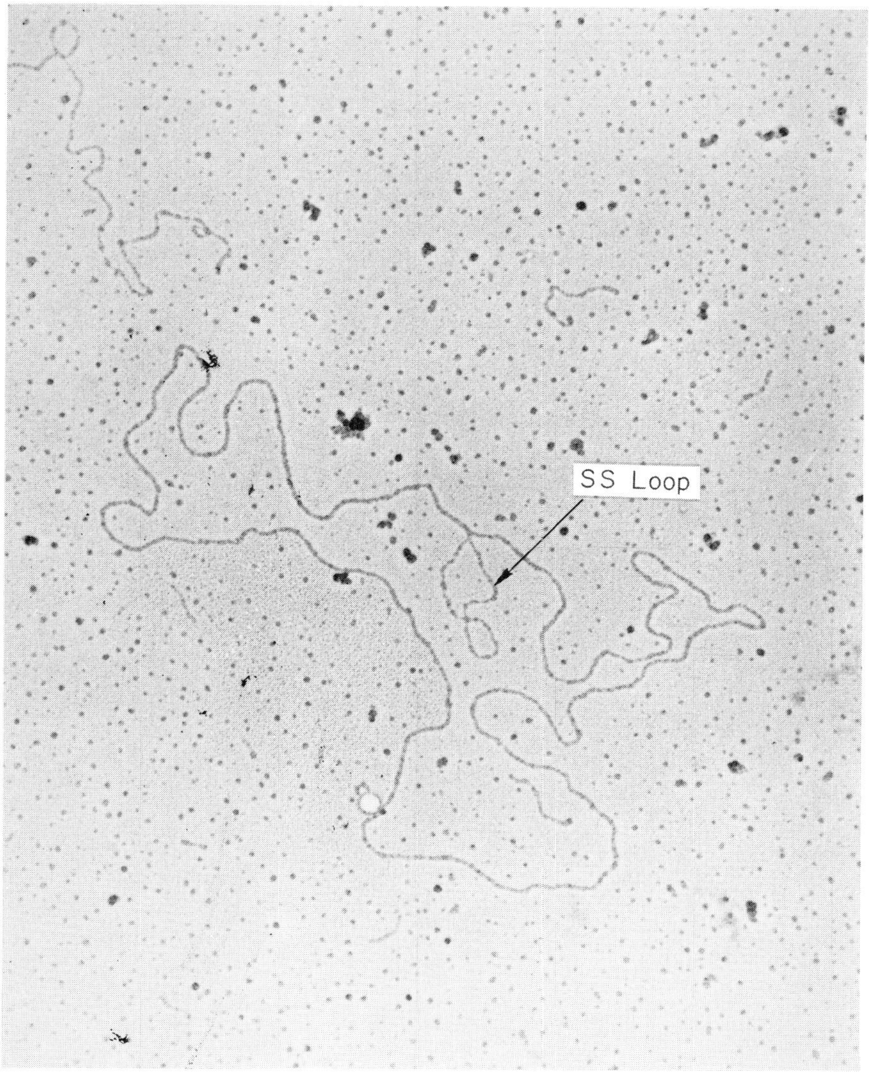

Fig. 1 *Heteroduplex molecule formed between one strand of the R plasmid Sa and one strand of Sa-1. Sa is a 24 MDal R plasmid conferring resistance to sulphonamide, streptomycin, kanamycin and chloramphenicol. Sa-1 is identical in all respects except for a single insertion loop of DNA, TnA, which contains TEM β-lactamase genes received from another plasmid. Sa-1 has a molecular size of 27.2 MDal*

single-stranded DNA appears as a lighter staining and somewhat "kinky" region. The molecule shown in Fig. 1 is totally homologous except for a single loop of single-stranded DNA. This loop of DNA represents the common 3 MDal segment common to R plasmids containing the TEM β-lactamase.

The complete details of our molecular findings are only summarized here, as they will appear in detail elsewhere (Heffron, Rubens and Falkow 1975). Simply stated, the data show that the genes specifying the TEM β-lactamase reside upon a sequence of DNA which can be translocated from plasmid to plasmid independently of the genes (*rec*) controlling normal host recombination. Although the precise genetic mechanism is still not clear, it appears that the ubiquity of the TEM β-lactamase segment, which we call TnA, is at least in part due to its ability to excise from one plasmid and become inserted into another. The plasmid receiving TnA does not lose or exchange any genetic information in the process but rather increases in size due to the insertion of TnA into its genome. The plasmid which donates TnA generally loses the DNA sequence *in toto*; in consequence, it loses the ability to synthesize the TEM β-lactamase (and the other as yet unknown proteins encoded by the TnA sequence) but is otherwise unchanged. Hence, the excision of TnA from the donor plasmid seems to be a rather precise mechanism. The insertion of TnA into a plasmid is also precise in that it does not occur simply at random. Nevertheless, it appears that the specificity of insertion is not high, since TnA can be found to insert into the 5.5 MDal plasmid in as many as twelve distinct sites.

Insertion of TnA may not be without consequence. If TnA inserts within the continuity of a structural gene, the gene is inactivated. If the gene happens to be essential for plasmid replication then the insertion event may be lethal. Insertion of TnA into a plasmid encoding for streptomycin and sulphonamide resistance sometimes occurs within one of the structural genes for antibiotic resistance; in this case the plasmid gains ampicillin resistance while giving up streptomycin or sulphonamide resistance. One can perhaps see how the translocation phenomenon can have rather profound structural and phenotypic effects.

The structural genes specifying many phenotypic characteristics of plasmids appear to have arisen independently from the essential transfer and replication regions of the plasmid. It is tempting to speculate that a large proportion of the non-essential plasmid-mediated determinants, such as the antibiotic resistance determinants of R factors which confer transient selective advantage, may be attributed to a limited pool of translocatable DNA segments. Thus translocatable sequences such as TnA could account for the observation that plasmids with identical transfer and replication genes may carry quite different antibiotic markers. Thus, even though R factors appear to be of diverse origin, the drug resistance genes carried by these plasmids may be of common origin. Until but a few months ago, ampicillin resistance (Heffron, Sublett *et al.* 1975) and tetracycline resistance (Kleckner, Chan and Botstein, personal communication) were the only known translocatable plasmid genes. However, it has become clear that two kanamycin resistance loci (Berg and Davies, personal communication) and chloramphenicol resistance genes (Rosener, personal communication) are also associated with a translocatable DNA sequence.

The R Plasmids of H. influenzae

The sudden emergence of ampicillin resistance in *H. influenzae* and its associated elaboration of β-lactamase suggested to us that a plasmid might be involved. We therefore examined 4 ampicillin-resistant clinical isolates and, rather as expected, plasmid DNA could be demonstrated in each (Elwell *et al.* 1975). Three of the strains contained a plasmid of approximately 30 MDal while one strain contained a much smaller plasmid with a molecular weight of only 3 MDal. To show definitively that the structural gene for β-lactamase was located on the plasmid DNA, we used purified plasmid DNA preparations to transform a typical antibiotic-sensitive *H. influenzae* to resistance. Both the 30 MDal and the 3 MDal plasmid species were effective in transformation, and we obtained absolute correlation between the presence of a plasmid species and ampicillin resistance. At the same time that these experiments were in progress we learned from W E Farrar and G Thorne of the Medical College of South Carolina that they had been successful in demonstrating the conjugal transfer of ampicillin resistance between strains of *H. influenzae*. We have found that the conjugative plasmid described by them is 30 MDal in size, while they have demonstrated (personal communication) that the 30 MDal plasmids seen in our isolates were conjugative. Not unexpectedly the smaller 3 MDal plasmid of *H. influenzae* has not been shown to be transmissible by conjugation.

The origin of the plasmids in *H. influenzae* is of critical epidemiological importance. Had we observed only a single plasmid species within the resistant Haemophilus strains a case might have been made that we were essentially dealing with a single clone of drug-resistant *H. influenzae* that had become widely disseminated throughout the world. The finding of the much smaller 3 MDal plasmid suggested, however, either that there have been at least two independent genetic events leading to the development of resistance or that a single plasmid had already undergone a series of recombinational interactions.

Table 3 summarizes our current genetic and molecular information concerning the two classes of Haemophilus R plasmids. Both plasmids possess a guanine + cytosine content of approximately 40% which is essentially identical to that of *H. influenzae* chromosomal DNA. We have been successful in transforming *E. coli* K-12 to ampicillin resistance using purified 3 MDal haemophilus DNA but have been unable to transform *E. coli* with the larger, 30 MDal, plasmid. This finding suggests that the two plasmid species of haemophilus are of independent origin. While the conjugative nature of 30 MDal plasmid species could be taken to indicate that this plasmic was of enteric origin it should be quickly pointed out that the G + C content of 40% is unlike that of any enteric R factor that has

Table 3

Summary of current genetic and molecular information of both classes of Haemophilus R factors

DNA	R7	R885
Molecular weight	30	3
Guanine + cytosine content ●	38.8	40.1
No. of copies per chromosome equivalent	3	28

● The guanine + cytosine content of the *H. influenzae* chromosome was 38.2 in these experiments

been previously described. We have, moreover, been unable to demonstrate any relationship between the *H. influenzae* plasmid and any known R factor classes found in enteric species.

The critical point to this discussion, however, was whether the TEM-like β-lactamase carried by the plasmids of *H. influenzae* was related to the TnA translocation sequence of enteric microorganisms. The data presented in Table 4 show unquestionably that in fact the TnA sequence is present *in toto* on the 30 MDal *H. influenzae* plasmid, while approximately one-third of the TnA sequences are present on the 3 MDal species. Since the TnA translocation sequence does not appear to be capable of independent autonomous replication it would seem that at some relatively recent point in time a genetic element carrying TnA must have been introduced into *H. influenzae*. Whether the plasmids carrying TnA now resident in *H. influenzae* were directly acquired from some unknown enteric species by conjugation or whether the plasmids were formed by the translocation of the ubiquitous Tn sequence into resident Haemophilus plasmid species is not clear from currently available data. Furthermore, the results of the hybridization studies show that the Haemophilus plasmids are of independent origin, since they share base homology only in the area of the TnA insertion sequence. It would appear, therefore, that R-factor-associated ampicillin resistance in *H. influenzae* has occurred by virtue of at least two separate genetic events.

Table 4

DNA-DNA hybridizations between labelled plasmid DNA and whole cell DNA

Source of unlabelled DNA	*Ampicillin resistance*	*Percentage relative DNA sequence homology*	
		With RSF 1030 ●	*With R885* ■
H. influenzae:			
G32: ampicillin-sensitive strain (MIC = 0.25 μg/ml)	–	1	1
G32(R885): ampicillin-resistant transformant strain containing 3 MDal Haemophilus plasmid (MIC > 1000 μg/ml)	+	23	100
G32(R7): ampicillin-resistant transformant containing 30 MDal Haemophilus plasmid (MIC > 1000 μg/ml)	+	45	27
E. coli:			
C600(RSF1030): ampicillin-resistant strain containing R-factor RSF1030	+	100	–
J53(RP4): strain containing P-class plasmid RP4, a 34 MDal R factor specifying ampicillin, tetracycline and kanamycin resistance	+	36	26
711 R^-: ampicillin-sensitive *E. coli* free of R factors	–	1	1.8

● RSF1030: 5.5 MDal plasmid containing entire TnA sequence
■ R885: 3 MDal Haemophilus plasmid containing approximately 33% of TnA sequence

Recently, Bouanchaud and his associates (Van *et al.* 1975) have documented that high-level tetracycline resistance in *H. influenzae* (reported for the first time in different countries in 1974) is also plasmid linked, although a single plasmid conferring both ampicillin and tetracycline resistance has yet to be isolated. Clearly, there has been a striking change in the origin and epidemiology of drug resistance determinants found in Haemophilus in a very short time.

This change is of considerable scientific import but, more significantly, has materially affected the clinical treatment of Haemophilus infection (Nelson 1974).

The Potential for the Acquisition of Plasmid-mediated Drug Resistance in the Gonococcus

It has been known for some time that the transmissible R plasmids of enteric species enjoy a very broad host range. The recent findings of our laboratory and of others that the drug resistance genes of plasmids are capable of host-independent, nonreciprocal, site-specific insertion demonstrate that the range of these genes may be even broader than that of the whole plasmid genome. Because *H. influenzae* have shown an epidemiological picture of drug resistance

Table 5

Plasmid species of *N. gonorrhoeae*

Plasmid	*Size (MDal)*	*Guanine + cytosine content*	*No. of copies per chromosome equivalent*
R1990	2.45 ± 0.15	50	27
R. Nix	23.5 ± 1.0	50	1–3

rather like that of the gonococcus it seems worth considering whether there is a possibility that we may eventually find ourselves faced with R plasmids in strains of *N. gonorrhoeae*. As noted earlier, there has been no documented incidence of plasmid-mediated antibiotic resistance in the gonococcus. It seems likely, therefore, either that R plasmids are not now resident in the gonococcus or that they are very rare. This is not to say that the gonococcus does not possess a plasmid gene pool. We demonstrated a few years ago (Mayer *et al.* 1974) that in fact the majority of clinical isolates possess a 3 MDal plasmid, and subsequently we have observed that a number of isolates also or alternatively possess a 24 MDal plasmid (Table 5). These gonococcal plasmids cannot be correlated, however, either with antibiotic resistance or with the striking transition in colonial morphology associated with the loss of pili. The gonococcal plasmids are, therefore, cryptic in the phenotypic sense. They are nevertheless important in the present context since it is likely that these plasmids could serve as very effective recipients for the insertion of TnA or other translocatable antibiotic resistance genes. This presupposes that these translocatable sequences are already present in gonococci (which seems unlikely) or that these genes could gain entry into the gonococcus. Is it plausible that the TnA and other plasmid-mediated antibiotic resistance genes could gain entry to the gonococcus? The answer is a qualified yes. R plasmids are well known for their promiscuity and one R factor class, P, derived from *Pseudomonas aeruginosa* shows a particularly broad host range. Olsen and Shipley (1973) have shown, and we have confirmed, that at least one P class R factor, R18222, can be transmitted by conjugation from *Pseudomonas aeruginosa* (and *P. fluorescens*) to a strain of *N. perflava. N. perflava* also possess a plasmid pool as do many other saprophytic Neisseria species and at the genetic level this species is related to *N. gonorrhoeae*. *N. perflava* receiving the R plasmid 1822 are stable if maintained under penicillin selection, but this R plasmid is rapidly segregated when the selection is relieved. The plasmid can be maintained in *N. perflava* long enough, however, to permit translocation of the TnA segment of R1882 to resident *N. perflava* plasmids. These experiments are cursory in nature but suffice, we think, to show that the possibility of entry of translocatable antibiotic resistance genes into gonococci is plausible. (We have not directly attempted to use *N. gonorrhoeae* as a recipient in these experiments since we believe the construction of a bona fide ampicillin-resistant strain of the gonococcus to be an unnecessary hazard). If one accepts the fact that the antibiotic resistance sequences can enter the gonococcus and become translocated onto resident neisserial plasmids it is not difficult to see how they might then become widely disseminated. Not only might the cells in which this sequence of events has occurred become disseminated by selection, but it has also been demonstrated that DNA liberated from gonococcal cells during the course of normal growth is capable of mediating transformation to other Neisseria strains and species.

In spite of this plausible sequence of events we do not know why the gonococcus does not already contain R plasmids. It is clear that the *in vivo* transmission of R plasmids does not occur at so high a probability as it occurs *in vitro*, and the translocation phenomenon itself occurs at a relatively low frequency. So the probability of the gonococcus acquiring plasmid-mediated resistance is low. Moreover, even if successful it is possible that, as in the case of *H. influenzae*, individual cells possessing a TEM type β-lactamase could still be killed by concentrations of penicillins only 1% the strength of those in which an *E. coli* cell with the enzyme could survive (Medeiros and O'Brien 1975). Thus, penicillin therapy may have already eliminated some infections caused by β-lactamase containing strains of the gonococcus. We can no more explain why this plausible phenomenon has not already occurred in the gonococcus any more than we fully understand why, after decades of not acquiring any significant level of penicillin resistance, *H. influenzae* suddenly developed resistant strains a few years ago. This seems possible only if we consider that recently some genetic event occurred which introduced the TnA sequence (and more recently, the Tet sequence) into this species. In much the same way the pneumococcus has suddenly begun to show plasmid-mediated chloramphenicol and tetracycline resistance (Y Chabbert, personal communication), and plasmid-mediated Ery resistance is becoming an important problem in Japan (Nakae *et al.* 1975). Perhaps we shall never see the day when we must deal with plasmid-mediated resistance in the gonococcus. If it does occur, however, whether by the mechanism we have discussed here or by some other genetic mechanism, it will surely dwarf the concern we now have about relatively insensitive gonococci.

Acknowledgments

We are grateful to the National Institute of Health, the US Army Research and Development Command and the National Science Foundation for their support.

References

Clymo, A. B. and Harper, I. A. (1974). *Lancet* **i**, 453

Crosa, J. H., Luttropp, L. K. and Falkow, S. (1975). *Proceedings of the National Academy of Sciences of the United States of America* **72**, 654

Dale, J. W. and Smith, J. T. (1974). *Journal of Bacteriology* **119**, 351

Elwell, L. P., Graaff, J. de, Seibert, D. and Falkow, S. (1975). *Infection and Immunity* **12**, 404

Farrar, W. E. and O'Dell, N. (1974). *Antimicrobial Agents and Chemotherapy* **6**, 625

Hedges, R. W., Datta, N., Kontomichalou, P. and Smith, J. T. (1974). *Journal of Bacteriology* **117**, 56

Hedges, R. W. and Jacob, A. (1974). *Molecular and General Genetics* **132**, 31

Heffron, F., Rubens, C. and Falkow, S. (1975). *Proceedings of the National Academy of Sciences of the United States of America* **72**, 3623

Heffron, F., Sublett, R., Hedges, R. W., Jacob, A. and Falkow, S. (1975). *Journal of Bacteriology* **122**, 250

Kahn, W., Ross, S., Rodriquez, W., Controri, G. and Saz, A. K. (1974). *Journal of the American Medical Association* **229**, 298

Maier, T. W., Zubryzycki, L. and Coyle, M. B. (1975). *Antimicrobial Agents and Chemotherapy* **7**, 676

Maness, M. J., Foster, G. C. and Sparling, P. F. (1974). *Journal of Bacteriology* **120**, 1293

Maness, M. J. and Sparling, P. F. (1973). *Journal of Infectious Diseases* **128**, 321

Martin, J. E. jr and Price, L. A. (1970). *Journal of Infectious Diseases* **122**, 459

Mayer, L. W., Holmes, K. K. and Falkow, S. (1974). *Infection and Immunity* **10**, 712

Medeiros, A. and O'Brien, T. F. (1975). *Lancet* **i**, 716

Nakae, M., Inoue, M. and Mitsuhashi, S. (1975). *Antimicrobial Agents and Chemotherapy* **7**, 719

Nelson, J. D. (1974). *Journal of the American Medical Association* **229**, 322
Olsen, R. H. and Shipley, P. L. (1973). *Journal of Bacteriology* **113**, 772
Richmond, M. H. and Sykes, R. B. (1972). *Nature* (*London*) **214**, 885
Sarrubi, F. A. jr, Blackman, E. and Sparling, P. F. (1974). *Journal of Bacteriology* **120**, 1284
Sparling, P. F. (1972). *Medical Clinics of North America* **56**, 1133
Tomeh, M. O., Starr, S. E., McGowan, J. E., Terry, P. M. and Nahmias, A. J. (1974). *Journal of the American Medical Association* **229**, 295
Van, A. D., Bieth, G. and Bouanchaud, D. H. (1975). *Comptes rendus hebdomadaires des séances de l'Académie des sciences* (*Paris*) **280**, 1321

Discussion

Professor Collier, in response to Dr Darougar's invitation to comment upon the results of trachoma vaccine trials, said that a trial by the MRC Trachoma Unit in The Gambia had confirmed that in vaccinated children who subsequently acquired the disease its severity was on average worse than in non-vaccinated controls. The effects of the trachoma vaccines used hitherto appeared to be complex and were possibly the resultant of two forces—an initial immunity that decreased comparatively quickly and a form of delayed hypersensitivity that might persist for much longer.

Professor Collier asked Dr Darougar what species of animal had provided the model for the experimental trachoma he had described, and also if he would regard as useful for routine diagnostic use any of the tests for serum antibodies to Chlamydia which he had reviewed. If any of these tests were thought useful, what would he accept as a significant titre?

Dr Darougar replied that he had used a cat. This animal's natural infection to Chlamydia produced pannus and scarring. Cats were sensitive to TRIC agents, both in the genital tract and in the eye.

Since chlamydial antibody remained for a long period, even after active disease was finished, it was not possible to say that any particular titre was diagnostic for chlamydial infection, but one could say that the presence of antibody over 1 : 64 might be suggestive of a present infection.

Dr Pavel Novotny (*Wellcome Research Laboratories, Beckenham*) was puzzled by the results obtained by Buchanan *et al.* 1973 (*Journal of Clinical Investigation* 52, 2896) using patients' sera and a pili antigen derived from strain 2868, since he had found that pili were usually strain-specific and cross-reactions between pili of different strains were rare (Novotny and Turner (1975) *Journal of General*

Microbiology 89, 87). Antiserum against strain 2868 (prepared in his laboratory) did not react with pili of any heterologous strain so far tested and none of the other sera which reacted with homologous pili reacted with the pili of the strain 2868. Sera from 3 patients suffering from septicaemia had been investigated using strains isolated from urethra and cervix of these patients. Pili antibodies were not found, but other antibodies (complement fixation, agglutination) were found including IgG reacting with gonococcal surface structures detected by immune electron-microscopy. The explanation for this discrepancy could be that the antigen used by Buchanan *et al.* and prepared from single strain was not pure pili antigen or that there are two classes of pili – some with shared and some with strain specific antigens. Two serological types of pili in one strain had been found, one common pili and the other pili with a knob on one end which are morphologically reminiscent of sex pili of *E. coli.*

Dr Gotschlich, in reply, said that in the sera under discussion T3 and T4 organisms were easily distinguishable from T1 and T2 organisms in the sense that only the pilated organisms gave rise to antibodies. One thing that had not been established by the present investigators was the degree of homology between different kinds of pili.

Dr Stanley Falkow (*Seattle*) said it was possible to locate the genes for pili; they could be seen and taken out and put in at will.

Dr Krause (*Chairman*) said that at the present, early stage of genetic analysis, differences of opinion in serological analyses would be expected. He would not be surprised at this stage if there was some discrepancy between serotypes in different laboratories, and particularly in how much cross-reaction was observed in the preparation from one laboratory to another. Much more standardization and exchange of materials would be needed before these difficulties could be overcome.

Dr Roberts asked if gonococci had surface polysaccharides and, if so, what was their biological function. He also asked if Neisseria membrane proteins had any cross-reaction.

Dr Gotschlich said there had not been any recent report concerning a capsular polysaccharide in gonococci. The serotypes of the gonococcus did not cross-react with the serotypes of the meningococcus.

Virus Diseases: I. Genital Herpes

Chairman

Dr John M Knox

Baylor College of Medicine,
Houston, Texas

Genital Herpetic Infection — The Old and the New

André J Nahmias, William E Josey, Zuher M Naib and
Aarolyn M Visintine
Departments of Pediatrics, Preventive Medicine,
Gynecology & Obstetrics and Pathology,
Emory University School of Medicine,
Atlanta, Georgia, USA

The subject of genital herpetic infection has evoked increasing interest over the past decade for the following major reasons: (1) It is a common venereal disease. (2) It is particularly troublesome in many individuals because of frequent recurrences. (3) Its occurrence in a pregnant woman may endanger her fetus or newborn. (4) It is associated with cervical cancer. These concerns have also been reflected in the lay press. Yet the first three of these aspects of genital herpetic infections have been recognized in humans for several decades, if not for centuries. Indeed, these same three aspects of genital infections have also been appreciated in several non-human species, including cows, horses and dogs infected with their own herpesviruses (Nahmias 1974).

A historical perspective of the clinicoepidemiological and laboratory aspects of genital herpetic infections (Table 1) provides a contrast between what is old and more recently confirmed or rediscovered, and what is really new. Thus, most of the clinical manifestations of genital herpetic infections in males and females, including children, have long been appreciated (Diday and Doyon 1886, Du Castel 1901, Lipschütz 1921, Baum 1920, Hutfield 1966, Nahmias and Dowdle 1968): what is new has been the recognition of herpetic cystitis (Masukawa *et al.* 1972, Person *et al.* 1973) and of asymptomatic urogenital herpetic infections (Naib *et al.* 1966, Josey *et al.* 1968, Centifanto *et al.* 1972). There is little question that the virus can be isolated from the urethra of asymptomatic males

Table 1

Historical perspective of genital herpetic infections

	First reported or suspected
Clinical	
Symptomatic infection:	
In males and females	1736
In children	1853
Asymptomatic infection:	
In females	1966
In males	1972
Involvement of:	
Urethra	1736
Vagina	1736
Cervix	1869
Bladder	1972
Anus	1736
Prostate, seminal vesicles, testes	1972 ●
Associated with:	
Arthritis	1886 ●
Neuralgias	1886
CSF pleocytosis and meningitis	1904
Radiculitis	1963
Myelitis	1973
Erythema multiforme	1966
Disseminated visceral disease	1974 ●
Epidemiological	
Common in VD clinics	1883
Associated with other venereal diseases	1886
Venereal transmission	1736
Autoinoculation to other body sites	1886
Recurrences:	1853
Associated with menses	1890
Exogenous reinfection with heterologous HSV type	1968
Exogenous reinfection with homologous HSV type	1968 ●
Latency in sacral ganglia	1974 ●
Intrapartum transmission to newborn	1934
Transplacental transmission to fetus	1963 ●
Postnatal transmission to newborn	1963
Associated with abortions	1970
Associated with congenital malformations	1969 ●
Associated with cervical cancer	1966 ■
Laboratory	
Transmission to humans	1886
Transmission to animals	1920
Histopathological changes	1896
Use of Papanicolaou smear for detection	1966
Differences between genital and non-genital herpes	1921
Antigenic differences (HSV-1 and HSV-2)	1961
Differences in pock size on chorioallantoic membrane	1967
Association of HSV type to body site and mode of viral spread	1967
Serological detection of HSV type antibodies	1968
Antigenic and biological differences within HSV-2	1973

● Unconfirmed
■ Causality unconfirmed

(Jeansson and Molin 1970); what is still unconfirmed are the isolations of HSV from the prostate, seminal vesicles and testes (Centifanto *et al.* 1972). Also unconfirmed is the relation reported in 1886 between genital herpetic infections and arthritis (Diday and Doyon 1886), made more cogent by the recent descriptions of the production of chronic arthritis with HSV in rabbits and guinea-pigs (Bacon *et al.* 1974). Of particular import is the increased clinical severity of genital herpes, including fatal viral dissemination, in immunocompromised hosts (Sutton *et al.* 1974).

The high frequency of genital herpes in venereal disease clinics had been reported in the nineteenth century (Unna 1883), but its frequent occurrence in private practice appears to be a more recent observation (Gardner and Kaufman 1972). The concepts of exogenous reinfection (Nahmias and Dowdle 1968) and evidence for latency of the genital virus in sacral ganglia (Baringer 1974) are also recent. The venereal transmission of genital infection (Diday and Doyon 1886, Lipschütz 1921) and intrapartum transmission to the newborn (Batignani 1934) have been suggested for a long time and more recently confirmed (Nahmias *et al.* 1969, Nahmias, Alford *et al.* 1970). The transplacental transmission of HSV and its role in congenital malformations remains to be corroborated (Nahmias, Alford *et al.* 1970, Nahmias, Visintine *et al.* 1975). The association of genital herpes with cervical cancer was only suspected a decade ago (Naib *et al.* 1966) and is the subject of Dr Roizman's presentation (p 151).

Even though the cytohistopathological changes of genital herpes were described close to a century ago (Lipschütz 1921, Unna 1896), and Papanicolaou cervicovaginal smears introduced for cervical cancer screening in the late 1940's, the usefulness of cytological techniques for detecting genital herpetic infections was not emphasized until 1966 (Naib *et al.* 1966). The differences between genital and non-genital herpes were suspected by Lipschütz in 1921, soon after the viral etiology of genital herpes was ascertained (Baum 1920). However, it was not until several decades later that Lipschütz was vindicated, when two antigenically distinct types of herpes simplex virus (HSV-1 and HSV-2) were recognized (Schneweis and Brandis 1961) and correlated with site of occurrence and usual mode of spread (Nahmias and Dowdle 1968, Dowdle *et al.* 1967). This differentiation also permitted the recent development of serological techniques to detect antibodies to the two HSV types (Rawls *et al.* 1970, Nahmias, Josey *et al.* 1970).

A review of our experience with the typing of HSV isolates from various body sites in over 1200 patients is now presented to emphasize certain clinicoepidemiological aspects. It should be noted that very recent studies suggest the existence of variants within each of the two HSV types (Seth *et al.* 1974, Pereira *et al.* 1975, Beck *et al.* 1974); however, their clinicoepidemiological correlates remain to be ascertained.

Clinicoepidemiological Correlates of HSV-1 and HSV-2

The most important conclusion which can be drawn from the data presented in Table 2 is that both HSV types can be isolated from almost any body site. Another point is that the same individual may have HSV-1 infection of one site concurrently with HSV-2 infection of another site, or have the same virus type isolated simultaneously from different body sites. It is of interest in this regard that HSV-1 has been isolated from the trigeminal ganglion and HSV-2 from the sacral ganglion of the same individual. Another point is that HSV-1 or HSV-2 can be acquired by accidental inoculation in laboratory personnel or as a nosocomial infection in medical, dental or nursery personnel.

The observation that all isolates from lip lesions and trigeminal ganglia have been HSV-1 may reflect the limited number tested thus far. For example, until relatively recently, all ocular or brain isolates, or those recovered from cases of eczema herpeticum, had been HSV-1. Exceptions to the general rules have important connotations. Thus, a different mode of viral spread might be suggested by those cases of HSV-2 infections of the mouth or brain or by cases of urogenital or neonatal HSV-1 infections.

It now appears that differences in the neurological manifestations most commonly associated with a particular HSV type, in individuals other than newborns, reflect different modes of internal virus spread (Craig and Nahmias 1973). HSV-2 seems more prone to cause a viremia and meningitis and HSV-1 to spread neurogenically to the brain. The two cases of HSV-2 encephalitis out of approximately 100 (Table 2) may be a result of oral HSV-2 also spreading neurogenically to the brain, although it is not possible to rule out blood dissemination to the brain with either virus type. Such hematogenous spread would be more likely in immunocompromised hosts, as recently reported in a woman with genital HSV-2 infection (Sutton *et al.* 1974).

More direct evidence of the various modes of transmission of genital HSV infections is summarized in Table 3. Thus, cases of fellatio or cunnilingus resulting in HSV-1 and HSV-2 infections of oral or genital sites of sexual partners have been observed. Similarly, genital-to-anal spread in male homosexuals has been reported. Still unrecorded, however, is sexual transmission of HSV of either type among lesbians. It should also be emphasized that autoinoculation

Clinical spectrum of infections caused by herpes simplex viruses 1 and 2 in newborns and older persons and the type isolated from different sites and clinical conditions. Typing is done by microneutralization or direct immunofluorescent tests (Dowdle *et al.* 1967, Nahmias *et al.* 1974)

	No. of individuals with HSV type		
Usually mild to moderately severe (persons over 1 month of age)	*Type 1*	*Type 2*	*Total*
Urogenital infections:			
Females (cervix, vulva, vagina, urethra)	35 (7●)	286 (5■)	321
Males (penis, urethra)	7 (1●)	199 (1▲)	206
Nongenital infections:			
Gingivostomatitis or asymptomatic (mouth)	142	3 (1○)	145
Herpes labialis (lips)	84	0	84
Keratitis and/or conjunctivitis (cornea and/or conjunctiva)	29	1	30
Dermatitis, skin above waist	89 (1○)	3	92
Dermatitis, skin below waist	4 (1●, 1○)	79 (6○, 1x)	83
Dermatitis, hands or arms	14 (1x)	12 (2x, 2○)	26
Latent infections, trigeminal or thoracic ganglia	21 (1●●)	0	21
Latent infections, sacral ganglia	0	5	5
Usually severe to fatal (persons over 1 month of age)			
Meningoencephalitis (brain, spinal cord CSF)	92	2	94
Multiple sclerosis (brain)	0	1	1
Eczema herpeticum (skin, lungs)	11	1	12
Generalized disease (visceral organs)	2	1 (1▼)	3
Newborns (localized or generalized infection affecting skin, eyes, brain, CSF, visceral organs)	43 (7■■)	90 (25■■)	133
Total	573	683	1256

● Simultaneous isolation of similar HSV type from mouth
■ Simultaneous isolation of type 2 HSV from cervix or vulva and type 1 HSV from lip or mouth
▲ Simultaneous isolation of type 2 HSV from penile lesion and type 1 HSV from eye
○ Simultaneous isolation of same HSV type from genitalia
x Laboratory- or hospital-acquired infection
▼ Isolated also from brain
●● Simultaneous isolation of type 2 HSV from sacral ganglia
■■ Same HSV type isolated from mother's genital tract

from mouth to genitalia with HSV-1, or from genitalia to mouth or other body sites with either virus type, can occur (Dolin *et al.* 1976, Nahmias *et al.* 1968).

The clinical manifestations of a virus type in an uncommon site do not appear to differ, although further studies are required to ascertain whether HSV-2 causes similar ocular manifestations in humans as HSV-1, or if they cause different clinical manifestations as with ocular infections in rabbits (Unna 1883, Oh and Stevens 1973). Similarly, the clinical spectrum of neonatal infection with HSV-1 or HSV-2 does not appear to differ. Both viral types can produce local skin, oral and CNS infections, as well as disseminated involvement to visceral organs (Table 4). The only exception, reflecting perhaps the small number of isolates, is in the case of chorioretinitis, so far associated only with HSV-2.

Table 3

Different modes of transmission of genital HSV-1 and HSV-2 infection

Modes of transmission	*Sex*	*HSV type*	
		HSV-1	*HSV-2*
Sexual transmission:			
Genital ⇌ genital	M ⇌ F	±	+
Genital ⇌ oral	M ⇌ F	+	+
Genital ⇌ anal	M ⇌ M	+	+
Non-sexual transmission (autoinoculation):			
Genital ⇌ Other body site (including oral)	M or F	+	+

We are thus faced with an interesting dilemma regarding the two HSV types. On the one hand, it appears that both virus types can spread to genital and extragenital sites, can produce similar clinical manifestations of the external sites and seem to be capable of remaining latent in sensory ganglia. On the other hand, the two viruses are different in many biochemical and biological characteristics (Nahmias and Dowdle 1968). We must therefore conclude that there must be some survival advantage for HSV-2 in the genital tract. A similar dilemma is exhibited by many other microorganisms, such as *Neisseria gonorrhoeae* and *Neisseria meningitidis*, which have a predilection for genital and extragenital sites respectively, although occasionally capable of infecting either site. Resolution of this important issue will require improved knowledge of the effect of the microenvironment of the genital tract on infectious agents (Dolin *et al.* 1976). That the central focus might be the female genital tract may be implied from several observations – the greater likelihood of

Table 4

Clinical spectrum and outcome of 90 cases of HSV-2 and 43 cases of HSV-1 neonatal infection

Clinical spectrum	*HSV-2 infection*				*HSV-1 infection*			
	No. of cases	*Died*	*With sequelae*	*Without apparent sequelae*	*No. of cases*	*Died*	*With sequelae*	*Without apparent sequelae*
Disseminated disease with or without encephalitis	46	32	4	10	24	19	3	2
Encephalitis:								
alone	21	5	12	4	5	2	3	—
with chorioretinitis	3	—	3	—	0	—	—	—
Keratitis and/or conjunctivitis:								
alone	3		1	2	7	—	2	5
with chorioretinitis	1	—	1	—	0	—	—	—
Skin vesicles and/or oral ulcers	16	—	4	12	7	1	—	6
Total	90	37	25	28	43	22	8	13

isolating HSV-1 from females than from males (Table 2) and the infrequent isolation of HSV-1 from the cervix in comparison to the vulva, in contrast to the frequent involvement of the cervix by HSV-2.

Clinical Aspects

The clinical descriptions of genital herpetic infections, recorded in the nineteenth century (Diday and Doyon 1886, Du Castel 1901), have rarely been surpassed by the more recent reports (Josey *et al.* 1968, Gardner and Kaufman 1972, Yen *et al.* 1965, Hutfield 1970, Poste *et al.* 1972) in their exquisite detail of the presentation and progress of the infection. With the newer laboratory technology, it has been possible more recently to define specific aspects of the infection. Thus, most cases of genital HSV-2 infections occur in individuals with prior HSV-1 infections (Nahmias, Josey *et al.* 1970). In general, genital HSV infections in individuals with no prior experience with either HSV type (primary infections) tend to have more severe symptoms than those occurring after a previous HSV-1 and/or HSV-2 infection (Nahmias, Josey *et al.* 1970). In either case, it is worth reemphasizing that the genital infection may be asymptomatic, particularly in case of cervical involvement. Primary cases are more likely to be associated with fever and constitutional signs, as well as with more marked regional adenopathy and dysuria. The lesions in primary infections, particularly during pregnancy, tend to persist for longer periods (up to three months) than in the case of recurrent infections (usually less than three weeks).

In women, HSV infection may involve, singly or in combination, the following urogenital sites: vulva, vagina, cervix, urethra and bladder, although isolations of HSV-1 from sites other than the vulva have been infrequent. It is still unclear whether the virus can also ascend to involve the endometrium, but it is well appreciated that the virus can spread to contiguous perineal areas and sometimes also to the thighs, buttocks and even the lower legs.

HSV vulvitis is commonly associated with cervical involvement (Du Castel 1901, Josey *et al.* 1968). After a prodrome of local irritation, typical single or multiple vesicles appear. The mucosal vesicles ulcerate earlier than those which affect the outer labial or perineal skin. Discrete vesicles or ulcers are less common in the vagina or cervix. Infection of the cervix, which often occurs in the absence of external genital lesions, is frequently asymptomatic. Even when clinically manifest, herpetic cervicitis may not be suspected, since it may resemble other types of cervical inflammation. The most severe manifestation is a necrotizing cervicitis.

In males, single but usually multiple vesicles and ulcers involve most commonly the glans, prepuce, balanopreputial sulcus and the shaft of the penis, and less frequently the scrotum, thighs or buttocks. The urethra may also be involved and cause symptomatic urethritis. As noted earlier, the recently reported high frequency of HSV isolation from the prostate, testes or seminal vesicles (Centifanto *et al.* 1972) awaits confirmation. It is still not as clear in men as it is in women that the virus can be transmitted between episodes of clinical recurrences.

Immediate complications of genital HSV infections are relatively infrequent and include secondary bacterial or mycotic infections, lymphatic suppuration and urethral stricture (Hutfield 1970). More serious, but usually self-limited, complications which can, however, recur with the herpetic recrudescences are neuralgias, meningitis, radiculitis, myelitis and erythema multiforme.

Genital herpes may be confused with various other conditions, especially other venereal diseases. External genital lesions may be misdiagnosed as chancroid, syphilis and the early lesions of lymphogranuloma venereum and granuloma inguinale. Herpetic urethritis and cervicitis may be clinically mistaken for gonococcal or chlamydial infections, and the more prominent cervical lesions may raise a suspicion of carcinoma. Other diseases to be differentiated include herpes zoster, Vincent's infection, Behçet's syndrome, impetigo, molluscum contagiosum, erythema multiforme and other dermatoses.

It has long been appreciated (Diday and Doyon 1886, Du Castel 1901, Lipschütz 1921, Unna 1883) that genital herpes is not infrequently found in association with other sexually transmitted infections, such as condyloma acuminatum and syphilis. Genital herpes has also been frequently associated with gonorrhea (Jeansson and Molin 1970, Beilby *et al.* 1968, Nahmias *et al.* 1973, Morse *et al.* 1974). We have emphasized (Nahmias *et al.* 1973) the possible value of information obtained on this association in providing some rough estimates on the frequency of genital herpetic infections, at least in women. This is because gonorrhea is a reportable disease, whereas genital herpes, at least in the US, is not. Realizing that there are differences in the types of patients attending VD clinics in various parts of the world, it is noteworthy that one patient with genital herpes has been identified for every 2 to 11 patients with gonorrhea (Table 5). In women seen in private practice genital herpes may actually be more common than gonorrhea (Gardner and Kaufman 1972). Also of interest is that 5 to 14 of every 100 patients with gonorrhea have been found to have evidence of a concomitant genital herpetic infection, which was most often asymptomatic. We have

Table 5

Association of genital herpes with gonorrhea in women •

	London			
	Middlesex	*St Mary's*	*Stockholm*	*Atlanta, Ga*
Herpes positive/ gonococcus negative	1/155 (0.6%)	12/168 (7.2%)	5/78 (6.4%)	3/52 (5.8%)
Herpes positive/ gonococcus positive	7/54 (13%)	4/29 (13.8%)	5/47 10.6%)	4/80 (5%)
Case ratio (herpes: gonorrhea)	1:7	1:2	1:5	1:11

• based on viral isolations, except for St Mary's which also includes cytological detection

also emphasized the VD clinic as a target site for a Papanicolaou screening program for the detection of cervical neoplasia (Nahmias *et al.* 1973).

Laboratory Diagnosis

Cytology

Most clinicians have greater access to cytological than to virological laboratory aids. The classical descriptions by Unna and Lipschütz many decades ago of the cellular changes associated with herpesvirus infection provided a simple and rapid means for confirming the diagnosis. Although similar changes can be produced by the varicella-zoster virus, these entities are usually readily distinguishable clinically. We do not believe it possible to differentiate by cytological techniques between primary and recurrent HSV infections, or between HSV-1 and HSV-2 infection.

The major cytological features are multinucleated giant cells with bland nuclei and eosinophilic intranuclear inclusions. These can be more readily appreciated with the fixative and stains used for Papanicolaou smears than with Wright or Giemsa stains in examination of exfoliated cells or scrapings, and with Bouin's fixative than with formalin in studying histological sections (Naib *et al.* 1973). In cervical smears, the cytological findings must be differentiated from those of other infections, from trophoblastic cells and from abnormal cells associated with dysplasia or carcinoma.

Exfoliative cytology has been particularly useful in detecting clinically inapparent cases of herpetic cervicitis (Naib *et al.* 1966). The technique has been found to be very specific and to be about two-thirds as sensitive as virological methods (Naib *et al.* 1973). Studies conducted in various populations in England and in the US

Table 6

Prevalence rates of cytologically detected genital herpetic infections

Locality	*Percentage positive for herpes*
London, VD clinic (Middlesex)	3.3
London, VD clinic (St Mary's)	4.6
London, gynecological outpatients	0.3
Chicago, not stated	0.5–1.5
Halifax, Canada, routine screening clinics	0.03
New York City, planned parenthood clinics	0.09
Cleveland, indigent patients	0.31
Cleveland, private patients	0.02
New Mexico, indigent patients	0.09–0.9
Atlanta, indigent patients	0.26

(reviewed in Morse *et al.* 1974 and Naib *et al.* 1973) have provided important information on the relative prevalence of this infection (Table 6). Thus the highest rates of 3.3–4.6% have been observed in VD clinics in London; the rate in London gynecological patients was about one-tenth as high. The rates in indigent patients in the US are at least ten times as high as in private patients. The rates in pregnant women were found in two US hospitals to be three times higher than in non-pregnant women. Using cytological methods, we have also found that the median age for detecting genital herpes in women is 22 years.

Virology

It is usually possible to identify HSV within one to three days by tissue culture methods available today in almost every virology laboratory. To facilitate handling of specimens by clinicians, we developed a transport medium (Leibovitz-Emory medium) which allows storage and transport at room temperature (Nahmias *et al.* 1971). Stuart's transport medium may also be satisfactory for this purpose (Rodin *et al.* 1971).

The means for futher differentiation into the two HSV types are becoming readily available (Nahmias and Roizman 1973). Various techniques can be used, including several serological tests (neutralization, complement fixation, passive hemagglutination, immunofluorescence and radioimmunoassays). Biological markers, such as plaque size or growth in certain tissue culture cells, or pock size on the chorioallantoic membrane of embryonated eggs, can also be employed, but are not as specific as serological methods.

The virus can be rapidly identified by electron microscopy; in addition, the presence of filaments would suggest HSV-2 (Couch and Nahmias 1969, Smith *et al.* 1973). HSV antigens can also be identified directly in clinical specimens by immunofluorescence within 1–2 hours (Nahmias *et al.* 1974). The virus type can also be ascertained directly by this method, although the technique is not as sensitive as viral recovery in tissue culture. In general, the ability to isolate the virus in tissue culture cells in a short time does not warrant use of the more rapid, though less accessible, immunofluorescent or electron microscopic methods.

As noted earlier, the recent finding of variants within HSV-2 has not yet been widely applied. Preliminary information suggests that there may be geographical differences, as well as differences in the oncogenic potential of HSV-2 variants to transform hamster embryonic cells (Seth *et al.* 1974, Aurelian *et al.* 1974).

Serology

A variety of serological tests have been developed to measure HSV antibodies, including neutralization, complement fixation, passive and inhibition passive hemagglutination, immunofluorescent tests and radioimmunoassays (Nahmias and Roizman 1973, Plummer 1973). In addition, the latter two techniques permit detection of IgM, IgG and IgA antibodies specific for HSV (Nahmias *et al.* 1974, Kurz 1974). The demonstration of HSV IgM antibodies in the serum of a newborn or in the CSF of a patient with HSV encephalitis has provided useful aids in diagnosis (Nahmias, Visintine *et al.* 1975, Nahmias *et al.* 1974). HSV IgM antibodies do not necessarily always reflect evidence of a primary herpetic infection. Similarly, a fourfold or greater rise of HSV antibodies by any of the serologic tests does not always signify a primary infection, since such antibody rises can be demonstrated occasionally with recurrent infections, particularly in immunosuppressed individuals.

None of the serological techniques currently available is totally specific in differentiating among the type-specific antibodies to HSV-1, HSV-2 or to both viruses (Plummer 1973, Adam *et al.* 1974). It is therefore not possible to be completely confident of the prevalence rates of HSV-2 antibodies in different populations. Studies reviewed elsewhere (Plummer 1973, Adam *et al.* 1974, Nahmias, Josey *et al.* 1975) indicate that the lowest rates of HSV-2 antibodies are found in children and nuns and the highest in prostitutes, and that the rates in low socioeconomic groups are higher than those in upper socioeconomic populations. A large variation in the frequency of HSV-2 antibodies (9% to 90%), as measured by various serological tests using different HSV strains, has been recorded from different geographical regions in women without cervical cancer. It is hoped that current attempts by European and American investigators to produce HSV type-specific antigens will improve the reliability of results obtained with current serological methodology.

Fetal and Neonatal Infections

The various aspects of fetal and neonatal HSV infections have been detailed previously (Nahmias, Alford *et al.* 1970, Nahmias, Visintine *et al.* 1975, Nahmias and Visintine 1975), but a few

Table 7

Clinical spectrum and outcome of 302 cases of neonatal herpetic infection

Clinical groups	*No. of cases*	*Outcome in infant (percent)*		
		Died	*Survived*	
			With sequelae	*Without apparent sequelae*
Disseminated				
Without CNS involvement	98	92	1	7
With CNS involvement	97	71	16	13
Localized: •				
CNS	52	38	46	16
Eye	16	—	37	63
Skin	34	3	24	73
Oral cavity	3	—	—	100
Asymptomatic	2	—	—	100
Total	302	60%	18%	22%

• Classified according to major site of involvement if more than one site infected

important points are worth emphasizing here in addition to the information related to HSV types noted earlier in Table 4. Our most recent review of 302 cases of neonatal HSV infections recorded since 1934 (Batignani 1934) is presented in Table 7. A wide clinical spectrum has been observed with the most severe outcome being noted in the disseminated and CNS forms of the disease. Unlike neonatal cytomegalovirus infections, neonatal herpes is rarely asymptomatic. Although it is still not well established whether the infection can be transplacentally transmitted or acquired postnatally, the increasing frequency of HSV-1 isolations in newborns is compatible with these pathways of transmission. In several cases of

HSV-1 neonatal infections the mother was also found to have a genital HSV-1 infection around the time of delivery (Table 1). It appears from current information that intrapartum infection is the major source of virus to the newborn. The data reviewed in Table 8 suggest that performing a Cesarean section prior to membrane rupture may prevent most infections. The need for individualization of every case and the guide-lines for the management of women with genital herpes during pregnancy are noted elsewhere (Nahmias *et al.* 1972).

Dr Juel-Jensen reviews current information on the treatment of HSV infection (see p 170) but some remarks regarding HSV vaccines might be desirable. Several old and new problems have to be considered in relation to HSV vaccines for the prevention of the initial or recurrent infection. One is the lack of evaluation under

Table 8

Risk of genital herpetic infection from mother with genital infection at delivery

Type of delivery	*No. of infants infected*
Vaginal	14/26 (54%)
Cesarean section:	
More than four hours after membrane rupture	18/19 (94%)
Before or within four hours of membrane rupture	2/30 (7%)

controlled conditions of the European (Diamant or Lupidon) or the American (Lilly) inactivated vaccines used primarily to alleviate the frequency of recurrences. A second problem is that the possible mechanisms of action of these vaccines have not been ascertained. In this respect, a large number of investigators recently have been studying immune responses to HSV in both *in vitro* and animal models, as well as in humans (Nahmias, Shore *et al.* 1975). These studies currently suggest a defect in lymphokines (MIF, leukocyte inhibitory factor, interferon) in those individuals with frequent recurrences. A third and major problem related to HSV vaccines is the fear that if the virus is indeed causally related to some human cancers, the widespread use of inactivated or live attenuated or mutant viruses would present great difficulties in terms of ascertaining freedom from a potential carcinogenic risk. Current approaches are therefore being pursued in the US with purified virus proteins free of DNA.

Conclusion

We have reviewed the clinicoepidemiological and laboratory aspects of genital herpetic infections. The historical perspective points to the large amount of information on the subject reported earlier by French and German investigators for over two centuries. Anglo-American investigators have finally caught up and perhaps made up for their deficiencies by their many recent contributions in the past decade. There are still many gaps in our knowledge. The association of genital herpes with fetal and neonatal disease, with cervical cancer, ocular disease, connective tissue and neurological diseases are still areas for investigators to pursue. The true incidence of these infections, which can only be ascertained by some reporting system, needs to be based on accurate methods of diagnosis. As regards prevention and treatment, work must go hand-in-hand between the clinical and laboratory investigators to provide the necessary knowledge of the biochemical, immunological and pathogenetic aspects related to these viruses. For us, as straddlers between the clinic and the laboratory, it has been an exciting ten years of research on these problems. We are eagerly awaiting the promise of the next decade in this field.

Acknowledgments

This work has been supported by grants from the National Institute of Dental Research, the USPHS and the National Foundation March of Dimes.

References

Adam, E., Rawls, W. E. and Melnick, M. J. (1974). *Preventive Medicine* 3, 122–141

Aurelian, L., Smerdel, I., Kessler, I. and Kulcar, Z. (1974). *Journal of Infectious Diseases* 129, 465–469

Bacon, P. A., Bluestone, R., Goldberg, L. S., Webb, F. W., Pearson, C. M., Cooke, M. and Stevens, J. G. (1974). *Annals of the Rheumatic Diseases* 33, 413–421

Baringer, J. R. (1974). *New England Journal of Medicine* 291, 823–830

Batignani, A. (1934). *Bollettino d'oculistica* 13, 1217–1220

Baum, O. (1920). *Dermatologische Wochenschrift* 70, 105

Beck, A., Fluker, J. L. and Platt, D. J. (1974). *British Journal of Venereal Diseases* 50, 367–369

Beilby, J. O. W., Cameron, C. H., Catterall, R. D. and Davidson, D. (1968). *Lancet* i, 1065–1066

Centifanto, Y. M., Drylie, D. M., Deardourff, S. L. and Kaufman, H. (1972). *Science* 178, 318–319

Couch, E. and Nahmias, A. (1969). *Journal of Virology* 3, 228–232

Craig, C. and Nahmias, A. (1973). *Journal of Infectious Diseases* 127, 365–372

Diday, P. and Doyon, A. (1886). "Les Herpès Génitaux". Masson, Paris

Dolin, R., Gill, F. A. and Nahmias, A. J. (1976). *Journal of the American Venereal Disease Association* (in press)

Dowdle, W., Nahmias, A., Harwell, R. and Pauls, F. (1967). *Journal of Immunology* 99, 974–980

Du Castel, P. (1901). "Herpès, Pratique Dermatologique". Masson, Paris: 2, 814–815

Gardner, H. L. and Kaufman, R. H. (1972). *Clinical Obstetrics and Gynecology* 15, 896–911

Hutfield, D. C. (1966). *British Journal of Venereal Diseases* 42, 263–268
(1970). *British Journal of Hospital Medicine* 3, 881–884

Jeansson, S. and Molin, L. (1970). *Laekartidningen* 231, 1–8

Josey, W., Nahmias, A. and Naib, Z. (1968). *American Journal of Obstetrics and Gynecology* 101, 718–729

Kaufman, R. H., Gardner, H. L., Rawls, W. E., Dixon, R. E. and Young, R. L. (1973). *Cancer Research* 33, 1446–1451

Kurz, J. B. (1974). *Journal of Medical Microbiology* 7, 333–341

Lipschütz, B. (1921). *Archiv für Dermatologie und Syphilis* 136, 428–482

Masukawa, T., Garaneis, J. C., Rytel, M. W. and Mattingly, R. F. (1972). *Acta cytologica* 16, 416–428

Morse, A., Coleman, D. V. and Gardner, S. D. (1974). *Journal of Obstetrics and Gynaecology of the British Commonwealth* 81, 393–398

Nahmias, A. (1974). *In* "Viruses, Evolution and Cancer". Ed. E. Kurstak and K. Maramorosch. Academic Press, New York and London; pp 605–622

Nahmias, A., Alford, C. and Korones, S. (1970). *In* "Advances in Pediatrics". Ed. I. Schulman. Year Book Publishers, Chicago; pp 185–226

Nahmias, A. and Dowdle, W. (1968). *Progress in Medical Virology* 10, 110–159

Nahmias, A., Dowdle, W., Naib, Z., Josey, W. and Luce, C. (1968). *Pediatrics* 42, 659–666

Nahmias, A., Dowdle, W., Naib, Z., Josey, W., McClone, D. and Domescik, G. (1969). *British Journal of Venereal Diseases* 45, 294–298

Nahmias, A., Josey, W. and Naib, Z. (1972). *Clinical Obstetrics and Gynecology* 15, 929–938

Nahmias, A., Josey, W., Naib, Z., Luce, C. and Duffey, C. (1970). *American Journal of Epidemiology* 91, 539–546

Nahmias, A. J., Josey, W. E. and Oleske, J. M. (1975). *In* "Epidemiology of Viral Infections". Ed. A. Evans. Plenum Press, New York (in press)

Nahmias, A. and Roizman, B. (1973). *New England Journal of Medicine* 289, 667–674, 719–725, 781–789

Nahmias, A., Shore, S. and Del Buono, I. (1974). *In* "Viral Immunodiagnosis". Ed. E. Kurstak and R. Morisset. Academic Press, New York and London; pp 157–172

Nahmias, A. J., Shore, S. L., Kohl, S., Starr, S. and Ashman, R. B. (1975). *Cancer Research* (in press)

Nahmias, A. and Visintine, A. (1975). *In* "Perinatal Infections". Ed. J. Remington and J. Klein. Saunders, Philadelphia (in press)

Nahmias, A., Visintine, A., Reimer, C., Del Buono, I., Shore, S. and Starr, S. (1975). *In* "Progress in Clinical and Biological Research". Ed. S. Krugman and A. A. Gershon. Liss, New York; pp 63–77

Nahmias, A., Von Reyn, C. F., Josey, W. E., Naib, Z. M. and Hutton, R. D. (1973). *British Journal of Venereal Diseases* 49, 306–309

Nahmias, A., Wickliffe, C., Pipkin, J., Leibovitz, A. and Hutton, R. (1971). *Applied Microbiology* 22, 451–454

Naib, Z., Nahmias, A. J. and Josey, W. E. (1966). *Cancer* 19, 1026-1030
Naib, Z., Nahmias, A., Josey, W. and Zaki, S. (1973). *Cancer Research* 33, 1452-1463
Oh, J. O. and Stevens, T. R. (1973). *Archives of Ophthalmology* 90, 473-476
Pereira, E., Cassai, E., Honess, R., Roizman, B., Terni, M. and Nahmias, A. (1975) *Infection and Immunity* (in press)
Person, D. A., Kaufman, R. M., Gardner, H. L. and Rawls, W. E. (1973). *American Journal of Obstetrics and Gynecology* 116, 993-995
Poste, G., Hawkins, D. F. and Thomlison. J. (1972). *Obstetrics and Gynecology* 40, 871-890
Plummer, G. (1973). *Cancer Research* 33, 1469-1477
Rawls, W. E., Owamoto, K., Adam, E. and Melnick, J. L. (1970). *Journal of Immunology* 104, 599-606
Rodin, P., Hare, M. J., Barwell, C. F. and Withers, M. J. (1971). *British Journal of Venereal Diseases* 47, 198-199
Schneweis, K. E. and Brandis, H. (1961). *Zentralblatt für Bakteriologie, Parasitenkunde, Infektionskrankheiten und Hygiene* 183, 556-558
Seth, P., Rawls, W. E., Duff, R., Rapp, F., Adam, E. and Melnick, J. L. (1974). *Intervirology* 3, 1-14
Smith, I., Pentherer, J. F. and Robertson, D. H. H. (1973). *British Journal of Venereal Diseases* 49, 385-390
Sutton, A. L., Smithwick, E. M., Seligman, S. J. and Kim, D. (1974). *American Journal of Medicine* 56, 545-553
Unna, P. G. (1883). *Journal of Cutaneous and Venereal Diseases* 1, 321-334
Unna, P. G. (1896). "The Histopathology of the Diseases of the Skin". Trans. N. Walker. Clay, Edinburgh
Yen, S. S. C., Reagan, J. W. and Rosenthal, M. S. (1965). *Obstetrics and Gynecology* 25, 479-492

Does Genital Herpes Cause Cancer? — A Midway Assessment

Bernard Roizman and N Frenkel
Division of Biological Sciences,
The University of Chicago, Chicago, Illinois 60637

Introduction

The only answer currently appropriate to this seemingly simplistic question is that we have no evidence that refutes the hypothesis that genital herpes causes cancer. To those who have spent many years wrestling with this question this estimate of the situation is not a signal to rejoice for we have no compelling affirmative evidence either. In this article we shall attempt to summarize briefly what we do know, and examine the problems that beleaguer attempts to obtain an unequivocal answer.

No analysis of a complex problem is complete without a history of how herpes simplex virus type 2 (HSV-2) came to be associated with cervical carcinoma. The personal perception of how Nahmias and his colleagues came to suspect genital herpes infections as a cause of cancer is detailed elsewhere (Nahmias *et al.* 1970*b*, Nahmias and Roizman 1973). From a more current point of view, epidemiological studies have suggested that women with cervical carcinoma possess characteristics which predict that they run a higher probability of acquiring venereally transmitted infections than other women (Rotkin 1967, 1973, Martin 1967, Pridan and Lilienfeld 1971). Implicit in these predictions is that acquisition of venereal infections and development of cervical carcinomas are covariant properties. From the point of view of virologists, HSV-2 genital infections appear to satisfy many of the requirements of a covariant to the development of cervical carcinomas. First, the infection is venereally transmitted. Second, because of its topological distribution, recurrent genital infections satisfy the added requirement of adequate contact with the tissues in which malignancy appears. This evidence is insufficient to indict the virus as a causative agent, but is sufficient to cast suspicion on it; and we can now turn to the problem of how we can go about verifying our suspicions.

The Rules of Evidence: The Problems

We should state at the outset that any inquiry into the suspicion that HSV causes cervical carcinoma must take into consideration the relevant biologic properties of the virus. In an absolute sense the fact that herpesviruses appear to cause tumors in certain animals under both natural (Biggs 1973, Mizell *et al.* 1969) and experimental (Melendez *et al.* 1972) conditions attests to the potential oncogenicity of the herpesvirus group, but has no real bearing on our central question. We must deal in the same summary fashion with the evidence that both HSV-1 and HSV-2 transform a number of mammalian cell lines (Rapp and Duff 1974). In this instance, the transformed cells are very useful in that they indicate what we could expect to find in human cervical carcinomas if they are indeed caused by HSV. The biologic property of considerable significance is the ability of HSV to persist in nerve tissues and to innervate the site of primary and recurrent infections. Although the virus has been consistently associated with nerve tissues, we cannot preclude the possibility that it is also harbored in other types of cells. This property of HSV places a serious limitation on the interpretation of findings of HSV in patients with cervical carcinoma and, in effect, requires that we discriminate between covariant and causative roles of HSV as one of the earliest steps in our investigations.

Operationally, the inquiry into the role of genital herpes infection, whether by chance or design, took three directions. The first was to inquire whether the epidemiology of cervical carcinoma clearly associated herpesvirus infection with cervical cancer above all other factors. In this instance, the factors investigated to date were limited only by the imagination of the investigator and have included the age of first intercourse, number of partners, and just about anything else related to sexuality and venereal transmission. The second direction, also epidemiologic, has sought not only a more global reaffirmation that genital herpes and cervical carcinoma are covariant properties but also the evidence that would discriminate between covariant and causal roles of genital herpetic infections. Whereas proof of covariation requires little more than evidence of spatial clustering of cervical carcinoma in women with genital herpetic infections, demonstration of a causal relation requires as a first step evidence that infection invariably precedes the evolution of cervical carcinoma. Evidence that infection precedes development of malignancy is essential to the thesis that the virus is the causative agent but, alas, it does not prove it. The third direction, superficially at least, seeks evidence of a molecular nature for the putative causal role of HSV-2 in cervical carcinoma.

Epidemiology of Cervical Carcinoma

Even on a casual survey of the literature of the past decade one cannot fail to be impressed by the comprehensive attempts to elicit and verify information on patterns of sexual behavior of patients with carcinoma of the cervix, and by the amount of effort expended to secure appropriately matched controls whose cervices, at least at the time they presented themselves to the attention of the epidemiologist, were free of carcinomas. The emerging pattern is that the incidence of cervical carcinoma is higher in women who engage in sexual activity early in life. According to Rotkin (1973), "onset of sexuality before age 17 is the most powerful discriminating variable in virtually all studies where this has been investigated". To this list one could add early pregnancy as well (Naguib *et al.* 1966, Moghissi *et al.* 1968). These findings if true, do not exclude the involvement of HSV. It has been suggested that both the period after puberty and youthful first pregnancy are associated with marked cervical metaplasia, i.e. conversion of the columnar epithelium into squamous epithelium (Coppleson *et al.* 1971). Morphologically, the immature metaplastic cell is said to be less differentiated than cells from other areas of the cervix and more vulnerable to the action of carcinogens.

Implicit in this hypothesis is that genital herpes infection furnishes the carcinogen.

Seroepidemiologic Studies on the Association of HSV with Cervical Carcinoma: Surveys of Incidence of Neutralizing Antiviral Antibody

Most analyses of the association of HSV with cervical carcinoma are based on seroepidemiologic studies whose main thrust is assays for antibody to HSV in patients with malignancy as compared with suitable control populations of similar age, sexual experience, socio-economic groups, &c. Since neutralizing antibody should be the most unequivocal evidence of infection, most epidemiologic studies were based on measurements of this activity. These studies have been reviewed elsewhere in detail (Adam *et al.* 1974, Melnick *et al.* 1974, Nahmias *et al.* 1973, Rawls *et al.* 1973). Although the results are impressive, they also make apparent the fallacy of this approach. For example, numerous studies (Royston and Aurelian 1970*a*, Nahmias *et al.* 1970*a*, *b*, Rawls *et al.* 1969, 1970, 1973, Catalano and Johnson 1971) have shown a higher incidence of neutralizing antibody in patients with cervical carcinoma than in control populations. The problem arises from the fact that, contrary to our requirements, the association of cervical cancer and HSV is at times difficult to demonstrate, largely because of lack of evidence of past infection in some patients with cervical carcinoma. Whereas in the study of Royston and Aurelian (1970*a*) 100% (32/32) of women with cervical carcinoma had antibody to HSV-2 as compared with 57% (17/32) of women in the control group, only 32% (14/44) of women with malignancy were positive in the study of Rawls *et al.* (1970). A lower incidence of antibody in women with malignancy was also noted in the studies of Catalano and Johnson (1971), Rawls *et al.* (1969), Plummer and Masterson (1971) and Pridan and Lilienfeld (1971), although again the incidence was higher in women with malignancy than in the control group. *A priori*, the finding of women with cervical carcinoma lacking demonstrable neutralizing antibody would seem to violate our requirement that infection precede development of cervical carcinoma. Before we accept the conclusions of this finding, it is necessary to evaluate the test itself and the implications arising from its application.

To begin with, HSV-2 is neutralized by antibody to HSV-1 and vice versa. For this reason, it is difficult to measure low levels of anti-HSV-2 antibody in the face of high anti-HSV-1 antibody titers. This would explain the absence of HSV-2 antibody in patients with high anti-HSV-1 antibody but not the absence of both HSV-1 and

HSV-2 antibody in such patients. The situation is rendered even more complex by two factors. First, there is considerable variability in the structural polypeptides of type 1 strains (Pereira, Cassai, Honess, Roizman, Terni and Nahmias 1976; Heine *et al.* 1974) and preliminary studies indicate that a similar situation may prevail among type 2 strains as well (Cassai, Sarmiento and Spear 1975). It could be expected that variability in structural polypeptides should be reflected in antigenic specificity as well and, in fact, this has been reported (Heine *et al.* 1974, Seth *et al.* 1974). Apart from the question whether cervical carcinoma may be specifically related to a strain with a unique viral phenotype, the validity of neutralization tests on sera collected from Africa or South America with virus isolated in the United States remains somewhat doubtful. Second, there are several types of neutralization tests on record. One recent study compared the results of two such tests and found the correlation between assays rather poor (Kessler 1974). The problems could be solved by availability of a type-specific antigen or of a simple technique for rendering the serum type specific. There are at the moment no type-specific antigens available. Although the homologous reaction is generally stronger, the antibody made against HSV-2 appears to be somewhat less specific than anti HSV-1. Moreover, although type-specific sera can be prepared by cross-absorption and there are reports that rabbit 19S antibody has a much higher specificity for the immunizing virus than late 7S antibody (Hampar *et al.* 1968, 1970, Stevens *et al.* 1968), to our knowledge none of the findings has been extended to actual field tests of human sera. Whether this is worth the effort is not clear: the antibody response to HSV-2 may be diminished or absent in an individual who had responded well to a previous HSV-1 infection (Smith, Adam *et al.* 1972, Smith, Lowry *et al.* 1972). Since primary HSV-1 infection generally precedes HSV-2 infection, it may well be the stronger. Furthermore, to interject a purely theoretical note, since a tumor could only arise from an abortively infected cell, it would be fallacious to expect that every abortive infection leading to carcinogenesis was invariably preceded by virus multiplication extensive enough to stimulate virus-specific neutralizing antibody. Herein lies the major pitfall of using neutralizing antibody as an indicator of past infection. Nevertheless, the existing data have been interpreted (perhaps erroneously) to show that the neutralizing antibody patterns in women with cervical carcinoma differ from those of the control population in at least two respects. First, the antibody titers appear higher in women with malignancy (Skinner *et al.* 1971, Adam *et al.* 1972, 1973); second, the presence of neutralizing antibody to HSV-2 appears to be age dependent in women in the control population but not in women with malignancy (Royston and Aurelian 1970*a*, Adam *et al.* 1972). This suggested that women with cancer are infected earlier in life than the women in the control population. Again we must point out the evidence that the incidence of cervical carcinoma is higher in women who engage in sexual activity early in life.

Before we leave seroepidemiologic studies based on surveys of neutralizing antibody for greener fields, several more points should be made. Coincident with expectations, a higher incidence of neutralizing antibody was also found in women with preinvasive lesions than in women with controls (Royston and Aurelian 1970*a*, Nahmias *et al.* 1970*b*). Other studies reported that infection precedes cervical lesions (Catalano and Johnson 1971), or at least predisposes the women with genital herpetic infections to develop cervical dysplasias and in-situ carcinoma (Naib *et al.* 1969, Nahmias *et al.* 1973).

The Search for a Tumor Antigen

Seroepidemiologic studies based on the presence of neutralizing antibody as evidence of past infection take advantage of the specificity of the reaction but make the unnecessary assumption that the virus multiplied to an extent sufficient to induce large amounts of neutralizing antibody which persisted to the date of the test. Another approach is based on the assumption that, by analogy with the experimentally induced viral tumors, the putative cells transformed from normal into malignant by HSV would express continuously a portion of the viral genome coding for specific polypeptides – tumor antigens – which could be identified immunologically. In one instance, notably in papova-transformed cells, these antigens are nonstructural viral proteins. Although this approach seems both logical and straightforward, the results obtained by several laboratories were all but clear cut, and divergence in both approach and results were soon apparent.

Not necessarily in a chronologic order, Royston and Aurelian (1970*b*), sought the antigen in cancer cells directly and reported finding HSV antigens by immunofluorescence in atypical exfoliated cells from women with preinvasive and invasive lesions. This antigen has not been fully characterized further. Parenthetically, the same laboratory (Aurelian *et al.* 1971, Aurelian 1972, 1973) reported the "induction" of HSV-2 in a cell line derived from a lesion of carcinoma-in-situ and maintained at high pH. However, since the induction was limited to a few passages of the cells and could not be reproduced in parallel cultures of the same line, chance contamination of the culture with virus being passaged in the laboratory cannot be excluded, although a valiant attempt to discredit this hypothesis was made (Aurelian and Strandberg 1974).

Sabin's laboratory took a different approach, followed subsequently by Hollinshead and by Aurelian. In a series of publications, Tarro and Sabin (1970, 1973) and Sabin and Tarro (1973) described the preparation and properties of a "non-virion antigen" and, ultimately, the reactivity of this antigen with sera from cancer patients. Briefly, the Sabin-Tarro antigen possessed three fundamental properties which determined the mode of its utilization in serologic tests. First, the antigenic acitivity was lost following extensive manipulation and on storage even at low temperatures, suggesting that it was probably due to a very labile substance or to a state of aggregation. Second, the rate of accumulation of this antigen in infected cells varied considerably. In HEp-2 cells, the antigen accumulated throughout infection. In guinea-pigs, the antigen accumulated early (three hours post infection). Third, virus strains differed in the amounts of the antigen they produced. Antibody to the non-virion antigen was detected in a two-step test. First, the test sera were absorbed with stable antigens in infected cell lysates stored until all non-virion antigen reactivity disappeared. Second, the absorbed sera were then tested in complement fixation tests with freshly prepared cell lysates containing both the unstable and stable antigens. Since the antibody to the virion antigens was removed by absorption, the test measured only antibody to non-virion antigens. In the initial studies (Sabin and Tarro 1973) antibody to the non-virion antigens was detected in patients with cancer of the lip, mouth, nasopharynx, pharynx, kidney, bladder, prostate, cervix uteri and vulva, but not in a variety of other cancers. Alas, subsequent and more extensive analyses by Sabin (1974) failed to confirm these data.

It is no accident that we discuss a study which was subsequently retracted. The design of the experiments executed in the Sabin-Tarro studies cited above is among the most careful and systematic on record. The failure of these tests to stand up to repeated experimental onslaughts reflects at least in part the complexity of the problem which has not been recognized with equal candor by the two other laboratories engaged in this work. Specifically, Hollinshead *et al.* (1972, 1973) reported finding antibody to their HSV-1 and HSV-2 complement-fixing antigens in sera of patients with cancer of the head, neck, larynx and cervix of the uterus. Aurelian, Schumann *et al.* 1973, and Aurelian, Davis *et al.* 1973 reported a high incidence of antibody to their complement-fixing antigen in women with malignancy and at least a decrease in the antibody levels following treatment of the cancers. The nature of the complement-fixing antigen used by Hollinshead *et al.* has not been fully described and is, in the final analysis, unknown. The antigen employed by Aurelian *et al.* and designated as AG-4 is prepared from 4 hour infected HEp-2 cells freeze-thawed in veronal-buffered saline containing $CaCl_2$, $MgCl_2$, and gelatin and then centrifuged for 30 minutes at 1550 g (Aurelian *et al.* 1974). In a more recent paper Aurelian and Strnad (1976) attempted to relate AG-4 to a polypeptide made in infected cells and designated by Spear and Roizman (1972) as virion polypeptide No. 4 (VP4). A careful analysis of the reports describing AG-4 indicates that its properties are deduced from rather circumstantial evidence. There is no convincing evidence, for example, that AG-4 and the antigen claimed to be present on the surface of abnormal exfoliated cells are identical or that it corresponds to VP4 (Aurelian and Strnad 1976). According to Aurelian *et al.* (1974), productively infected cells make AG-4 in a single major burst between 3 and 4 hours post infection. The antigen remains at a relatively constant level to about 8 hours post infection and declines to insignificant levels by 12–14 hours post infection. The same report indicates that AG-4 makes an equally dramatic appearance in the extracellular fluid between 4 and 5 hours post infection and totally disappears by 16 hours. VP4 on the other hand is made very early in infection, becomes phosphorylated and accumulates in the nucleus of the infected cell (Honess and Roizman 1974, 1975, and unpublished data). Although Aurelian *et al.* (1974) attempted to exclude the possibility that AG-4 is a structural antigen, the data are not very convincing. Specifically, not all structural viral polypeptides binding to membranes induce neutralizing antibody; hence, failure of AG-4 to compete with virions for neutralizing antibody (Aurelian *et al.* 1974) does not exclude the possibility that it is a structural polypeptide. In fact, HSV-1 and HSV-2 polypeptides very likely related to structural glycosylated polypeptides have been reported to be excreted from infected cells (Kaplan *et al.* 1975), and might in fact be the antigens detected in these studies.

The Search for Viral Nucleic Acids in Cancer Cells

We have so far examined the implication of the timing of genital infection relative to the development of cancer but not that of finding viral antigens or of viral nucleic acids in cancer cells. Several points bear on this issue. First, productive infection with HSV is invariably lethal to the cell. The viral functions which ultimately destroy the cell are expressed early in infection (Roizman 1972). Hence, for the cell to survive and become transformed the infection must abort, and only those viral functions which are compatible with cell survival could be expressed. Second, if the virus in the cancer tissue is an innocuous passenger, if it merely induces a host function, or if the expression of a viral gene function is not required for the maintenance of the transformed state, we might expect that the viral gene expression might be absent or variable. If, on the other hand, a viral gene expression were required for the maintenance of the transformed state, we might expect that all cancer cells in all patients would share this function. We have already described the search for a tumor-specific antigen and the problems associated with this work. In essence, current technology does not permit us to perform experiments which would unequivocally show that a putative "tumour antigen" is virus specific, i.e. genetically determined by the viral genome. Since a "tumor antigen" has not been purified, the number, function and diversity of gene products which might constitute it are also not known. Furthermore, simplistic calculations indicate that, in order to be visualized, the antigen must be present in concentrations of hundreds per cell. Theoretically at least, the maintenance of transformed state need not require a high concentration of viral gene products. In the light of these considerations, examination of cancer cells for viral nucleic acid seems particularly rational since viral specificity and uniqueness can be readily established and, in some cases, the sensitivity could be increased to ensure detection of one copy per many cells.

In the first phase of this work, reported more than two years ago (Frenkel *et al.* 1972, Roizman and Frenkel 1973), we deliberately selected the largest tumor available; the 70 g exophytic tumor was trimmed to yield tissue which consisted largely (80%) of cancer cells. Analyses of the nucleic acids extracted from the tumor by renaturation kinetics with viral DNA labeled by repair synthesis revealed three interesting findings. First, the data showed that the tumor contained viral DNA and RNA, but that only a fragment of the genome was present. Moreover, only a small portion of the fragment contained in the tumor was transcribed. Lastly, application of a new technique led to the demonstration that viral DNA was probably covalently linked with host DNA.

These studies also presented us with some unexpected problems. First, the labeled probe did not reassociate properly; specifically 16% of the DNA reassociated more rapidly than the remainder. If we were to ignore the fact that the probe reassociated as if it consisted of both unique and reiterated sequences, we could estimate that the tumor contained viral sequences homologous to 39% of viral DNA. The second problem concerned the sensitivity of the assay. The only precedent in the herpesvirus field at that time were analyses of lymphoblastoid cells transformed by EBV; they were found to contain numerous copies of apparently intact viral DNA per cell (Zur Hausen and Schulte-Holthausen 1970, Nonoyama and Pagano 1971). Assuming that we did have 39% of the viral DNA, we calculated that only one copy of the fragment was present per cancer cell.

The anomalous reassociation of the probe was of special concern to us for several reasons. First, HSV DNA has a high guanine + cytosine (G + C) content. For this reason we hybridized the DNA in 1M Na+ at 79°C, i.e. approximately 25 below the Tm. Since the hybridization lasts weeks on end, the deviations from the second order kinetics could be due to degradation of the DNA at that temperature. Alternatively, our probe could have been contaminated by reiterated defective DNA sequences of the kind reported in papovavirus infected cells (Martin *et al.* 1973). Analyses of the HSV-1 and HSV-2 DNAs have revealed several interesting findings. First, we found that HSV does generate defective DNA on serial propagation. These molecules consist of tandem repeats of a small region and reassociate more rapidly than normal DNA (Frenkel *et al.* 1975, Roizman *et al.* 1974). Second, degradation of the DNA also contributes to the anomalous renaturation kinetics. Thus the reassociation of DNA extracted from virus passaged at low multiplicity and renatured in formamide over a long period of time, to permit a lower temperature of hybridization, followed second order kinetics until at least 60% of the viral DNA was renatured. Parenthetically, portions of HSV-DNA from the left end and 4.5% from the right end of the HSV-DNA molecule are inverted and repeated internally in the DNA (Wadsworth *et al.* 1975). Although this reiteration (Fig. 1) does not account for and probably could not be detected by renaturation kinetics, it is probably responsible for many of the unusual structural features of the DNA molecule (Hayward, Frenkel *et al.* 1975, Hayward, Jacob *et al.* 1975, Roizman *et al.* 1974).

The finding of a fragment of HSV-2 DNA in the cancer cells was consistent with the hypothesis that the expression of viral functions would be lethal to the cell, but presented us with a problem. Specifically, we could now expect that all cells transformed by HSV would contain a fragment rather than the entire genome. The problem concerns the sensitivity of the technique for detection of viral nucleic acid and since it is crucial to many other studies in progress it should perhaps be discussed in detail. Fundamentally, two techniques are available for the detection of viral DNA sequences. The first, and least reliable, involves preparation of RNA transcribed *in vitro* from viral DNA with a bacterial or mammalian polymerase. This transcript, usually referred to as cRNA, is then hybridized to tumor cell DNA fixed on filters. The basic flow of this technique arises from the fact that the extent to which the viral DNA is transcribed is not readily apparent, there is a limit to the amount of tumor cell DNA which can be placed on a filter, and RNA hybridizing to the DNA tends to pull the hybrid off the filter (Haas *et al.* 1972). An illustration of this type of study is a recent

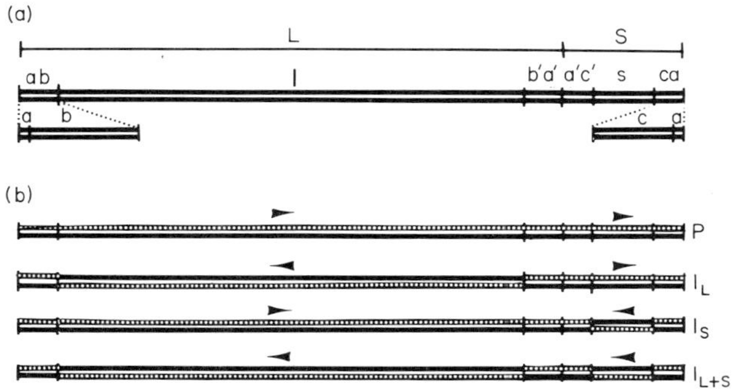

Fig. 1 *The anatomy of HSV DNA.* (a) *Arrangement and relative dimensions of regions in segments* L *and* S *of the linear structure of viral DNA. The regions were identified by electron microscopy of* (*i*) *single-stranded DNA allowed to self anneal* (*Sheldrick and Berthelot 1974, Roizman* et al. *1974, Wadsworth* et al. *1975*), (*ii*) *partially denatured DNA* (*Wadsworth* et al. *1975, Roizman* et al. *1974*) *and* (*iii*) *circularized DNA following exonuclease digestion of HSV DNA* (*Roizman* et al. *1974, Sheldrick and Berthelot 1974*). (b) *Arrangements of regions in the 4 kinds of molecular forms of HSV DNA. Note that the 4 molecules differ in the orientation of the* L *and* S *regions relative to each other. In the figure, one of the two strands is shown as a dotted line. Note that inversion of the* L *or* S *segments does not change the orientation of the* ab, b'a'a'c' *and* ca *regions of the DNA molecule. Thus, even though the entire segment inverts, the nucleotide sequences in these regions retain the orientation of the prototype molecule. P – parental or prototype molecule.* I_S *– molecule with* S *region inverted.* I_L *– molecule with* L *region inverted.* I_{L+S} *– molecule with inversion in both* L *and* S *regions.*

publication by Zur Hausen *et al.* (1974) in which cRNA obtained from transcription of HSV-2 DNA with *E. coli* polymerase was hybridized to 50 μg of cervical cancer DNA fixed to a filter. According to the authors, the extent of transcription of viral DNA with *E. coli* polymerase, although unknown, was probably small (Zur Hausen, personal communication); hence, hybridization could not be expected if the regions transcribed by the *E. coli* polymerase were not those present in the cancer cell. Parenthetically, this problem does not arise if the whole viral genome is present in the cancer cells

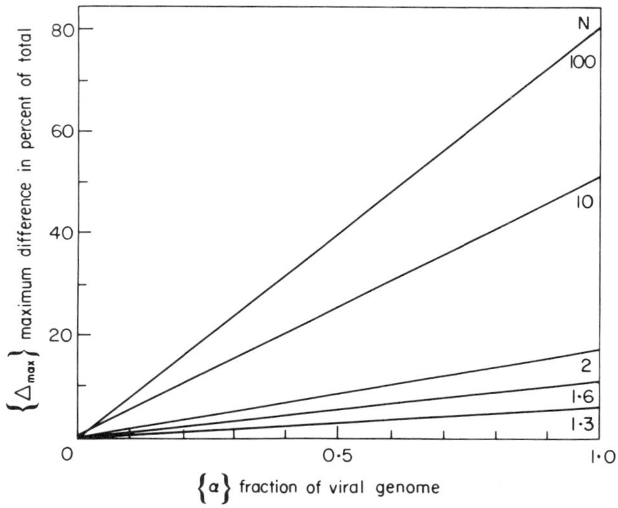

Fig. 2 *The sensitivity of the molecular hybridization assay for detection of viral genomes in DNA extracted from cells and tissues. In principle, the presence of viral DNA in cancer tissue is determined from the absolute difference between the reassociation of viral DNA probe by itself given by*

$$\frac{Dt}{D_0} = \frac{1}{1 + \tau} \qquad (1)$$

and that of the probe in the presence of cancer tissues containing a fragment of viral DNA and given by

$$\frac{Dt}{D_0} = \frac{1}{1 + N\tau} + \frac{1 - \alpha}{1 + \tau} \qquad (2)$$

where Dt/D_0 *is the fraction of the labeled probe remaining single stranded and* α *is the fraction of the viral DNA present in the cells.* τ *is defined by* KC_0t *where* K *is the reassociation rate constant, (liter moles nucleotides*$^{-1}$ *sec*$^{-1}$*),* C_0 *is the concentration of viral DNA (moles nucleotides per liter) in the probe and* t *is time of hybridization (in seconds).* N *is defined by*

$$\frac{f \cdot C_0^c + C_0^p}{C_0^p}$$

where C_0^p *and* C_0^c *are the concentrations of labeled viral DNA (probe) and of cancer tissue DNA, respectively, in moles nucleotides per liter, and* f *is the fraction of the DNA being analysed that is homologous to the probe. For example, the* N *value, assuming one genome equivalent per cancer cell, in a hybridization mixture of 2 mg of DNA from cancer tissues containing 50% cancer cells with 3.0 x 10*$^{-5}$ *mg of labeled viral DNA per ml can be calculated from*

$$N = \frac{(2.0 \times 10^{-5} \times 0.5 + 3.0 \times 10^{-5})}{3.0 \times 10^{-5}} = 1.3$$

as in the case of lymphoblastoid cells carrying EBV. The authors claim that in reconstruction experiments they were able to detect one genome equivalent per cell. This is equivalent to detecting unique, non-reiterated cellular sequences by filter hybridization – a difficult, if not impossible, task. Our calculations suggest that the limit of detection of this study was closer to tens of genome equivalents per cell.

The second technique for detection of viral DNA sequences involves hybridization of denatured excess cancer tissue DNA with trace amounts of labeled viral DNA in a liquid phase. The test is based on the fact that the rate of renaturation of the labeled probe is dependent on DNA concentration. If the cancer tissue contains viral DNA sequences, the rate of renaturation of the probe will be faster in the presence of the cancer tissues DNA than in the presence of unrelated DNA. The detection and quantitation of viral DNA sequences in cancer tissues hinge on the magnitude of the difference between the renaturation of the probe in the presence of test and control DNAs. In principle, two factors affect the magnitude of this difference. The first, which we shall designate as N, is the ratio of the molar concentration of viral sequences hybridizing in the presence and absence of the DNA extracted from cancer tissues. The second factor, designated as α, is the fraction of the genome present in the cancer tissue. The figure of interest to us is the *maximal difference* expected between the renaturation of the probe DNA in the presence and absence of the cancer tissue DNA. It is obvious from the calculated values shown in Fig. 2, that the differences between the two renaturation rates are strongly affected by both N and α and

---

where 10^{-5} *is the ratio of the molecular weights of viral DNA* (10^8, *Kieff* et al. *1971*) *to human cancer cell DNA* (10^{13}, *Leuchtenberger* et al. *1954*) *assuming one genome equivalent per cell, and 0.5 is the fraction of cancer cells in the cancer tissue being analysed. Of interest to us is the difference between the hybridization of the probe in the presence and absence of cancer cell DNA given by the differences in equations (1) and (2) i.e.,*

$$\Delta = \frac{\alpha}{1 + N\tau} - \frac{\alpha}{1 + \tau}$$

and especially in the maximum difference that can be observed during the reassociation given by

$$\Delta_{max} = \frac{\alpha(1 - \sqrt{N})}{(1 + \sqrt{N})}$$

The values in Fig. 2 were calculated from this equation. Data from Cox, Frenkel and Roizman (in preparation) that at low levels of N the differences in the renaturation of the probe DNA in the presence and absence of tumor DNA become very small. Whether, for example at $N = 1.3$, it is possible to detect one intact ($\alpha = 1.0$) viral genome equivalent per cell, which gives a maximum predictable difference of 6.5%, hinges on the standard error of the assay. This can be as small as 1% in assays employing single strand specific nucleases to monitor the extent of renaturation (Frenkel *et al.* 1972) to perhaps 2 or 3 times this value in assays using hydroxy-apatite chromatography for this purpose. The sensititivy of the hybridization assay can be improved by increasing the ratio N or by substituting restriction enzyme fragments in place of the entire genome as the probe. N can be increased in two ways: by increasing the concentration of the DNA extracted from tumor tissues, which is not always feasible because of the size of the tumor; or by decreasing the concentration of the DNA in the labeled probe. The amount of viral DNA in the probe is fixed by the specific activity of the DNA. Thus, increasing the specific activity of the labeled DNA probe allows a reduction in the concentration of the probe DNA in the hybridization mixture, thereby increasing the N value.

The value of N plays a particularly significant role if the cancer cell contains only a small portion of the viral genome. For example, as illustrated in Fig. 3, no viral DNA sequences were detected in the DNA of transformed hamster cell (Rapp and Duff 1974) in tests constructed to yield an N value of 1.9. Hybridization tests designed to allow N values of 10.6 and 26.5 readily demonstrated the presence of a fragment of viral DNA in the transformed cells. Parenthetically, the failure to grasp the significance of the ratio N may well explain the failure of Zur Hausen's laboratory to detect viral DNA sequences in cervical tumor biopsies. These workers hybridized DNA from 17 tumors with HSV-2 DNA with a specific activity $1-2 \times 10^5$ ct min^{-1} μg^{-1} and DNA from 9 biopsies with viral DNA of specific activities of 2×10^6 ct min^{-1} μg^{-1}. In the best situation involving the high specific activity probe, the test mixture contained 2 mg of tumor DNA and 3×10^{-5} mg of viral DNA probe per ml (Zur Hausen, personal communication). Assuming that the estimate that cancer cells constituted 50% of the biopsy is correct, N can be calculated to be 1.3 (*see* legend to Fig. 2). As indicated in Fig. 2, this value barely allows detection of one viral genome per cancer cell assuming the standard error of the hydroxyapatite chromatography assay was low. Molecular hybridizations (Frenkel, Locker, Roizman and Rapp 1976) constructed to maximize the value of N have shown that hamster embryo cells transformed with HSV-2 and one tumor obtained by injecting transformed cells into a newborn hamster

(Rapp and Duff 1974) contain from 5% to 40% of the viral genome. The data, interestingly enough, revealed that sublines of the same transformed cell lines differed in the size of the fraction of viral genome they contain.

Replacement of the entire viral DNA in the probe with individual fragments generated by restriction endonuclease cleavage of viral DNA will not only increase the sensitivity of the assay but also help

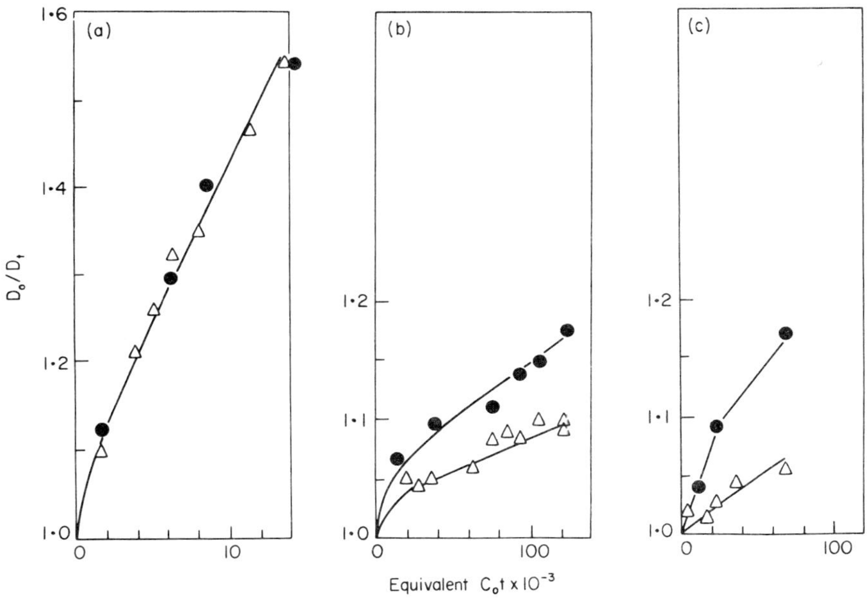

Fig. 3 *Hybridization of labeled HSV-2 labeled* in vitro *by repair synthesis in the presence of unlabeled DNA extracted from transformed hamster cell lines or in the presence of calf thymus DNA.* (a), (b) *HSV-2 DNA was labeled with ^{3}H TTP to a specific activity of 2×10^{6} ct min^{-1} μg^{-1}.* (c) HSV-2 DNA was labeled with *^{32}P CTP to a specific activity of 5×10^{8} ct min^{-1} μg^{-1}. Based on the assumption that the cells contain only one genome equivalent of HSV-2 DNA per genome equivalent of host DNA, the hybridization tests were constructed to yield values of* N = *1.9 for* (a), *10.6 for* (b), *and 26.5 for* (c). (*Details on the hybridization assay are given in Frenkel* et al. *1972*)

clarify the significance of the findings of viral DNA in transformed cells. It is obvious from the foregoing discussion that the significance of the finding would hinge on whether the HSV-DNA sequences present in the transformed cell lines and in the cancer tissues are totally random or share a unique region of viral DNA. To answer this question we began some time ago to construct a restriction endonuclease map of HSV DNA for the purpose of hybridizing the restriction endonuclease fragments with DNA extracted from cancer tissues.

This would allow us to identify specifically the viral DNA regions contained in the transformed cells. Parenthetically, studies of the restriction endonuclease fragments revealed that, unlike all other DNA viruses infecting humans, HSV-1 and HSV-2 DNA exist in four molecular configurations differing only in the orientations of the regions S and L (Fig. 1) (Hayward, Frenkel *et al.* 1975, Hayward, Jacob *et al.* 1975, Roizman *et al.* 1975) and not in the nucleotide sequence content. Analyses of hamster transformed cell lines with HSV-2 restriction endonuclease are in progress.

Perspectives

The accumulated information on the relationship between genital herpes and human cancer is insufficient to determine if the association is causal. However, some of the landscape of genital herpes and of cervical cancer, as research areas, has become apparent and some of the ground rules are set down. We are confronted now with two questions. The first is what needs to be done to prove that the association is causal. Since this will undoubtedly call for specific experiments, the question arises as to what are the possible alternative results of such experiments and their significance.

Table 1

HSV-2 DNA sequences in the transformed hamster cell lines and in hamster tumor.[a]

Hamster transformed[b] cell line and tumor	*Fraction of viral DNA[c]*	*Number of copies of viral DNA[c] per polyploid cell[d]*
333-2-39 line A	0.37 ± 0.02	3.1
333-2-29 line B	0.10 ± 0.04	1.5
333-8-9 Tl-P32	0.09 ± 0.01	N.D.[e]
333-8-9 P80	0.16 ± 0.02	0.7
333-8-9 Tumor	0.08 ± 0.02	3.0
Col 6-1	0.14 ± 0.04	1.8
MS-4-1	0.09 ± 0.02	1.9
333-2-26	0.10 ± 0.03	2.4

(a) Data from Frenkel, Locker, Roizman and Rapp (1976)
(b) 333-2-29 line A and 333-2-29 line B are parallel passages of the same line. 333-8-9 Tl-P32 is the 32nd passage in culture following explantation of a tumor derived by inoculation of 333-8-9 cells into a newborn hamster. 333-8-9 P80 is passage 80 of the original clone.
(c) The fraction of viral DNA and number of copies per cell were determined by non-linear least square repression of a line specified by equation (2) in legend to Fig. 2 to best fit the experimental data.
(d) Estimated to contain 16pg DNA per cell.
(e) Number of copies could not be determined because the first points were done at C_0t values at which the hybridization was already leveling off.

To establish criteria of proof, we must first establish the range of non-trivial hypotheses among which we wish to discriminate. These are: (1) HSV, or fragments of its DNA, are occasional, innocuous passengers. (2) Cervical cancer is induced by a number of factors of which HSV-2 is a major and significant contributor. (3) HSV-2 uniquely causes cervical cancer. Based on what we think we know about viral oncology, we might be tempted to predict that finding no viral genome in occasional cancers, or only random bits and pieces of it, would tend to refute hypothesis (3). However, we cannot exclude the "hit and run" hypothesis, i.e. that HSV-DNA is not required to maintain the transformed state and could be lost. The "hit and run" hypothesis is not trivial because is lacks precedent. On the other hand, the finding of a specific region of the viral DNA in cancer cells is very meaningful, but again it is not absolute evidence to refute hypotheses (1) and (2) since it could be argued that the particular region is required for the maintenance of the DNA fragment in cells, but does not involve their transformation, i.e. similar fragments occur in normal cells as well, but in too few to be detected. Obviously the information on the status of viral genes in human cancers is necessary but it will not provide definitive evidence. In the final analysis the most dramatic proof that genital herpes causes cancer is to preclude genital herpes, and this should be our major objective.

Acknowledgments

These studies were done under the auspices of the Chicago Cancer Research Center Project (CA 14599), and were aided by grants from the American Cancer Society (VC 103J) and the National Science Foundation (GB 38270) and Public Health Service Grant No. CA 08494 from the National Cancer Institute.

References

Adam, E., Kaufman, R. H., Melnick, J. L., Levy, A. H. and Rawls, W. E. (1972). *Americal Journal of Epidemiology* **96**, 427–442

Adam, E., Kaufman, R. H., Melnick, J. L., Levy, A. H. and Rawls, W. E. (1973). *American Journal of Epidemiology* **98**, 77–87

Adam, E., Rawls, W. E. and Melnick, J. L. (1974). *Preventive Medicine* **3**, 122–141

Aurelian, L. (1972). *Federation Proceedings* **31**, 1651–1659

Aurelian, L. (1973). *Cancer Research* **33**, 1539–1547

Aurelian, L., Davis, H. G. and Julian, C. G. (1973). *American Journal of Epidemiology* **98**, 1–9

Aurelian, L., Schumann, B., Marcus, R. L. and Davis, H. J. (1973). *Science* **181**, 161–164

Aurelian, L. and Strandberg, J. D. (1974). *Archiv für die gesamte Virusforschung* **45**, 27–38

Aurelian, L., Strandberg, J. D. and Marcus, R. L. (1974). *Progress in Experimental Tumor Research* 19, 165–181

Aurelian, L., Strandberg, J. D., Melendez, L. V. and Johnson, L. A. (1971). *Science* 174, 704–707

Aurelian, L. and Strnad, B. C. (1976). *Cancer Research* 36, 810–820

Biggs, P. M. (1973). *In* "Herpesviruses". Ed. A. S. Kaplan. Academic Press, New York and London; pp 557–594

Cassai, E., Sarmiento, M. and Spear, P. G. (1975). *Journal of Virology* 16, 1327–1331

Catalano, L. W. and Johnson, L. D. (1971). *Journal of the American Medical Association* 217, 447–450

Coppleson, M., Pixley, E. and Reid, B. (1971). *In* "Colposcopy, A Scientific and Practical Approach to the Cervix in Health and Disease". Ed. L. A. Gray. Thomas, Springfield, Ill.; p 65

Frenkel, N., Jacob, R. J., Honess, R. W., Hayward, G. S., Locker, H. and Roizman, B. (1975). *Journal of Virology* 16, 153–167

Frenkel, N., Locker, H., Roizman, B. and Rapp, F. (1976). *Journal of Virology* 17 (in press)

Frenkel, N., Roizman, B., Cassai, E. and Nahmias, A. (1972). *Proceedings of the National Academy of Sciences of the United States of America* 69, 3784–3789

Haas, M., Vogt, M. and Dulbecco, R. (1972). *Proceedings of the National Academy of Sciences of the United States of America* 69, 2160

Hampar, B., Martos, L. M., Chakrabarty, M. and Burroughs, M. A. K. (1970). *Journal of Immunology* 104, 593–598

Hampar, B., Notkins, A. L., Mage, M. and Keehn, M. A. (1968). *Journal of Immunology* 100, 586

Hayward, G. S., Frenkel, N. and Roizman, B. (1975). *Proceedings of the National Academy of Sciences of the United States of America* 72, 1768–1772

Hayward, G. S., Jacob, R. J., Wadsworth, S. C. and Roizman, B. (1975). *Proceedings of the National Academy of Sciences of the United States of America* 72, 4243–4247

Heine, J. W., Honess, R. W., Cassai, E. and Roizman, B. (1974). *Journal of Virology* 14, 640–651

Hollinshead, A. C., Lee, O. B., Chretien, P. B., Tarpley, J. L., Rawls, W. E. and Adam, E. (1973). *Science* 182, 713–715

Hollinshead, A. C., Lee, O. B., McKelway, W., Melnick, J. L. and Rawls, W. E. (1972). *Proceedings of the Society for Experimental Biology and Medicine* 141, 688–693

Honess, R. W. and Roizman, B. (1974). *Journal of Virology* 14, 8–19

Honess, R. W. and Roizman, B. (1975). *Proceedings of the National Academy of Sciences of the United States of America* 72, 1276–1280

Kaplan, A. S., Erickson, J. S. and Ben-Porat, T. (1975). *Virology* 64, 132–143

Kessler, I. I. (1974). *Cancer Research* 34, 1091–1110

Kieff, E. D., Bachenheimer, S. L. and Roizman, B. (1971). *Journal of Virology* 8, 125–132

Leuchtenberger, C., Leuchtenberger, R. and Davis, A. (1954). *American Journal of Pathology* 30, 65–85

Martin, E. M. (1967). *American Journal of Public Health and the Nation's Health* 57, 803–814

Martin, M. A., Gelb, L. D., Fareed, G. C. and Milstein, J. B. (1973). *Journal of Virology* 12, 748–757

Melendez, L. V., Hunt, R. D., Daniel, M. D., Fraser, C. E. O., Barahona, H. H., King, N. W. and Garcia, F. G. (1972). *Federation Proceedings* 31, 1643-1650
Melnick, J. L., Adam, E. and Rawls, W. E. (1974). *Cancer* 34, 1375-1385
Mizell, M., Toplin, I. and Isaacs, J. J. (1969). *Science* **165**, 1134-1137
Moghissi, K. S., Mack, H. C. and Porzak, J. P. (1968). *American Journal of Obstetrics and Gynecology* **100**, 607-614
Naguib, S. M., Lundin, F. E. and Davis, H. J. (1966). *American Journal of Obstetrics and Gynecology* **28**, 451
Nahmias, A. J., Josey, W. E., Naib, Z. M., Luce, C. and Duffey, C. (1970*a*). *American Journal of Epidemiology* **91**, 539-546
Nahmias, A. J., Josey, W. E., Naib, Z. M., Luce, C. and Guest, B., (1970*b*). *American Journal of Epidemiology* **91**, 547
Nahmias, A. J., Naib, Z. M., Josey, W. E., Franklin, E. and Jenkins, R. (1973). *Cancer Research* 33, 1491-1497
Nahmias, A. J. and Roizman, B. (1973). *New England Journal of Medicine* **289**, 667-674, 719-725, 781-789
Naib, Z. M., Nahmias, A. J., Josey, W. E. and Kramer, J. H. (1969). *Cancer* 23, 940-945
Nonoyama, M. and Pagano, J. S. (1971). *Nature New Biology* 233, 103-106
Pereira, L., Cassai, E., Honess, R. W., Roizman, B., Terni, M. and Nahmias, A. (1976). *Infection and Immunity* 13, 221
Plummer, G. and Masterson, J. G. (1971). *American Journal of Obstetrics and Gynecology* **111**, 81-84
Pridan, H. and Lilienfeld, A. M. (1971). *Israel Journal of Medical Sciences* 7, 1465-1470
Rapp, F. and Duff, R. (1974). *Cancer* 34, 1353-1362
Rawls, W. E., Adam, E. and Melnick, J. L. (1973). *Cancer Research* 33, 1477-1482
Rawls, W. E., Iwamoto, K., Adam, E., Melnick, J. L. and Green, G. H. (1970). *Lancet* ii, 1142-1143
Rawls, W. E., Tompkins, W. A. F. and Melnick, J. L. (1969). *American Journal of Epidemiology* **89**, 547-554
Roizman, B. (1972). *In* "Oncogenesis and Herpesviruses". Ed. P. M. Biggs, G.de The and L. N. Payne. International Agency for Research on Cancer, Lyon; pp 1-20
Roizman, B. and Frenkel, N. (1973). *Cancer Research* 33, 1402-1416
Roizman, B., Hayward, G., Jacob, R., Wadsworth, S. W. and Honess, R. W. (1974). *Excerpta Medica, International Congress Series* No. 350, 2, 188-198
Rotkin, I. D. (1967). *American Journal of Public Health and the Nation's Health* **57**, 815-829
Rotkin, I. D. (1973). *Cancer Research* 33, 1353-1367
Royston, I. and Aurelian, L. (1970*a*). *American Journal of Epidemiology* **91**, 531-538
Royston, I. and Aurelian, L. (1970*b*). *Proceedings of the National Academy of Sciences of the United States of America* **67**, 204-212
Sabin, A. B. (1974). *Proceedings of the National Academy of Sciences of the United States of America* 71, 3248-3252
Sabin, A. B. and Tarro, G. (1973). *Proceedings of the National Academy of Sciences of the United States of America* **70**, 3225-3229
Seth, P., Rawls, W. E., Duff, R., Rapp, F., Adam, E. and Melnick, J. L. (1974). *Intervirology* 3, 1-14
Sheldrick, P. and Berthelot, N. (1974). *Cold Spring Harbor Symposia on Quantitative Biology* 39, 667-678

Skinner, G. R. B., Thouless, M. E. and Jordon, J. A. (1971). *Journal of Obstetrics and Gynaecology of the British Commonwealth* **78**, 1031–1038
Smith, J. W., Adam, E., Melnick, J. L. and Rawls, W. E. (1972). *Journal of Immunology* **109**, 554–564
Smith, J. W., Lowry, S. P., Melnick, J. L. and Rawls, W. E. (1972). *Infection and Immunity* **5**, 305–310
Spear, P. G. and Roizman, B. (1972). *Journal of Virology* **9**, 143–159
Stevens, D. A., Pincus, T., Burroughs, A. K. and Hampar, B. (1968). *Journal of Immunology* **101**, 979–983
Tarro, G. and Sabin, A. B. (1970). *Proceedings of the National Academy of Sciences of the United States of America* **65**, 753–760
Tarro, G. and Sabin, A. B. (1973). *Proceedings of the National Academy of Sciences of the United States of America* **70**, 1032–1036
Wadsworth, S. W., Jacob, R. J. and Roizman, B. (1975). *Journal of Virology* **15**, 1487–1489
Zur Hausen, H. and Schulte-Holthausen, H. (1970). *Nature* (*London*) **227**, 245–248
Zur Hausen, H., Schulte-Holthausen, H., Wolf, H., Dorries, K. and Egger, H. (1974). *International Journal of Cancer* **13**, 657–664

Antiviral Compounds with Special Reference to Genital Herpes

B E Juel-Jensen
Department of the Regius Professor of Medicine, University of Oxford

A considerable number of compounds will destroy viruses. Infusion of formaldehyde in large amounts into the vascular tree will certainly kill any virus with which man may happen to have become infected. Such a procedure has certain regrettable disadvantages. This crude example is, of course, a gross caricature of the problem which, nevertheless, is real for the clinician who wants to rid his patient of a virus disease. Most viruses share vital metabolic steps with the cells of the host and unfortunately very few of the compounds that to date *in vitro* have proved active against viruses and non-toxic to tissue cultures have also been non-toxic and effective when tried in infected animals (where suitable animal models exist). The very few substances that have passed these hurdles have, with few exceptions, been equally disppointing when used in man, for the same reasons. The few that are of use have sometimes been condemned, perhaps too lightheartedly, as "inactive" or "disappointing" because we as doctors traditionally have been unable to count up to more than two. We expect a pill or an injection either not to work at all or to cure the patient, often with too little reference to the natural history of the illness we are trying to eliminate and with little regard for the admirable defence mechanisms with which man is provided, which in most situations we can at best only hope to support.

There is no time to review the use of current antiviral compounds in general, nor would it be appropriate to do so. Rather, I have chosen to discuss the problem of the treatment of one condition, infection with herpes simplex virus (HSV), which has already been dealt with so ably by Dr Nahmias and Dr Roizman. No doubt many other virus diseases may be transmitted sexually. Most clinicians who practice hebeatrics would have little doubt that another herpesvirus disease, infectious mononucleosis, caused by the Epstein-Barr virus, may be what Hoagland (1955) called the "kissing disease"; but as it is usually a short-lived benign disease, which is probably diagnosed only after the main virus replication has taken place, it is hardly ever worth treating with specific antiviral compounds. It is not wise for the intrepid youth who thumbs his way along the modern pilgrim's trek via the Middle East to Katmandu to indulge in indiscriminate sexual intercourse without a reasonable awareness of the high carriage rate of HBsAg in, say, Greek or Turkish ladies of easy virtue. It is of theoretical interest at present for most that it might be relatively safe to indulge in the Ethiopian Highlands (Ross and Juel-Jensen (1976) found an incidence of HBsAg of 2.7%). The possible usefulness of antiviral chemotherapy (ribavirin) in hepatitis A, B, and perhaps now also C, is still very much *sub judice*. Prevention is better than cure. If abstinence is not possible in high-risk areas, passive inmmunization with hyper-immune immunoglobulin is theoretically possible, but this must surely come low on the list of priorities. Active immunization is a possibility but still not a reality (WHO Technical Report Series 1975).

Treatment of Genital Herpes

Herpes simplex virus is a DNA virus which can be divided into at least two types. The DNA of the virus is polymerized from thymidine, formed by a series of enzymatic steps from relatively simple aliphatic compounds. The few antiviral compounds that in clinical trials have so far been shown to be effective and to have low toxicity are pyrimidine analogues which act mainly by entering the synthetic chain and causing the formation of false DNA which either does not replicate or causes miscoding. One of the first of these analogues to be tried in man was 5-iodo-2′-deoxyuridine (idoxuridine, IUDR) which is thymidine where the methyl group in the 5 position has been replaced by iodine, first synthesized by Prusoff in 1959. Though bromine and fluorine analogues are active *in vitro*, BUDR has been suspected of being potentially mutagenic (Kaback *et al.* 1964) and the fluorine of FUDR has too short a van der Waal's radius to be incorporated. The latter is active as an enzyme poison but is too toxic for use clinically. Trifluorothymidine has been shown to be active in HSV eye infections (Wellings *et al.* 1972). Unfortunately idoxuridine is very insoluble in most solvents and is inactive except in the eye in watery solution or in cream (0.1% and 0.5% respectively) when topically applied; it does not penetrate the skin (Burnett and Katz 1963, Juel-Jensen and MacCallum 1964, Kibrick and Katz 1970). Idoxuridine should not be given systemically. Doses that theoretically should be effective are so large that severe side-effects on the bone marrow, gut and liver are inevitable. Systemic idoxuridine was until recently used occasionally in HSV encephalitis without evidence that it was effective, but a well-conducted double-blind controlled trial (Boston Interhospital Virus Study Group 1975) showed no benefit and severe side-effects, and should finally have put an end to parenteral administration of the drug. We overcame the problem of the insolubility of idoxuridine in topical use by dissolving it in dimethyl sulphoxide (DMSO) and proved in a double-blind trial that a 5% solution was effective in recurrent HSV lesions of the face when given early in the eruption (MacCallum and Juel-Jensen 1966). Subsequent work demonstrated (Juel-Jensen *et al.* 1970) that a stronger solution (40%) continuously applied to the affected area for four days was very active in segmental zoster of recent onset, and concurrently that certain primary forms of HSV infection, such as herpetic whitlows, could be cured and did not relapse when followed in some instances for more than five years. In one particularly well-documented case (otherwise apparently immunocompetent) so little antigen was left that only traces of neutralizing antibody could be detected.

Cytosine arabinoside (cytarabine, Ara-C), another pyrimidine analogue, has the great advantage of being easily soluble in water. It is used as a cytotoxic drug, particularly in neoplastic disorders of the lymphoid tissue, but if given rapidly intravenously in modest doses ($\leqslant$3 mg/kg per day) it is rarely possible to detect any adverse effect on the marrow (occasionally very transient macrocytosis occurs in the second week after treatment). Slow infusion of the same amount is more likely to affect the marrow. High doses, such as 10 mg/kg per day, have been used in HSV encephalitis and practically always give transient suppression of reticulocytes, platelets, and, to a lesser extent, leukocytes, but apparently always with full recovery (Juel-Jensen 1973*a*). Cytarabine has been used in serious primary and recurrent HSV infections. These occur too rarely in any one centre to allow double-blind controlled studies to be carried out, but it is possible to measure the period during which virus can be isolated, for instance in primary HSV stomatitis, and apart from often dramatic clinical improvement (a subjective measurement) the excretion of virus is reduced to two to five days when one might have expected to recover it for two to three weeks in the untreated case. We have not seen recurrences in patients with primary infections treated early and some have been followed over many years, when a proportion could have been expected to have relapsed had they not been treated. In an occasional patient the virus does not appear to be affected by cytarabine. Prusoff has suggested (personal communication) that there are people who produce an abnormal amount of pyrimidine kinase and metabolize the cytarabine very rapidly. Unfortunately assay of this enzyme is still cumbersome. If we could measure its activity readily the optimum dosage of cytarabine in the individual might be arrived at with greater sophistication.

I have deliberately mentioned varicella/zoster infection – for there is increasing evidence that HSV infections behave in a similar manner, if differently in degree: they recur in those who get relapses more frequently than does the latent virus in those who have had chickenpox. The latent HSV probably resides in the nerve cells of nerves that innervate the site where the primary infection took place. We know with some certainty that one-third of patients who have had a primary infection with Type 1 virus are likely to relapse. The majority of patients with genital herpes have been infected with Type 2 virus – 95% in Oxford; Naib *et al.* (1970) found a similar figure. To my knowledge there are no certain figures for whether the relapse rate is the same as for Type 1 or higher. It is intriguing that the majority do not relapse. A knowledge of the immunological determinants might help us towards more rational treatment. Once the primary infection has run its course it is unlikely that more than a proportion of the latent virus replicates during a recurrence. There is no doubt that the local visible lesion can be treated effectively with topical chemotherapy. In recurrent genital HSV we use a 35% solution of idoxuridine in DMSO applied about five times a day for not more than three days. It is important not to continue for longer, for we have never been able to grow the virus for more than at most 48 hours from the local lesion. The DMSO will macerate the skin in the patient who continues treatment for longer, and he thinks his lesion is getting worse. But we are only treating the visible lesions and will not eradicate virus along the nerve fibres and in the cells, let alone the latent virus. Experience suggests that some patients, by treating each eruption, eventually cease getting recurrences. Certainly the duration of the lesion is cut significantly and the interval between recurrences beomes longer. Ideally, one would like to get all patients early in the primary infection. We have a group of women with extremely unpleasant early primary vulvovaginitis, some with evidence of generalized spread, in whom systemic cytarabine was given with rapid relief and disappearance of the virus; so far none of those followed for several years has relapsed.

Unfortunately, the physician rarely has the opportunity of seeing the patient in the primary attack, and I believe this is also the experience of venereologists and gynaecologists. However, all may not be lost. We have, over the last few years, had the opportunity of seeing a group of patients with proven Type 2 genital herpes. The history was almost identical. Each recurrence (which happened with varying intervals, from one to three months) was preceded by pain corresponding to a distribution of S1 to S5. After an interval of 24–72 hours these patients would invariably get an eruption, in the males usually on the penis and on the skin of the buttock-thigh corresponding to S3–S5 (where, in 4 cases, lesions had not been present in the first attack). To one highly intelligent young male patient, extremely distressed by his condition, as are most with recurrent genital herpes, who was prepared to try anything that offered a hope of relief, I have now on three occasions over the last eighteen months given intravenous cytarabine, 3 mg/kg per day for four days, within 24 hours of the onset of the premonitory symptoms. No lesions appeared and the pain disappeared within hours. The intervals between attacks (which used to happen about once a month) have become longer, but on one occasion he was away and could not have cytarabine; after the usual interval one small eruption appeared on the penis only – in a different site – accompanied by pain. Constant monitoring for side-effects on blood, hepatic and renal function failed to reveal abnormalities.

Another pyrimidine analogue, adenosine arabinoside (vidarabine, Ara-A) is practically non-toxic but fairly insoluble and therefore impossible to administer except on an inpatient basis, for it must be given intravenously in normal saline. It is very effective against severe chickenpox and severe zoster, particularly awkward to treat by topical application when it affects the sacral dermatomes. Anyway, local treatment does not affect the involvement of the bladder (retention due to bladder atony) and bowel. There is hope that soluble variants such as cyclic Ara-AMP shortly may become available. The advantage of vidarabine over cytarabine is that although it is metabolized within half an hour like cytarabine, its metabolite hypoxanthine arabinoside, which is as active as cytarabine, is excreted slowly – over 24–36 hours – and active levels remain throughout the 24 hours of the day. This type of drug may indeed have a place in the treatment of wart-virus. We have reported elsewhere (Juel-Jensen

1973*b*) how a child went into remission from laryngeal papillomata (virus was found on electron microscopy of a biopsy) and now has remained clear for three years. It may be that venereal warts will respond to Ara-A. In conjunction with surgical colleagues we are at present investigating its effect on urethral papillomata.

For the reasons given, photosensitization of recurrent HSV with dyes such as neutral red, though interesting as a form of topical treatment (Felber *et al.* 1973), as with topical antiviral drugs in recurrent genital herpes, will probably not provide more than a partial answer to the patient's problems. The aim must be to kill all replicating virus and hope that eventually so little antigen remains that recurrences cease. I would venture a guess that an effective safe sytemic drug alone will provide an effective solution. We must aim not only at treating spots and ulcers we can see but also the replicating virus in the depths we cannot see.

Time does not allow me to consider the particular problems that arise in HSV infection around the period of conception, during pregnancy, and in the neonate. Tobin (1975) has ably discussed the position recently at a meeting in the Royal Society of Medicine.

Of necessity this paper has been brief and incomplete. I hope I may have left you with a few thoughts, however speculative, on the problems that face the clinician who has to treat virus disease.

References

Boston Interhospital Virus Study Group and the NIAIB-sponsored Cooperative Antiviral Clinical Study (1973). *New England Journal of Medicine* **292**, 599

Burnett, J.W. and Katz, S.L. (1963). *Journal of Investigative Dermatology* **40**, 7

Felber, T. D., Smith, E. B., Knox, J. M., Wallis, C. and Melnick, J. L. (1973). *Journal of the American Medical Association* **223**, 289

Hoagland, R. J. (1955). *American Journal of the Medical Sciences* **229**, 262

Juel-Jensen, B. E. (1973*a*). *Postgraduate Medical Journal* **49**, 375

Juel-Jensen, B. E. (1973*b*). *British Journal of Hospital Medicine* **10**, 402

Juel-Jensen, B. E. and MacCallum, F. O. (1964) *British Medical Journal* **ii**, 987

Juel-Jensen, B. E., MacCallum, F. O., Mackenzie, A. M. R. and Pike, M. C. (1970). *British Medical Journal* **iv**, 776

Kaback, M. M., Sakseal, E. and Mellman, W. J. (1964). *Experimental Cell Research* **34**, 182

Kibrick, S. and Katz, A. S. (1970). *Annals of the New York Academy of Sciences* **173**, 83

MacCallum, F. O. and Juel-Jensen, B. E. (1966). *British Medical Journal* **ii**, 805

Naib, Z. M., Nahmias, A. J., Josey, W. E. and Wheeler, J. H. (1970). *Obstetrics and Gynecology* **35**, 260

Prusoff, W. H. (1959). *Biochimica et biophysica acta* **32**, 295

Ross, D. and Juel-Jensen, B. E. (1976). *Oxford University Medical School Gazette* (in press)

Tobin, J. O'H. (1975). *Proceedings of the Royal Society of Medicine* **68**, 371
Wellings, P. C., Awdry, P. N., Bors, F. H., Jones, B. R., Brown, D. C. and Kaufman, H. E. (1972). *American Journal of Ophthalmology* 73, 932
World Health Organization Technical Report Series (1975). "Viral Hepatitis". No. 570, p 44

Discussion

Dr Catterall asked Dr Nahmias how accurate and specific he thought the typing of herpes virus to be. He also asked Dr Nahmias if they were seeing an increasing amount of anorectal herpes simplex in the United States as there appeared to have been an increase in this condition in Europe. He enquired whether there was any indication that the herpes virus could cross the placenta from the maternal circulation to the fetal circulation and produce either stillbirth or serious damage to the fetus. Finally he asked Dr Nahmias to give further details about cerebral complications such as meningitis and encephalitis.

Dr Nahmias replied that he thought the typing was moderately accurate but that recently variants of the two main types of virus were being recognized.

With regard to the neurological complications of herpetic infection he had noticed that meningitis appeared to be a relatively benign process whereas the encephalitis was one of the most serious infections of the central nervous system. It required brain biopsy for diagnosis and the mortality and morbidity were very high. With regard to chronic meningitis he thought it was just possible that the virus might remain latent in the brain but there was no direct evidence yet of this happening in human beings.

With regard to transplacental infection he thought there was an interesting contrast with the cytomegalovirus, which was definitely transmitted transplacentally, whereas evidence that the herpes virus was transmitted in this way was small.

Dr Krause asked whether there was an unusual distribution of HL-A antigen in patients who developed carcinoma of the cervix and those who developed herpetic infections as compared with those who had never had herpes.

Dr Nahmias replied that this was a growing and exciting area of study. At the Sloane-Kettering Institute Dr R J O'Reilly and his colleagues, using the same dose of virus among different inbred strains, had found a genetic difference in the ability of herpes simplex to kill mice. In Canada Dr A S Russell had reported a greater frequency of HL-A 1 in people with frequently recurring manifestations of herpes simplex.

Dr Frank Young (*Rochester, NY*) asked whether the terminal redundancies or terminal sequences were similar in Type 1 and Type 2 infections usually looked at by either hybridization technique or restriction nucleases. He also asked whether the degree of homology between Type 1 and Type 2 virus precluded the use of DNA probes to distinguish between those types of viruses.

Dr Roizman replied that Types 1 and 2 could not be differentiated with respect to terminal reiterations or inversion of the terminal sequences since the overall arrangement of the sequences in the DNAs appeared to be similar. The HSV-1 and HSV-2 DNA appeared to differ in the localization of restriction endonuclease cleavage sites. The DNAs could therefore be readily identified on the basis of the number of electrophoretic mobilities on Hin III, Eco R1, Hpa 1, or Sal 1 restriction endonuclease digests of the DNAs. Although very likely one could devise a method for identification of HSV-1 and HSV-2 DNAs based on hybridization with a type specific fragment, this technique would probably be beyond the capability of most diagnostic laboratories.

Dr Parker thought that there was a tendency to overlook the possibility of neonatal herpetic infection and asked Dr Juel-Jensen how he would manage a patient with active genital herpes who was 38 weeks pregnant.

Dr Juel-Jensen replied that if it was a primary infection the danger to the fetus was considerable and he would discuss with the obstetrician the possibility of delivery by Caesarean section. If it was a recurrent manifestation then the risk to the fetus would be less. He had no experience of the use of antiviral drugs in pregnant women and he thought that the dangers to the fetus of the majority of the available drugs were too great to justify their use.

Dr Nahmias suggested that the figures for neonatal herpes in Britain were on the low side.

Dr Juel-Jensen said that, in the Oxford region, the incidence of neonatal herpes was extremely low, and that this low incidence was genuine, for intensive search had been going on for the last fifteen years.

Dr Roizman, commenting on the typing of strains of herpes virus, pointed out that there were discrepancies between the results from different virus laboratories and said that there were considerable difficulties in accurate typing of strains as well as considerable variation between strains.

Virus Diseases: II. Genital Warts

Virological Aspects of Genital Warts

June D Almeida
Wellcome Research Laboratories,
Langley Court, Beckenham, Kent BR3 3BS

A consideration of the microbiology of the genital region reveals that three possible types of organisms can be implicated. First, there are organisms that infect the genitals specifically: although they give rise to infections on other sites these are rare. An example of this group would be *N. gonorrhoeae*. Secondly, there are ubiquitous organisms such as *Candida albicans* that infect both the genitals and general body sites. Thirdly, there is a group of organisms that can give rise to both general and genital infections, but those recovered from the genital region show either morphological or serological variations from those on non-genital areas. For example, *Trichomonas vaginalis* differs considerably from either the oral or gut varieties of this species. Turning to virus infections, herpes simplex hominis can be subdivided into Type 1 and Type 2, depending on whether the virus is recovered from a general body site or from the genitals (Roizman *et al.* 1970). Yet another example of this type of variation would seem to be supplied by the human wart virus, a member of the papillomavirus group. Examination of common skin warts (verruca vulgaris) and genital warts (condyloma acuminatum) show that both lesions contain morphologically identical virus (Oriel and Almeida 1970). However, serological studies using immune electron microscopy have shown that the two viruses are not antigenically identical, the genital virus appearing to be a variant of the common wart virus (Almeida *et al.* 1969).

Materials and Methods

Surgically excised common and genital warts were examined electron-microscopically by the thin section technique. Extracts of the warts were used for recognition of virus by negative staining and also as antigen for immune electronmicroscopy (IEM). Sera from individuals with common warts, genital warts or both were used as antiserum in IEM tests.

Results

It is known from light microscope studies that genital warts vary histologically from the common skin wart. The genital lesions are more cellular, have separate cell nests and can on occasion present an

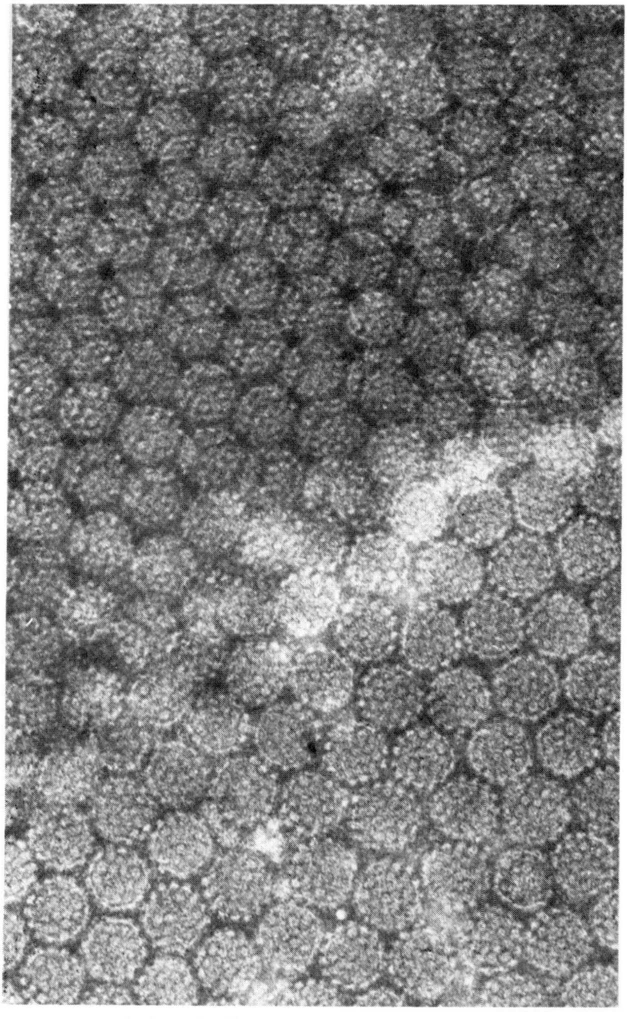

Fig. 1 *The amount of virus in human common warts is so great that even after simple concentration procedures it is possible to obtain preparations such as this. The curious superimposition pattern at the top left of the micrograph occurs because there is more than one layer of virus particles.* × *170 000*

appearance verging on neoplasia (Lever 1967). The histopathological appearance is partially reliant on the thinner structure of the genital epidermis and the general lack of keratin which, by contrast, is the main structural feature of the common skin wart. However, there would seem to be other differences between the two lesions not so easily explained by the nature of the epidermis. By thin sectioning,

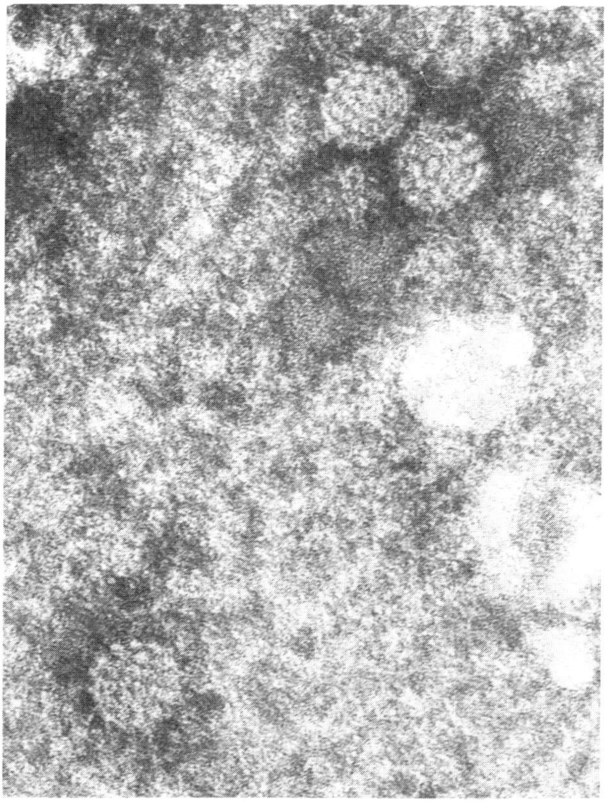

Fig. 2 *An exceptionally good micrograph of genital wart virus, as it contains three virus particles. Morphologically these virus particles are identical to the common skin wart virus but more usually there is only one virus particle present in a micrograph.* × *250 000*

the common wart, in and above the level of the stratum granulosum, contains many cells with numerous intranuclear virus particles, until at the level of the keratin the only remaining traces of the cells are large aggregates of virus (Almeida *et al.* 1962). Thin section examination of the genital wart shows a highly cellular structure with so little recognizable virus that only rare micrographs of intranuclear virus can be obtained (Oriel and Almeida 1970).

Thin section findings were confirmed by the results obtained with the negative staining method. Crudely prepared extracts of common warts yield such vast quantities of virus that three-dimensional arrays of virus can be obtained with ease (Fig. 1). The corresponding genital wart extract contains so little virus that two or three particles is the

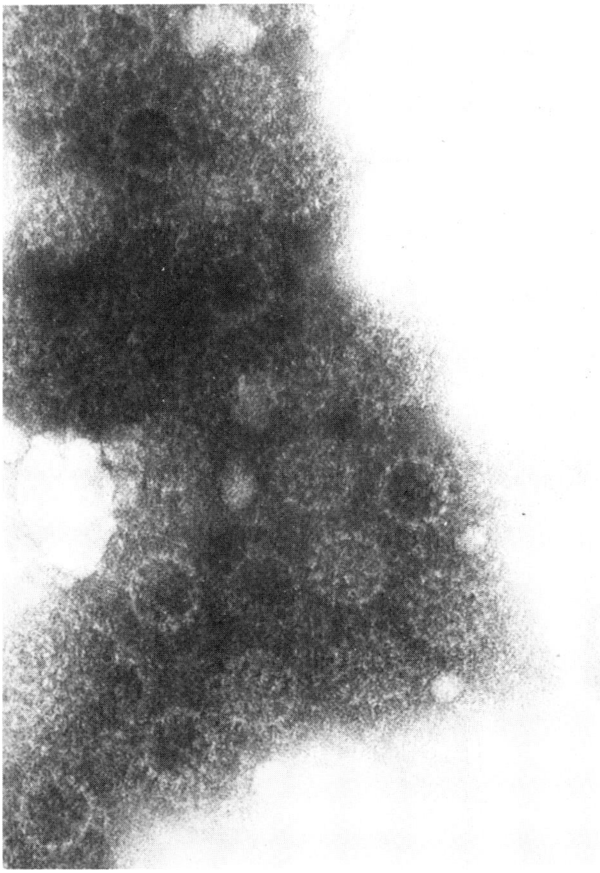

Fig. 3 *A group of common wart virus that have been treated with serum from a patient with skin warts. The virus is aggregated and obscured by antibody molecules. This appearance represents a positive result by the technique of immune electronmicroscopy.* x *250 000*

maximum ever obtained on one photographic plate, and the majority of micrographs contain only one virus particle (Fig. 2).

Immune electronmicroscopy (IEM) is now an accepted technique for establishing the presence of either viral pathogens or virus associated antibody (Almeida and Waterson 1969). It is of particular

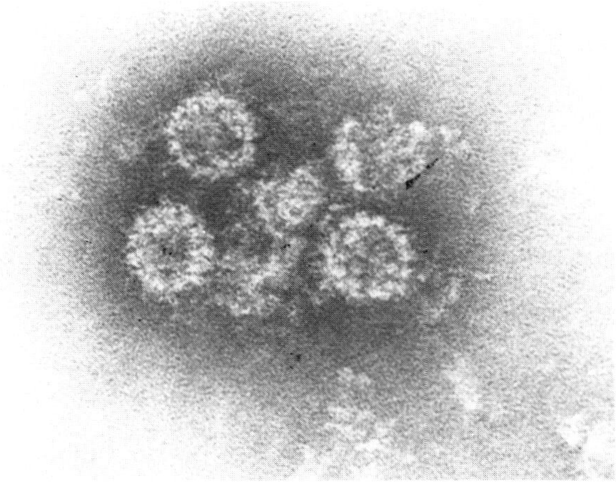

Fig. 4 *When the same skin wart antiserum used in Fig. 3 was reacted with genital wart virus a positive result was obtained. The virus is clumped and attached antibody molecules can be seen.* x *250 000*

use in situations where a virus cannot be grown *in vitro* or obtained in quantitities sufficient for grosser serological techniques. Since both these criteria apply to genital wart virus, IEM proved the most successful means of establishing the presence of antibody in patients' serum. A positive result is obtained when the patient's serum clumps previously unaggregated virus preparations and antibody molecules are seen attached to the particles.

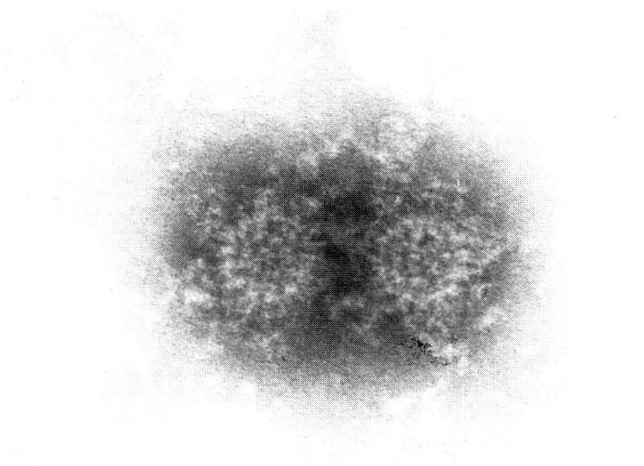

Fig. 5 *This micrograph shows that serum from a patient with genital warts when reacted with genital wart virus yields a positive reaction. However, the same serum used against common skin wart virus does not react with the virus.* x *250 000*

Sera from patients with common warts all gave a positive reaction against common wart virus (Fig. 3). Using these same sera against virus from genital warts, a positive reaction was once again obtained (Fig. 4). However, when sera from genital wart patients were used in this test aggregation was achieved with genital wart virus (Fig. 5) but there was no aggregation when common wart virus was used as antigen. It might have been argued that the titre of anti-wart antibody in these sera was low and that the discrepant amounts of wart virus in the two preparations could have given a positive result with homotypic virus and a negative one with the heterotypic preparation. To compensate for this factor the common wart virus was diluted to a level where the virus was present in amounts comparable to that present in the genital wart preparations. Even after this adjustment the sera from genital wart patients were unable to aggregate the skin wart particles.

Discussion

Virologically, the virus associated with common skin warts is problematical as it has proved impossible to grow it in an *in vitro* system even although pure preparations of high titre virus can be obtained. Without an *in vitro* cultivation method it is impossible to carry out many classical virological experiments that would establish parameters such as the nature of neutralizing antibody to the virus. If one then considers that genital warts have the same problems associated with them but in addition contain so little virus that only the most sensitive techniques can identify its presence it will be seen that information about this virus-induced lesion will not be readily obtained.

Using the more amenable common wart system it has been shown that circulating antibody to wart virus is produced, particularly around the time when warts resolve (Goffe *et al.* 1966, Ogilvie 1970, Matthews and Shirodaria 1973, Pyrhonen and Johansson 1975). It has also been postulated that cell-mediated immunity has a role to play in wart regression (Morison 1974). Greenberg *et al.* (1973), among others, have cured warts by stimulating local cellular immunity (Tagami *et al.* 1974, Russo *et al.* 1975). Our studies have shown that patients with genital warts produce humoral antibody to the homotypic virus. However, by itself, this may not be enough to produce resolution of the lesion and information on cell-mediated immunity is required. Unfortunately, the amount and state of viral antigen that can be obtained from lesions would almost certainly be inadequate to carry out these experiments. Once again there is a requirement for greater amounts of genital wart virus, but without a culture technique these cannot be obtained.

The results of immune electronmicroscopy suggest that a one-way antigenic cross exists between the virus of the common skin wart and that of the genital wart. Sera from patients with common warts react with both the common skin and the genital wart virus, while serum from patients with genital warts appears to react only with the homotypic genital wart virus. This finding is of interest, as it follows a pattern established by several other organisms infecting both general and genital sites. Among mycoplasmas it is possible to distinguish serologically between *M. hominis* Types 1 and 2, Type 1 being an oral organism and Type 2 a genital one (Taylor-Robinson *et al.* 1963). Herpes simplex virus is a well-known example of this phenomenon, HSV 1 being the general herpes simplex infection of man while HSV 2 is associated with infection of the genital area.

The shift in antigenicity associated with organisms infecting the genital region has two likely explanations. First, it might be postulated that initially there was one type of wart virus. This virus would occasionally infect the genitals, an area that offers a considerably different environment from the rest of the epidermis. In turn this new environment might select a substrain of the original virus, and an organism better suited to the limited area of the genitals might establish itself. On the other hand, a mutation of the original wart virus may have occurred and the resulting mutant be confined to the genital area as the only suitable environment. Unfortunately, the results that we have obtained do not allow us to differentiate between these two probabilities. The explanation that there have always been two distinct and separate wart virus types seems unlikely as this would imply that the same antigenic structures had evolved on two separate and unrelated occasions.

Genital warts are of considerable virological interest. The causative virus belongs to the papovavirus group, which contains several truly oncogenic animal viruses. Genital warts, although only rarely implicated in malignant transformation, are nevertheless lesions where a high degree of cellular proliferation occurs. In addition, while virus in both types of warts is found in the upper layers of the epidermis, cell proliferation occurs in the basal layer. A better understanding of the interaction between wart virus and host cell would obviously be of the greatest interest in the general context of virally induced oncogenic change.

Another problematical aspect of wart viruses is their inability to grow in cell culture. There is as yet no explanation for this phenomenon although it might be remarked that another skin-associated virus, molluscum contagiosum, is also refractory. The simplest explanation would be that epidermal viruses have special metabolic requirements. A great many attempts have been made to find suitable *in vitro* conditions for these viruses and it is hoped that a breakthrough might be obtained in the next few years. As Dr Oriel reports (*below*), the incidence of genital warts has increased considerably in recent years, making them a not unimportant clinical condition. This importance from a practical viewpoint, taken together with their undoubted but poorly understood viral etiology, makes both skin warts and genital warts strong candidates for further investigation. A better understanding of the interaction between wart virus and host cell could well shed light on other, seemingly more spectacular, clinical problems.

References

Almeida, J. D., Howatson, A. F. and Williams, M. G. (1962). *Journal of Investigative Dermatology* **38**, 337

Almeida, J. D., Oriel, J. D. and Stannard, L. M. (1969). *Microbios* 3, 225

Almeida, J. D. and Waterson, A. P. (1969). *Advances in Virus Research* **15**, 307

Goffe, A. P., Almeida, J. D. and Brown, F. (1966). *Lancet* **i**, 607

Greenberg, J. H., Smith, L. and Katz, R. M. (1973). *Archives of Dermatology* **107**, 580

Lever, W. F. (1967). "Histopathology of the Skin". 4th edn. Lippincott, Philadelphia

Matthews, R. S. and Shirodaria, P. V. (1973). *Lancet* **i**, 689

Morison, W. L. (1974). *British Journal of Dermatology* **90**, 531

Ogilvie, M. M. (1970). *Journal of Hygiene* **68**, 479

Oriel, J. D. and Almeida, J. D. (1970). *British Journal of Venereal Diseases* **46**, 37

Pyrhonen, S. and Johansson, E. (1975). *Lancet* **i**, 592

Roizman, B., Keller, J. M., Spear, P. C., Terni, M., Nahmias, A. and Dowdle, W. (1970). *Nature (London)* **227**, 1253

Russo, L., Russo, A. and Russo, V. (1975). *Lancet* **i**, 921

Tagami, H., Ogino, A., Takigawa, M., Imamura, S. and Ofuji, S. (1974). *British Journal of Dermatology* **90**, 147

Taylor-Robinson, D., Somerson, N. L., Turner, H. C. and Chanock, R. M. (1963). *Journal of Bacteriology* **85**, 1261

Genital Warts — The Clinical Problems

David Oriel
University College Hospital,
Gower Street, London WC1E 6AU

The management of patients with genital warts is a problem only too familiar to clinicians. The disease is common, and seems to be becoming commoner; genital warts have appeared in the statistics compiled by the Department of Health and Social Security in England since 1971, and between 1971 and 1973 there was a 30%

increase in new cases of the disease per 100 000 population seen in hospital clinics for sexually transmitted diseases (Table 1). Throughout the world the amount of time spent on the treatment of patients with genital warts must be enormous.

The commonest clinical presentation of genital warts is the familiar condylomata acuminata. Contact-tracing studies have shown that this is a sexually transmitted disease with an incubation period of about two months (Oriel 1971), and presumably the "genital wart virus" is the agent which is sexually transmitted. Condylomata acuminata appear first on the penis (Fig. 1) and vulva (Fig. 2), and at the anus in passive homosexuals. Rarely, lesions appear within the mouth after orogenital contact with an infected partner. Since they are sexually transmitted condylomata acuminata are often associated with other sexually transmitted diseases, and in hospital practice in England approximately 50% of patients with warts have other genital infections, of which non-gonococcal urethritis is the commonest in men and candidosis in women. Clearly, careful screening, with treatment of any associated infections, is necessary before therapy of genital warts is undertaken.

Table 1

New cases of genital warts per 100 000 population at all ages seen in hospital clinics for sexually transmitted diseases in England 1971–1973

Year	*Male*	*Female*	*Male and female*
1971	39.81	20.32	29.79
1972	45.54	23.42	34.17
1973	51.19	26.48	38.50

Condylomata acuminata often spread to adjacent sites, no doubt through the shedding of virus. Approximately 10% of men and 20% of women with genital warts develop anal warts subsequently. In men, warts may involve the distal urethra, and in women the cervix. In contrast with this local extension, which may occur quite rapidly, involvement of areas remote from the genitals does not seem to occur.

Immunological factors affect the growth of condylomata acuminata. Defective cell-mediated immunity is probably the reason for the particularly florid genital warts which are seen in some patients with Hodgkin's disease (Morison 1974). In pregnancy, where cell-mediated immunity is likewise depressed, large lesions may develop whose management often gives difficulty at the time, although they usually regress in the puerperium.

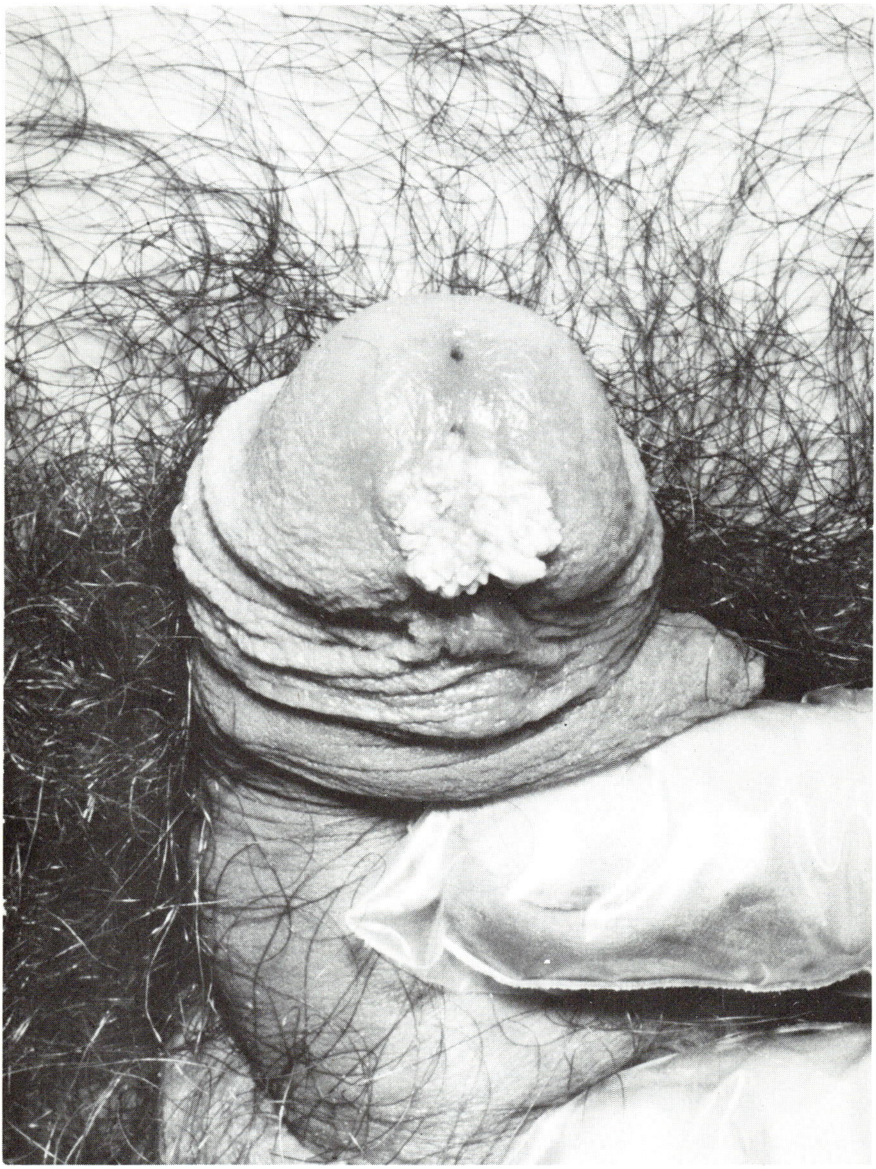

Fig. 1 *Early condylomata acuminata of the penis. The frenum is one of the commonest sites affected*

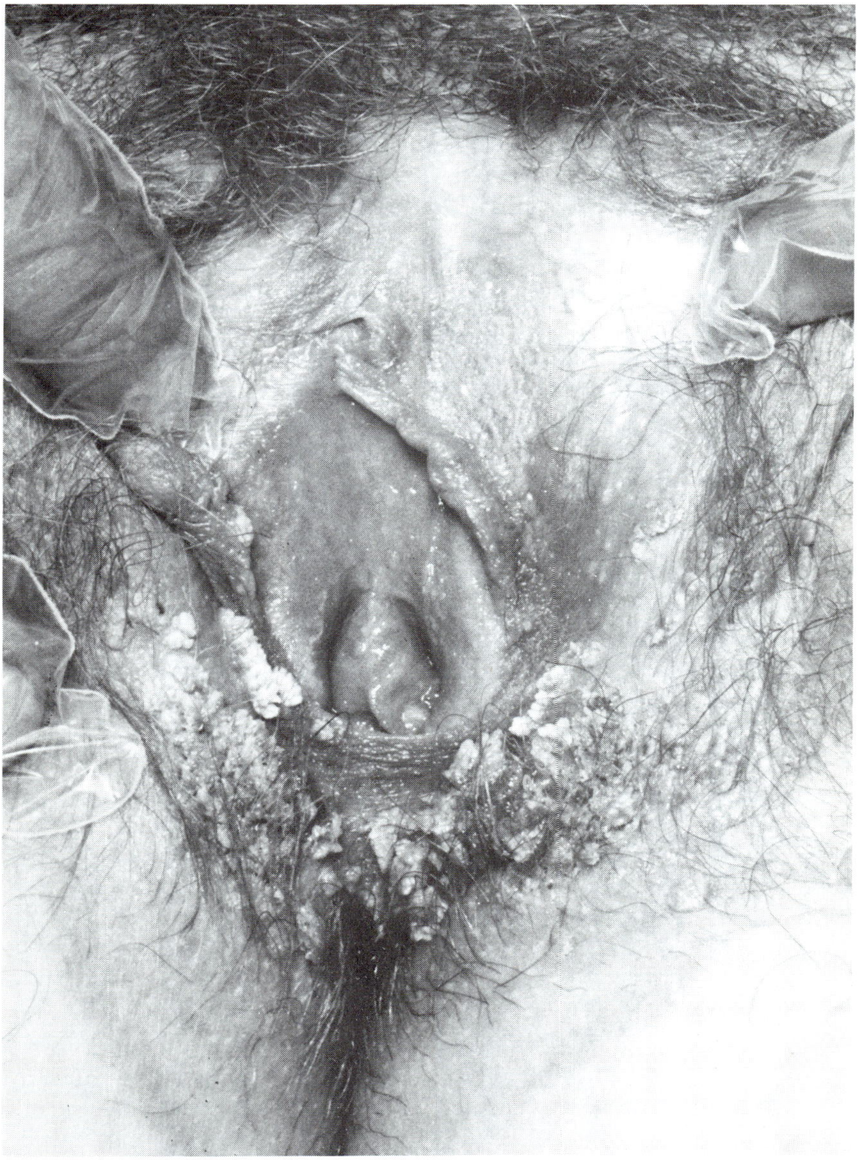

Fig. 2 *Condylomata acuminata of the vulva of two weeks' duration. This patient's sexual contact also had genital warts*

Malignancy is an occasional complication of condylomata acuminata, and has been described in penile, vulval and anal lesions, either as carcinoma-in-situ or as a squamous cell carcinoma (Oriel and Whimster 1971, Fitzgerald and Hamit 1974). Although this complication is fortunately rare, any lesions of atypical appearance or behaviour should be excised early for histological examination.

There is a second variety of genital wart which is quite different in its natural history and clinical appearance from condyloma acuminatum. Common skin warts, verruca vulgaris, occur on most parts of the skin, including that of the genital area (Figs 3, 4). Genital warts of this type are seen much less often than condylomata acuminata. There is no evidence that they are sexually transmitted, and very often the patient is found to have common skin warts elsewhere on the body (Fig. 5), which are presumably the source of the virus (Oriel 1971). These observations accord well with Dr Almeida's description of the virology of warts in the preceding paper (p 179), and we may envisage a "skin wart virus" which may be accidentally transferred to the genitals, probably by the patient's own hands, and a distinct sexually transmitted "genital wart virus". Thus, in terms of natural history and perhaps also in oncogenic potential, there are interesting resemblances between genital herpes and genital warts.

The differential diagnosis of genital warts includes normal states such as coronal papillae and Fordyce's syndrome, molluscum contagiosum and the condylomata lata of secondary syphilis. Distinction of genital warts from carcinoma in older patients may be difficult, and the importance of biopsy has already been stressed.

The treatment of genital warts is notoriously unsatisfactory, and recurrences are common. These may occur either because the original lesions were not destroyed completely or because shedding of virus has already occurred, with the resulting appearance of new warts. It is possible that in some patients defective cell-mediated immunity facilitates this process. A direct surgical attack by cautery, diathermy, cryocautery or the application of corrosives such as trichloracetic acid is favoured by some clinicians; however, the lesions must be destroyed down to the basement membrane if recurrences are to be avoided, and this may involve an unacceptable amount of genital trauma – even then, seedling warts may appear subsequently. More usually, cytotoxic agents are applied, of which podophyllin is the best known (Kaplan 1942). Podophyllin acts against rapidly growing virus-transformed cells. Success with the agent clearly depends in part on its ability to penetrate into the substance of the lesions down to the basement membrane, and for this reason it is more effective in recent, rapidly growing condylomata acuminata; these have only a layer or two of parakeratotic epithelium, and

penetration is relatively easy. Unfortunately, warts which have already been treated several times, and verruca vulgaris, are hyperkeratotic and thus not readily penetrated by podophyllin; lesions of this kind do not respond well and may therefore require cautery. Severe toxic effects have followed the application of large amounts of podophyllin to genital warts; this is particularly likely to occur during pregnancy, when the use of podophyllin is best avoided (Chamberlain *et al.* 1972). A possible alternative to podophyllin is 5-fluorouracil, another antimetabolite which undoubtedly causes regression of some genital warts (Nel and Fourie 1973, Dretler and

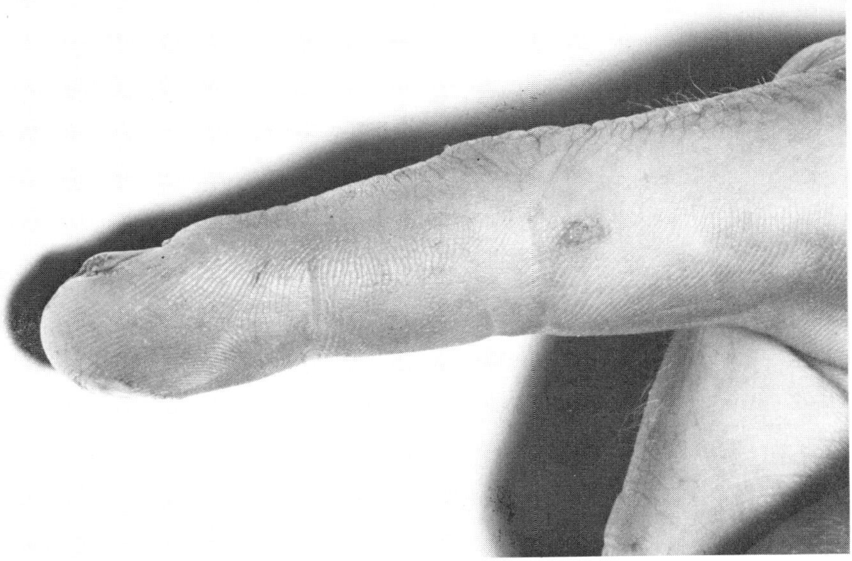

Fig 5 *Common warts on the index finger of the patient illustrated in Fig. 3*

Klein 1975), but the best vehicle and treatment schedule for this agent have yet to be decided, and again it should not be used during pregnancy.

Since wart viruses contain DNA, the use of anti-DNA agents in the treatment of warts has been considered. Theoretically, their action might reduce the appearance of seedling warts, and some of these agents, for instance idoxuridine (IUDR), have a cytotoxic action as well. In a limited clinical trial Morison (1975) has reported favourable on the action of IUDR against skin warts, but little information is available on its effect against genital warts.

Genital warts, like skin warts, have a tendency towards spontaneous cure. This process is complex, and the part played in it by humoral antiviral and antitumour antibodies, and by cell-mediated immunity, is not fully understood. Nevertheless, in an attempt to reproduce natural regression, systemic vaccines have been used in the treatment of genital warts, and some success has been claimed (Nel and Fourie 1973). Evaluation of the results of these procedures is difficult, and the wisdom of systemic administration of a virus of possible oncogenic potential might be questioned.

After a long period of neglect the virology and immunology of warts is now being increasingly studied. The reappraisal of methods of treatment is long overdue, and should be considered in the light of what is already known of the natural history of genital warts. Existing therapeutic procedures must be refined, and new ones introduced, if this increasingly common disease is to be managed satisfactorily.

References

Chamberlain, M. J., Reynolds, A. L. and Yeoman, W. B. (1972). *British Medical Journal* **iii**, 391

Dretler, S. P. and Klein, L. A. (1975). *Journal of Urology* **113**, 195

Fitzgerald, D. M. and Hamit, H. F. (1974). *Annals of Surgery* **179**, 328

Kaplan, I. V. (1942). *New Orleans Medical and Surgical Journal* **94**, 388

Morison, W. L. (1974). *British Journal of Dermatology* **90**, 531

Morison, W. L. (1975). *British Journal of Dermatology* **92**, 97

Nel, W. S. and Fourie, E. D. (1973). *South African Medical Journal* **47**, 45

Oriel, J. D. (1971). *British Journal of Venereal Diseases* **47**, 1

Oriel, J. D. and Whimster, I. W. (1971). *British Journal of Dermatology* **84**, 71

Discussion

Dr Knox (*Chairman*) pointed out that the skin in the genital area was anatomically, physiologically and histologically similar to that of other areas of the body, and asked whether there were two different strains of virus producing the venereal type of wart and the plain wart.

Dr Nahmias said that he had been struck by the difference in behaviour between genital and non-genital warts. He also asked whether it was possible that a baby born to a mother with genital warts might develop clinical wart-like conditions. He had noticed an interesting correlation with laryngeal papillomas and a history of genital warts in the mother at the time of delivery.

Dr Almeida pointed out that there was a strange phenomenon in which the earliest age at which warts were seen in children was about the age of 2, despite the fact that many infants came into contact with people with warts from birth. She asked what happened to the wart virus in infants at this early stage.

Dr Parker asked if there was any evidence that individuals with a history of non-genital warts possessed any immunity to genital warts and whether those with genital warts were less likely to develop non-genital warts.

Dr Oriel replied that there was some evidence to support the first point but no available data on the second point.

Dr Juel-Jensen asked if there was any information about passively transferred antibodies in the newborn or very young. Could passive immunity play a role in preventing early manifestations and could these antibodies disappear at about the age of 2?

Dr Almeida replied that this was a very reasonable explanation of the facts and said that there had been several reports of warts being cured by stimulating local cellular immunity. It was probable that cellular immunity was more important than humoral immunity.

Dr Juel-Jensen asked why some so-called wart cures worked. He thought that some of them just stimulated cell-mediated immunity.

Dr K W M Fulford (*London*) said that in their large series of patients investigated for hepatitis there were about 15 chronic carriers of hepatitis antigen, and among these there was a higher incidence of warts than in the normal population. He thought that the carrier state both for hepatitis virus and for genital wart infection might be due to deficient cell-mediated immunity.

Dr King Holmes asked whether Dr Almeida had experience with organ culture, and how Dr Oriel treated and managed patients with genital warts.

Dr Almeida replied that organ culture had been employed on more than one occasion for the propagation of wart virus, but there had not been clear-cut results.

Dr Oriel said that he used podophyllin but thought it was sometimes left on the lesions for too short a time. It was his practice to use 25% podophyllin in spirit and leave it on for about four hours after the first application, but later to leave it on for a full twenty-four hours. The patients were treated twice a week and if the warts had not cleared within a month he thought there should be a full reassessment of the situation. He was against the ritualistic application of podophyllin for months on end.

Virus Diseases: III. Hepatitis

Australia Antigen-positive Hepatitis as a Sexually Transmitted Disease (*preliminary communication*)

K S Lim
Department of Sexually Transmitted Diseases, The Middlesex Hospital, London W 1
V Taam
The Royal Free Hospital, London NW 3
K W M Fulford and R D Catterall
Department of Sexually Transmitted Diseases, The Middlesex Hospital, London W 1,
Moya Briggs and D S Dane
Department of Virology, The Middlesex Hospital Medical School, London W 1,
and Philippa Simpson
Queen Mary College, London E 1

The association of serum hepatitis with Australia antigen (HBsAg) (Blumberg *et al.* 1965, Prince 1968, Giles *et al.* 1969) was followed within two years by the observation (Prince *et al.* 1970) that a majority of antigen-positive cases gave no history of exposure to infected blood or serum. Occasional case reports suggested that the infection might be transmitted between sexual partners, but there was no evidence that sexual transmission was an important factor in maintaining the prevalence of the disease in the general population.

In 1973 we reported a series of 974 patients attending the Department for Sexually Transmitted Diseases at the Middlesex Hospital (Fulford *et al.* 1973). In this study the incidence of both Australia antigen and Australia antibody was shown to be about 10 times that found in a population of new blood donors tested by identical means. Analysis of information from the case notes showed that antigen-positive patients were mostly heterosexual men of Mediterranean or Middle Eastern origin who were thought to be chronic carriers. By contrast, the distribution of the antibody, which is a marker of previous antigen-positive hepatitis, was associated with promiscuity and with homosexuality among men of British or Western European origin. In a parallel but independent study from the Royal Free Hospital, Heathcote and Sherlock (1973) reported a high incidence of male homosexuality and of previous venereal infection among patients who had had antigen-positive hepatitis and in whom parenteral infection had been excluded. Furthermore, many of the sexual partners of these patients were also positive either for antigen or antibody.

The suggestion was made, therefore, that not only was it possible for Type B hepatitis to be transmitted sexually, but that this method of transmission, at least in the London area, made an important contribution to the general prevalence of the disease. However, certain reservations were necessary in interpreting the results at this stage. First, although we had shown a strong association of the disease with homosexuality we had not identified the precise mechanism of sexual transmission. Secondly, the clinical features of hepatitis as a sexually transmitted disease were undefined. In particular, we had no information on the severity of the acute illness, the proportion of subclinical cases, the incidence of chronic carriers or on the characteristics of infectious cases. Thirdly, neither study was performed under adequately controlled conditions and possible effects of observer bias and case selection could not be excluded.

The present investigation, which was performed as a cooperative study between the groups at the Middlesex Hospital and the Royal Free Hospital, was designed to avoid as far as possible these methodological deficiencies and to extend the range and detail of our clinical and epidemiological information.

Detailed interviews and examinations were carried out by two of the authors (KSL, VT) on 200 male patients attending the Department for Sexually Transmitted Diseases at the Middlesex Hospital between November 1974 and May 1975. Patients of Mediterranean origin were excluded but otherwise cases were selected on a random basis and only 4 refused to take part in the study. Clinical and epidemiological information relating to possible liver disease was obtained by one examiner (KSL) and the histories of sexually transmitted diseases and sexual practices by the other (VT). At the time of interview neither examiner was aware of the other examiner's findings and the results of the laboratory investigations were not available. The study was thus of an unselected population and every attempt had been made to exclude bias. HBsAg and HBsAb were identified by haemagglutination techniques that were more sensitive than the immunodiffusion method used in the original series.

Three antigen-positive patients were identified: all were homosexual and all three had clinical signs of hepatitis. There were 29 antibody-positive patients, and subsequent statistical analyses of the differences between these and the remaining 165 antibody-negative patients revealed information of interest in three main areas: (1) On the possibility that some factor other than sexual practice might explain our original findings. (2) On the clinical course of Type B hepatitis as a sexually transmitted disease. (3) On the distribution of the antibody in relation to differences in sexual practice.

Non-sexual Sources of Infection

Enquiries were made about a wide variety of non-sexual possible source of infection; these are shown in Table 1. No significant differences were found between the antibody positive and negative groups for histories of social jaundice contacts, hospital visiting, engagement in traumatic sports, tattooing, either current or past, blood transfusions, dental treatment, drug abuse, both oral and by injection, inoculations and injections. The sharing of toilet facilites was positively associated with the presence of the antibody and this

Table 1

Non-sexual sources of infection: no significant differences were found for a wide variety of non-sexual possible sources of infection. (The sharing of toothbrushes and razors was shown to be associated with homosexuality but within this group these two factors were equally distributed between antibody positive and negative patients)

Source	*HAb negative (%)*	*HAb positive (%)*	*Statistical significance*
Social contacts:			
Hospital visits	59.3	42.3	NSD
Jaundice	18.0	26.9	NSD
Sports	51.3	53.8	NSD
Parenteral:			
Tattoo	3.3.	–	NSD
Transfusion	1.3	–	NSD
Dental	80.7	76.9	NSD
Drug abuse (injection)	0.7	–	NSD
Inoculations	49.3	34.6	NSD
Injections	70.7	76.9	NSD
Employment:			
Hospitals	25.2	19.2	NSD
Middle East	53.5	50.0	NSD
Tropics	24.5	23.1	NSD
Shared toilet:			
Bathroom	88.7	84.6	NSD
Toothbrush	20.7	3.8	*P*0.07
Razor	14.7	30.8	*P*0.08

NSD: No significant difference

effect was found to be due to sharing toothbrushes and razors. However, this practice was commoner among homosexuals and within this group there was no association with the antibody. Sharing razors and toothbrushes therefore seems to be associated with homosexuality but not to be implicated as a mechanism of transmission of the infective agent. An analysis of occupations, both current and previous, that might be expected to increase the risk of infection, also showed no significant differences between the groups. It should be emphasized that quite different results might be anticipated in other parts of the world where other routes of infection, particularly in childhood, may be important.

Clinical Course

In our previous study we had noted the virtual absence in the clinical records of reference to overt hepatitis. This appeared to contradict the inference from the rate of antibody-positive results that, at least among homosexual men, the disease was common. We had been told by some of our patients that hepatitis was a risk that was well recognized among homosexuals, but it had not been apparent in routine clinical practice. However, under-reporting or under-recording might have accounted for this result. In the present study all patients were interviewed and examined by a doctor with experience of liver disease, and of the 29 who were antibody positive, 7 gave a history compatible with a diagnosis of hepatitis. This result was not significantly different from the rate for the antibody-negative group of whom 21 had a history suggestive of hepatitis and 140 had none. It seems likely, therefore, that if Australia antigen positive hepatitis is acquired sexually the acute stage of the disease is often mild and frequently subclinical.

Sexual Activity

The present study confirmed our previous finding of a strong association between HBsAb and homosexuality. Thus, 21 (30%) of homosexual or bisexual patients were antibody positive as opposed to 50 (70%) who were antibody negative; while in the heterosexual group 7 (5.4%) were antibody positive and 122 (94.6%) were antibody negative. This difference is significant at $P < 0.01$. We were able to confirm also that promiscuity, at least in men, is not associated strongly with the antibody. An analysis of the numbers of sexual partners, regular, casual or professional, reported by heterosexual, homosexual or bisexual men showed that for men with homosexual experience the antibody tended to be associated with increased numbers of casual or professional partners but there were no groups in which the difference reached the 5% level of significance.

Qualitative differences in sexual practice were examined also. For the group as a whole, vaginal intercourse was negatively, and rectal intercourse positively associated with the antibody, but these differences disappeared when the three sexual orientation groups were considered separately. These associations therefore reflected only the sexual orientation of the subjects. A point of particular interest was that we found no association, either for the group as a whole or for heterosexual men alone, between intercourse during menstruation and the presence of the antibody. This would suggest that menstrual blood is not in practice an important vector for the infectious agent. Finally, we examined orogenital intercourse which was found to be associated with the presence of the antibody in the group as a whole at $P < 0.05$. Thus, of the patients who were antibody positive 5 (18.5%) had not had orogenital contact, and 22 (81.5%) had; while of the patients who were antibody negative 69 (44.2%) had had no orogenital contact compared to 87 (55.8%) who had. A breakdown of these figures by sexual orientation, however, showed the effect to be confined to homosexual and bisexual men. This suggests that some element peculiar to homosexual rather than heterosexual orogenital contact is important in the transmission of the disease. Two possible vectors would of course be semen and anal secretions. Unfortunately, our data are incomplete on oral-anal contact, but thus far no significant difference has been demonstrated between those who practise this form of sexual contact and those who do not. On the other hand, the practice of swallowing semen during orogenital contact, although widespread among homosexual men in general, does show a positive association with the antibody. Of the patients who were antibody positive, 14 (50%) had swallowed semen and 14 (50%) had not; of those who were antibody negative, on the other hand, 31 (20%) had swallowed semen, and 124 (80%) had not. This difference is significant at $P < 0.005$.

Australia antigen has been shown (Heathcote *et al.* 1974) to be present in semen when it is present in the blood, and serum known to be infectious parenterally is infectious also, though in larger doses, by oral administration. However, the antigen is present also in saliva (Heathcote *et al.* 1974) and in other body fluids (Sherlock 1972), so that some explanation for the particular infectivity of semen would have to be provided if indeed further epidemiological studies confirm our findings. It may be, for example, that semen is relatively more infectious than other secretions during sexual intercourse simply because it is transferred in, as it were, larger doses. Similar considerations might apply to the route of transmission, that swallowing semen, although a common mechanism of infection, is not the only possible mechanism and that rectal or even vaginal intercourse may also result in transmission of the disease, though less readily or less commonly. None the less, our results may be taken to suggest that semen may be an important vector and that it is infectious particularly when swallowed during orogenital sexual contact.

Summary

A preliminary analysis of the data from 200 unselected male patients attending a clinic for sexually transmitted diseases confirmed the strong association reported previously between male homosexuality and serological evidence of previous Australia antigen positive hepatitis. There were 29 patients with positive serological tests for Australia antibody and 21 of these were either homosexual or bisexual. There was evidence that the acute stage of the disease in its sexually acquired form may be mild in many cases and frequently subclinical. The precise mechanism of transmission of the disease remains undefined but there was no evidence to implicate non-sexual routes, such as drug abuse or tattooing, or, among various aspects of sexual behaviour, promiscuity and rectal intercourse or intercourse during menstruation. However, significant associations were demonstrated with homosexual orogenital contact, and with the practice of swallowing semen. It is suggested that semen itself may be an important vector in the transmission of the infective agent between sexual partners.

References

Blumberg, B. S., Alter, H. J. and Visnich, S. (1965). *Journal of the American Medical Association* **191**, 541

Fulford, K. W. M., Dane, D. S., Catterall, R. D., Woof, R. and Denning, J. V. (1973). *Lancet* **i**, 1470

Giles, J. P., McCollum, R. W., Berndtson, L. W. jr. and Krugman, S. (1969). *New England Journal of Medicine* **281**, 119

Heathcote, J., Cameron, C. H. and Dane, D. S. (1974). *Lancet* **i**, 71

Heathcote, J. and Sherlock, S. (1973). *Lancet* **i**, 1468

Prince, A. M. (1968). *Proceedings of the National Academy of Sciences of the United States of America* **60**, 814

Prince, A. M., Hargrove, R. L., Szmuness, W., Cherubin, C. E., Fontana, V. J. and Jeffries, G. H. (1970). *New England Journal of Medicine* **282**, 987–991

Sherlock, S. (1972). *British Medical Bulletin* **28**, 109

Discussion

Dr King Holmes congratulated Dr Fulford on an extremely important study. He thought that if it could be established that the virus of hepatitis was transmitted among homosexual men by swallowing semen, then it would be possible for the first time to make practical recommendations for prophylaxis against a venereal disease. He pointed out that semen also contained other viruses including the cytomegalovirus.

Dr Fulford's paper should cause the public health authorities to reflect on the methods used to try to control the spread of hepatitis. The data suggested that this was a disease of young urban males who acquired it by homosexual activity or by drug abuse. Since Dr Fulford's first paper on the subject, investigations had been carried out into men attending steam baths and homosexual social functions in Seattle and it had been found that antibody was present in 35% of the homosexual men, which was nearly ten times as high as in a control group of heterosexual men. Antigen had been present in 6% of homosexuals, which was again ten times higher than in heterosexual males. If the Kinsey data indicating that at least 4% of men in a given population were actively homosexual at any time were still true, then in a community like that in Seattle one could conclude that nearly 29% of all hepatitis B would be in homosexual males.

Dr Fulford pointed out that they had not excluded the possibility that oro-anal or other forms of sexual contact might be involved in transmission of the disease. All he could say was that in the present study there was a positive association with the practice of swallowing semen.

He also pointed out that in their original study, in which there were approximately equal numbers of men and women, there were very few homosexual women. However, those women who had had more than 3 sexual partners in a six-month period were ten times as likely to have the antibody than women who had less than 3 sexual partners in a similar period. This was quite different from the situation among the men in the study, for whom homosexuality was of major importance and promiscuity of only minor significance. He thought it was just possible that women who were promiscuous were also women who were more likely to have orogenital sexual contact, including swallowing of semen, and therefore more likely to get infected by this route.

Finally, he was interested that Dr King Holmes had found similar results in the United States and that other people had confirmed the findings in Europe; but the situation was quite different in other parts of the world, particularly in the Eastern Mediterranean and the Middle East.

Dr Almeida asked Dr Fulford to comment on the fact that although he found semen highly infectious, if one looked at vertical transmission it seemed to depend on the mother being positive rather than the father being positive.

Dr Fulford replied that in vertical transmission the factors were completely different and perhaps in this instance it was blood itself that was infectious and was being swallowed. He said he would be surprised if it was found that antibody-positive mothers produced positive children. He thought it was antigen-positive mothers who produced positive children and he thought this was probably due to the swallowing of blood during the process of birth.

Dr Waugh said that a similar study on 600 homosexual male patients had been carried out at the West London Hospital and had produced results comparable with the study at the Middlesex Hospital. He had found that 5.3% of homosexual males were antigen positive and that 40% were antibody positive. He had also found that several members of the group investigated by him had had sexual contact with patients in Dr Fulford's group and also with those from St Mary's Hospital.

Dr Willcox asked whether it was necessary to postulate that the semen was swallowed. He wondered whether the virus could get through abrasions in the lips, diseased gums and other lesions in the mouth.

Dr Fulford replied that he and his colleagues had asked in detail about the swallowing of semen as opposed to merely receiving it into the mouth. He pointed out that homosexual men regarded these practices quite differently. The patients had been divided into 3 groups: those who never swallowed semen, those who did so occasionally, and those in whom it was a regular practice.

Dr Sven A Kvorning (*Copenhagen*) asked whether there was any history of recent infestations with blood-sucking insects.

Dr Fulford replied that he had not found any significant association with scabies or with pediculosis pubis.

Dr P Rodin (*London*) said that he was puzzled why there was a much higher incidence of gonococcal pharyngitis in the United States and Scandinavia than in this country when there seemed to be a similar incidence of Australia antibody and when orogenital sexual practice among homosexuals in both countries seemed to be similar to that in Britain.

Dr Fulford replied that he thought the methods of diagnosing pharyngeal gonorrhoea were not as well developed in the United Kingdom as in some areas of the world but that there might be biological factors responsible as well.

Dr Kvorning said that in Denmark they had found the incidence of pharyngeal gonorrhoea to be as high as 20% of infected patients at one time but the figures had recently gone down and were now about 3% of the total number of infections. He thought this might be due to change in fashions in sexual practices.

Dr Waugh said that he thought that the techniques used in Copenhagen for diagnosing pharyngeal gonorrhoea were superior to those in London and that in Britain we should take note of the techniques used in Copenhagen. He asked Dr Fulford whether there were any age differences between patients with Australia antigen and those with antibody.

Dr Fulford replied that there was no striking difference but that the antibody group had a slightly higher mean age.

Dr E Stolz (*Rotterdam*) said that in his clinic 10% of females and 4% of males were found to have pharyngeal gonorrhoea. Investigations on 2000 patients resulted in 41 being found to have been positive for Australia antigen. In those with antigen-positive sera there was a marked difference between homosexuals and heterosexuals but this was not found in those patients with pharyngeal gonorrhoea. He asked Dr Fulford how he would explain the difference.

Dr Fulford thought this was probably due to the practice of swallowing semen and that this had very different biological implications from simple orogenital contact.

Dr Morton asked whether Dr Fulford was carrying out any serial tests on the patients to see whether antibody and antigen were sustained for months or years or whether there were peaks from time to time.

Dr Fulford replied that he and his colleagues were carrying out serial studies and had only limited data at the present time. He thought that the antigen appeared in the blood three to four weeks before the clinical disease or before biochemical changes occurred and it was probable that the most infective period was immediately prior to the disease becoming clinically manifest. Once the clinical disease disappeared the antigen also started to disappear from the blood and in all but a few cases it had completely gone by the end of six months. Antibody appeared immediately in some cases, but in others only after a latent period and, so far as was known, it was likely to remain positive for the rest of the patient's life. This data was based on transfusion hepatitis and it was possible that the sexually transmitted type might behave differently.

Syphilis

Chairman

Dr Harry J Robinson

President, Royal Society of Medicine Foundation Inc

The Change in Clinical Manifestations

John M Knox
Baylor College of Medicine, Texas Medical Center, Houston, Texas 77025

Data on this important subject are sparse, and many of my comments will be of a personal nature and not necessarily confirmed by observers. However, in an attempt to approach it from a broader base than my own locale, letters were sent to a cross-section of expert clinicians in the United States, Great Britain, and Europe, resulting in a somewhat broadly-based perspective. Specific individuals are not quoted, and only consensus of opinion or thought-provoking concepts are mentioned.

When one speaks of "the change in clinical manifestations", a period of time must be specified – the past twenty-five years, from the early 1900s, or since the initial recognition of the disease at the close of the fifteenth century. I shall begin by reviewing classic primary and secondary syphilis lesions. The classic hunterian chancre is regularly seen today, just as it has been since early times. Also, in most patients the early lesions of secondary syphilis still appear much as they were described in Fracastor's poem, *Syphilis sive morbus gallicus*. Cases of tertiary syphilis – gummas, cardiovascular syphilis, and central nervous system syphilis – are still with us, as is congenital syphilis.

At the beginning of the sixteenth century, syphilis was rampant throughout Europe. Secondary syphilis was referred to as "the great pox", in contrast to smallpox. Systemic manifestations were frequently severe and fatalities were not uncommon. In many instances skin lesions were extensive, destructive and disfiguring. As late as 1935, during the International Congress of Dermatology meeting in Budapest, a number of patients with widespread and severe secondary syphilis were exhibited. Fortunately, physicians now see little or no syphilis of this severity. There have, therefore, been changes in the clinical manifestations of syphilis.

The original severe and often fatal virulent syphilis of the early years gradually and progressively became less severe, as a result either of decrease in virulence of the organism to a more benign form, or of host response; this occurred during three to four hundred years, with most of the attenuation concentrated in the first hundred years.

However, coincident with the introduction of penicillin and other highly effective antibiotics, another evolution has apparently transpired. Armed with a nontoxic, rapid cure, physicians launched an all-out attack on infectious syphilis in the late 1940s and early 1950s. Incidence fell rapidly and it was thought that the disease would soon be eradicated. Such optimistic hopes soon proved to be unrealistic. Syphilis remains endemic throughout most of the world.

As mentioned earlier, the classic signs and symptoms are usual; however, I want to emphasize that clinicians are diagnosing earlier and more subtle manifestations of syphilis. This phenomenon is not limited to early disease, for atypical cases of tertiary syphilis are being discovered and reported. Perhaps it is an educated public that is responsible for the current evolution rather than a change in the disease itself. Most people, at least in the developed countries and in the cities of underdeveloped areas, seek medical care when signs or symptoms suggesting disease appear and persist or progress.

A second change has been the recognition of large numbers of patients with extragenital chancres. There has been an apparent change in morals and behavior within the last two decades. Sexual freedom, including experimentation, is accepted by many. Homosexuals are particularly prone to have anal and oral lesions. Fortunately, the incidence of tertiary and congenital syphilis has decreased. Many believe that this decline has occurred because most cases of infectious syphilis are being diagnosed and treated effectively. Others mention that the lower incidence could be a beneficial effect of widespread indiscriminate use of antibiotics. Perhaps both factors play a role.

Indiscriminate use of antibiotics may have contributed to the fact that atypical and unusual cases of syphilis (all types) are not uncommon. Several authorities mentioned this possibility. Also, corticosteroids and immunosuppressants are quite capable of altering the course of an infectious disease. The following two case histories are illustrative.

Case 1

A 34-year-old white male consulted his dermatologist because of a 4 cm reddish-brown, plaque-like nodule on the left forearm. The disorder began as a small nodule four weeks earlier. Because the lesions suggested a granuloma or a lymphoma, a biopsy was performed. The histology was nonspecific, yet the differential diagnosis included syphilis. A serologic test for syphilis was obtained; the VDRL was reactive at a titer of 1 : 64. This lesion rapidly disappeared following penicillin thereapy.

A retrospective history revealed that the patient often took tetracycline for minor upper respiratory infections and almost any low-grade fever of undetermined origin. There had been no chancre.

Case 2

A 45-year-old petroleum engineer working in a remote area of Mexico suddenly developed pruritic erythematous papules which rapidly became crusted. He had a total of about 12 lesions on the scalp, face, arms, and feet. These were initially treated with Benadryl, without improvement, then with prednisone 15 mg daily, bringing symptomatic relief, but no particular improvement in the lesions.

About four weeks following onset, he returned to the United States and entered the hospital for the annual physical examination required by his employer. Physical examination was unremarkable except for 8–10 erythematous crusted nodules on the face, scalp, left arm, and sole of right foot, Although the lesions were atypical, the clinical differential diagnosis included secondary syphilis. However, the RPR was nonreactive and a biopsy was done. The histology was compatible with syphilis, and VDRL and FTA-ABS tests were obtained which were reactive 1 : 128 and reactive, respectively. The patient was treated with 2.4 megaunits benzathine penicillin with prompt clearing of all lesions. No follow up was carried out.

Conclusion

As a general rule, diseases do not change appreciably and when they do it is primarily the result of environmental factors, technological advances and new knowledge. Syphilis does appear to have evolved from its original virulent stage into a more stable and predictable course; then came penicillin, and syphilis as we have it today. Perhaps the disease has not changed as much as have people and technology: a more educated public that consults a physician earlier, a public that has undergone something of a sexual revolution, and a population that is being diagnosed and treated by highly-trained physicians equipped with sophisticated diagnostic procedures and highly effective antimicrobial agents.

Autoantibodies in Syphilis and in Chronic Biological False Positive Reactors

Professor Deborah Doniach
Department of Immunology,
Middlesex Hospital Medical School,
London W1

Syphilitic patients do not show an increased prevalence of the tissue antibodies found in the "primary" autoimmune disorders (Table 1). However, the Wassermann antibodies which react with cardiolipin, the diphospholipid specific to the mitochondrial inner membranes, may be considered as true autoantibodies, although they arise as a direct result of infection with the treponeme. The treponeme probably has a related phospholipid in its structure which stimulates antibody

Table 1

Tissue antibodies in 75 syphilitic patients

Type of antibody	*Postive reactions (%)*
Antinuclear (ANA)	5
Mitochondrial (AMA)	0
Liver/kidney microsomal (LKM)	0
Smooth muscle	4
Thyroid microsomal	7
Gastric parietal cell	5

synthesis and this leads to cross-reacting antibodies with the host's cardiolipin. This is difficult to prove because *Treponema pallidum* can only grow in living tissues which contain mitochondria, and treponemal extracts are all contaminated with tissue cardiolipins.

Wassermann antibodies are complement fixing and agglutinating but do not produce immunofluorescence (IFL) reactions on tissue sections, probably because the antigenic site is in a hydrophobic part of the molecule. In active secondary syphilis, we described a second type of cardiolipin antibody (CLF) which does stain all mitochondria in tissues (Wright *et al.* 1970, Wright and Doniach 1971). CLF may be present in the serum as early as the first month after appearance of the primary chancre, and is detectable in practically all cases during the active secondary phase where titres vary between 1 and 80 (Fig. 1). At first the antibody is of IgM class, which makes it possible to distinguish between a reinfection and reactivation of an old infection in doubtful cases but it soon switches over and becomes mainly IgG. This antibody disappears within 2–7 weeks upon treatment with antibiotics, although the Wassermann and VDRL remain positive for much longer. We have recently had the opportunity of testing 2 cases of secondary syphilis complicated by syphilitic hepatitis in one case and HB virus hepatitis in the second, and both patients had unusually high titres of 160 and 320 respectively in the CLF fluorescence test. This is of interest in view of the possible confusion with the mitochondrial antibodies of primary biliary cirrhosis (AMA) (Doniach and Walker 1974). These antibodies are directed against an inner membrane lipoprotein which is quite distinct from cardiolipin although giving a similar staining pattern.

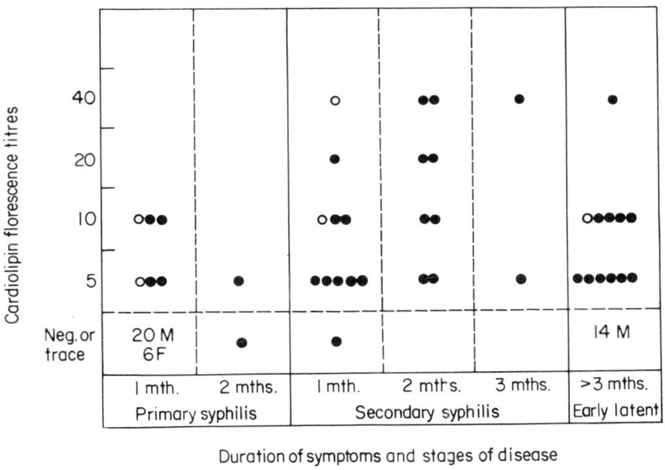

Fig. 1 *Distribution of cardiolipin fluorescence in untreated infectious syphilis*

The CLF can be absorbed with cardiolipin while the mitochondrial fluorescence in chronic liver diseases is unchanged by such treatment. In addition to syphilis, CLF antibodies have been found in the monoclonal IgM of a case of macroglobulinaemia who had VDRL titres of 4000–16 000 and in two other patients with extremely high serological tests for syphilis and no history or clinical evidence of the disease.

In the more usual chronic biological false positive (BFP) reactors the VDRL titre is low, there are often multiple autoantibodies and some of the patients, especially females, later develop collagen disorders (Catterall 1972). Results of our studies (Doniach *et al.* 1970) in 60 cases are shown in Table 2. The most unexpected finding was the high frequency of mitochondrial AMA reactions (56%). These were usually of IgM class and of titres between 2 and 80 but they could not be absorbed out with cardiolipin. Several of the sera gave atypical IFL patterns and at the time we were doubtful as to the relationship of these antibodies to those found in primary biliary cirrhosis. Since then Maas and Schubothe (1973) have described a new syndrome, pseudolupus, where mitochondrial antibodies are present in high titres instead of the more usual antinuclear reactions. Another unusual neurological syndrome associated with BFP reactions and mitochondrial IFL was described by Fulford *et al.* (1972). It now appears that a different mitochondrial antigen is involved in pseudolupus (Berg *et al.* 1975) although, as in the case of CLF, the staining pattern resembles that obtained with cirrhosis sera. It must be stressed that in these two collagen disorders there is no evidence

Table 2

Autoantibodies in 60 patients with chronic BFP reactions

Antibody	*Positive*		*Highest titre*
	No.	%	
Mitochondrial immunofluorescence	34	56	80
Mitochondrial CFT	27	45	512
Smooth muscle fluorescence	16	27	20
Antinuclear (ANA)	28	47	320
CFT rat kidney homogenate	32/41	80	512
Rheumatoid factors (latex FII)	6/58	10	40
Thyroid	16	27	TRC 1280 CFT 64
Gastric parietal cell	6	10	256
Total patients with antibodies	58	96	

of liver disease and most of the patients have normal liver function tests. The pseudolupus syndrome has been attributed to a drug called Venocuran (Knoll AG) given for vascular disorders mainly in Germany, Switzerland and Spain (Grob *et al.* 1975). This contains phenopyrazone, horse-chestnut extract and glycosides from several plants. However, it is thought that some cases arise spontaneously, as the disease has been observed in this country.

In BFP reactors complement fixation titres (CFT) with rat liver mitochondria did not always correspond to the IFL and similar discrepancies were noted in liver cases with classical AMA. When the test was done with whole homogenate of rat kidney, 80% of the BFP reactors gave positive CFT, which suggests antibodies to as yet uncharacterized subcellular components. In syphilis, on the other hand, mitochondrial and tissue extract CFT was proportional to VDRL titres (Fig. 2), which means that the reactions were due to the cardiolipin only.

Thus there are at least 4 autoantibodies reacting with mitochondria in human sera, including the two cardiolipin antibodies, the primary biliary cirrhosis antibodies which react with a dense submitochondrial fraction (specific gravity 1.2) and the pseudolupus antibodies reacting with a lighter fraction (sp. gr. 1.1). It would be interesting to know the exact nature of the AMA found in BFP reactors with this new information in mind.

Mitochondria have enzyme systems and a circular form of DNA which relate them to bacteria. An attractive evolutionary theory

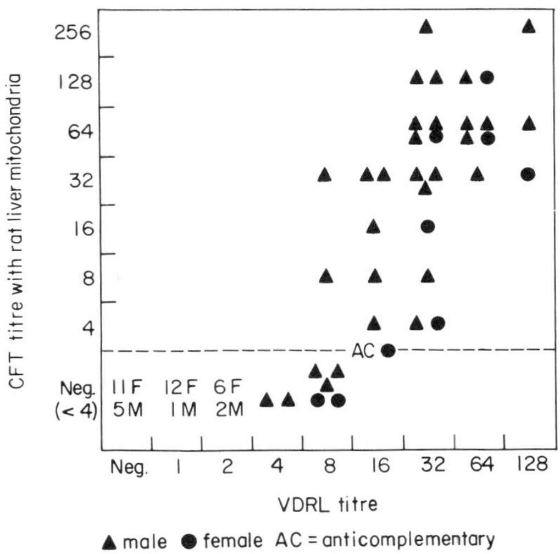

Fig. 2 *Correlation of mitochondrial CFT with VDRL titre in 75 syphilitic patients*

considers them as symbiotic organisms which became incorporated into primitive unicellular organisms and made it possible for them to evolve into more complex beings owing to the specialized ability of mitochondria to produce energy. Many patients with autoimmune disorders show positive leukocyte migration inhibition tests (LMT) when mitochondria are used as the antigen even though mitochondrial antibodies cannot be detected in their serum. These diseases include thyroiditis (Wartenberg *et al.* 1973), gastritis, adrenalitis and juvenile diabetes mellitus. It would be interesting to study syphilitic patients by LMT with mitochondria to see if they have cellular immunity to cardiolipin. The purified phospholipid has proved too insoluble and toxic to lymphocytes in this test.

References

Berg, P. A., Binder, T., Lindner, H. M., Bannaski, H., Maas, D., Hemming, H. and Brügel, H. (1975). *Deutsche medizinische Wochenschrift* **100**, 1123
Catterall, R. D. (1972). *British Journal of Venereal Diseases* **48**, 1
Doniach, D., Delhanty, J., Lindqvist, H. J. and Catterall, R. D. (1970). *Clinical and Experimental Immunology* **6**, 871
Doniach, D. and Walker, G. J. (1974). *Gut* **15**, 664
Fulford, K. W. M., Catterall, R. D., Delhanty, J. J., Doniach, D. and Kremer, M. (1972). *Brain* **95**, 373
Grob, P. J., Müller-Schoop, J. W., Häcki, M. A. and Joller-Jemelka, H. (1975). *Lancet* **ii**, 144
Maas, D. and Schubothe, H. (1973). *Deutsche medizinische Wochenschrift* **98**, 131
Wartenberg, J., Doniach, D., Brostoff, J. and Roitt, I. M. (1973). *Clinical and Experimental Immunology* **14**, 203
Wright, D. J. M. and Doniach, D. (1971). *Proceedings of the Royal Society of Medicine* **64**, 419
Wright, D. J. M., Lessof, M. M., Grimble, A. S., Doniach, D., Turk, J. C. and Catterall, R. D. (1970). *Lancet* **i**, 740

Some Aspects of Research on Syphilis: Serological Evidence of Activity of the Disease

A E Wilkinson
Venereal Disease Reference Laboratory (PHLS),
The London Hospital, London E1 2BL

Treponemal tests, such as the TPI, FTA-ABS and TPHA tests, will provide a diagnosis of treponemal infection with some certainty. But positive results do not show whether the disease process is active or whether they are merely a relic of a long past, adequately treated infection – a "serological scar" as Harrison termed it. Because most infections in this country are first diagnosed on serological evidence

Table 1

Serological tests as possible indications of recent or active infection

Antibody	*Occurrence*
Antilipoidal (reagin)	Rising titre. ? Persistent high titre after treatment (VDRL $\geq$ 16)
Cardiolipin F	Present in early infections
Antitreponemal (specific)	IgM as "early warning" test. IgM in neonatal syphilis. IgM in latent and late syphilis

in the latent stage, a laboratory test that provided evidence of activity would be of help to the clinician. Some work bearing on this is reviewed; the main approaches are summarized in Table 1.

Antilipoidal Antibody (Reagin)

Although the function of reagin is still uncertain, its level seems to be roughly related to the amount of tissue reaction by the host, rising rapidly with increasing numbers of treponemes in early syphilis and later falling as the number of organisms declines with developing immunity. Frederiksson *et al.* (1968) noticed this when they correlated the reagin and immobilizing antibody response with the histological changes in experimental syphilis in animals.

It is common practice to regard a rising reagin titre as evidence of a developing infection or of relapse. The interpretation of persisting high levels of reagin (VDRL $\geqslant 16$) in a minority of treated patients is uncertain. If treatment is thought to have been adequate, many would ignore them, but the suspicion remains that they might mean continued activity of the disease.

Cardiolipin F Antibody

This antibody reacts with the inner membranes of mitochondria and was demonstrated by an indirect fluorescence test with sections of kidney as substrate by Wright *et al.* (1970). Although it can be absorbed from serum by cardiolipin or VDRL antigen, its titre does not seem to be related to the VDRL titre. It is found mainly in primary, secondary and early latent syphilis and soon disappears after treatment; its presence is thought to suggest a fairly recent infection and to be of use in dating latent infections. Similar results have been reported by Andre *et al.* (1973).

IgM Specific Antitreponemal Antibody

In syphilis, as in many infections, the earliest humoral response is the production of IgM antibody, followed by IgG. This order of development has been found both in man and in experimentally infected rabbits. The FTA-ABS test with monospecific antiglobulin conjugates has proved a useful method for studying the contribution made by the immunoglobulin classes at different stages of infection.

The early appearance of IgM led to hopes that an FTA-ABS test for IgM might provide an "early-warning" test applicable to the prompt detection of syphilis in contacts. In practice, however, it is unusual to find IgM antibody alone without IgG also being present, but I have seen this pattern in a very few cases.

IgM Antibodies in Neonatal Syphilis

IgM antibodies do not cross the intact placenta. The presence of specific antitreponemal IgM antibody in cord blood or serum from a baby was thought (Scotti and Logan 1968) to indicate active infection of the child. Similar findings have been reported by a number of groups of workers (Alford *et al.* 1969, Scotti *et al.* 1969, Armenio and Cecil 1970, Mamunes *et al.* 1970, Kipnis *et al.* 1971, Johnston 1972) although Sepetjian *et al.* (1970) express some reservations. Serial tests may be needed to detect infection because some babies show a delayed onset, the FTA-ABS IgM test being negative at birth but becoming positive after an interval of up to several weeks. This could be due to infection having occurred late in pregnancy or to competition between IgG and IgM in the test.

Table 2

Reports of IgM FTA-ABS test reactivity at various stages of syphilis

Authors	*Sera IgM reactive/sera tested*		
	Early	*Latent*	*Late and congenital*
Atwood and Miller (1969) ● ■	3/3	0/3	2/5
Logan *et al.* (1969) ■		20/49	11/17
Julian *et al.* (1969) ●	33/33		
Atwood and Miller (1970) ● ■	23/23	47/94	20/30
Julian *et al.* (1971) ●		47/69	
O'Neill and Nicol (1972) ●	91/92	36/36	10/10

● Untreated or inadequately treated
■ Treated

IgM Antibody in Acquired Syphilis

Reports of the results of FTA-ABS IgM tests at different stages of syphilis are summarized in Table 2.

There is agreement in all these studies that IgM antitreponemal antibody is consistently present in untreated primary and secondary syphilis. From serial tests on the same groups of patients O'Neill and Nicol (1972) found that on average it persisted for three to six months after treatment of primary syphilis and for an average of eight months after treatment of secondary or early latent infections. They suggest that arrest of disease is associated with its disappearance; persistence may reflect recent or inadequate treatment or relapse. Its continued presence in a proportion of treated late infections is surprising; in the series reported by Logan *et al.* (1969) the patients had been treated thirteen years previously and about half were still positive. Atwood and Miller (1969) have suggested that its continued presence may reflect persistence of the antigen.

In all these studies the test was carried out with sorbent to remove group antitreponemal antibody. Some preliminary results of tests with a sonicate of Reiter treponemes for the removal of this antibody are shown in Table 3.

This work is incomplete, but the IgM FTA test has been found positive in a proportion of treated late infections.

The IgM FTA-ABS test requires careful control of the reagents used and it may be more complex than is apparent at first sight. Reimer *et al.* (1975) have recently reported that some syphilitic babies do not produce significant amounts of IgM antibody against *T. pallidum*, but instead make an antibody of IgM class which reacts against IgG – a rheumatoid factor-like antibody. This could react with treponemes in the antigen which have united with passively

Table 3

IgM reactivity at various stages of disease (FTA-ABS tests with Reiter sonicate)

Stage	*Sera IgM reactive/sera tested*	
	Untreated	*Treated*
Primary	3/3	1/3
Secondary	11/11	5/11
Latent	3/5	0/7
Late and congenital	—	5/14
Latent treponemal disease (?yaws ? syphilis) in patients from yaws areas	1/12	6/20

transferred maternal IgG antitreponemal antibody to give an apparent positive FTA-IgM test. Rheumatoid factor has been found in some early and late syphilitic sera, so that a similar process could occur at other stages of the disease. They also found some evidence of inhibition of IgM by excess IgG antibody, tending to a false negative result. This competition has also been demonstrated experimentally in the FTA system by Cohen *et al.* (1967). These findings suggest that further study of the FTA IgM test is necessary to eliminate these possible pitfalls before we use it as an indication of active disease.

References

Alford, C. A., Polt, S. S., Cassidy, G. E., Straumfjord, J. V. and Rimington, J. S. (1969). *New England Journal of Medicine* **280**, 1086

Andre, D., Salussola, D. and Trepo, C. (1973). *Pathologie et Biologie* **21**, 697

Armenio, L. and Cecil, A. (1970). *Pediatria* (*Napoli*) **78**, 246

Atwood, W. G. and Miller, J. L. (1969). *Archives of Dermatology* **100**, 763
Atwood, W. G. and Miller, J. L. (1970). *International Journal of Dermatology* **9**, 259
Cohen, I. R., Norins, L. C. and Julian, A. J. (1967). *Journal of Immunology* **98**, 143
Frederiksson, T., Hederstedt, B. and Rosengren, S. (1968). *Acta pathologica et microbiologica Scandinavica* **72**, 125
Johnston, N. A. (1972). *British Journal of Venereal Diseases* **48**, 464
Julian, A. J., Logan, L. C. and Norins, L. C. (1969). *Journal of Immunology* **102**, 1250
Julian, A. J., Logan, L. C., Norins, L. C. and Scotti, A. T. (1971). *Infection and Immunity* **3**, 559
Kipnis, J., Camargo, M. E., Netto, C. F., Ferreira, A. W. and Guarnieri, D. B. (1971). *Revista do Instituto de medicina tropical de São Paulo* **13**, 179
Logan, L. C., Norins, L. C., Atwood, W. G. and Miller, J. L. (1969). *Journal of Investigative Dermatology* **53**, 300
Mamunes, P., Cave, V. G., Budell, J. W., Anderson, J. A. and Steward, R. E. (1970). *American Journal of Diseases of Children* **120**, 17
O'Neill, P. and Nicol, C. S. (1972). *British Journal of Venereal Diseases* **48**, 460
Reimer, C. B., Black, C. M., Phillips, D. J., Logan, L. C., Hunter, E. F., Pender, B. J. and McGrew, B. E. (1975). *Annals of the New York Academy of Sciences* **254**, 77
Scotti, A. T., and Logan, L. (1968). *Journal of Pediatrics* **73**, 242
Scotti, A. T., Logan, L. and Caldwell, J. G. (1969). *Journal of Pediatrics* **75**, 1129
Sepetjian, M., Guerraz, F. T., Monier, J. C., Nivelon, J. L. and Thivolet, J. (1970). *British Journal of Venereal Diseases* **46**, 18
Wright, D. J. M., Doniach, D., Lessof, M. H., Turk, J. L., Grimble, A. S. and Catterall, R. D. (1970). *Lancet* **i**, 740

Discussion

Dr J R W Harris (*London*) asked Professor Doniach if she had any detailed results of liver function tests and fluorescent tests on patients with secondary syphilis.

Professor Doniach replied that liver function tests were usually normal in uncomplicated secondary syphilis. Syphilitic hepatitis was a rare disease and was associated with a rise in transaminases. The cardiolipin fluorescent antibodies (CLF) were present in nearly all secondary syphilis cases in titres up to 1 : 80 and disappeared within a few weeks of penicillin treatment. In 2 cases of syphilitic hepatitis studied so far, the CLF fluorescence had been of higher titre (160–320) and could be entirely absorbed out by cardiolipin. The mitochondrial antibodies (AMA) in primary biliary cirrhosis stained the same renal tubules as CLF but the antigen was quite different, being an inner membrane lipoprotein, so that the AMA fluorescence remained intact after mixing the serum with excess cardiolipin.

Dr Lawrence said that in central London he had seen an increasing number of patients with early syphilis presenting with neurological features. These were principally VIII nerve perceptive deafness, but one 50-year-old man had bilateral papilloedema only and one 35-year-old man developed a complete right facial palsy 24 hours after commencing penicillin therapy, probably as a Herxheimer reaction. The majority of them responded satisfactorily to anti-syphilitic treatment: he wondered whether Dr Knox had seen similar problems in Houston.

Dr Knox said that they had not seen many cases of this sort in Houston, where they diagnosed approximately 30 to 40 cases of primary and secondary syphilis each month. The total incidence of gonorrhoea in his clinic was now 18 000 cases a year.

Dr Nahmias said he had had similar problems to Dr Wilkinson with the IgM test producing false positive and false negative results. He suggested that one way of overcoming this was by using absorption with staphylococcus protein A. He asked Professor Doniach if the explanation for the antibodies to the mitochondria could be that there were micro-organisms and bacteria-like mitochondria inside the cells which might be associated with the disease.

Professor Doniach replied that this was a decided possibility and that an unknown virus or bacterium might have antigenic properties in common with mitochondria so that the patient's mitochondrial antibodies might represent a cross-reaction.

Dr Stolz asked if Professor Doniach had found antibodies against smooth muscle and mitochondria in the secondary stage of syphilis.

Professor Doniach replied that these two antibodies were not found in syphilitic patients as a rule. The incidence of thyroid, gastric and nuclear reactions was also the same in syphilitics as in normal controls.

Dr Stolz said that some of his colleagues had found in patients with secondary syphilis a high percentage of smooth muscle immunofluorescence.

Professor Doniach replied that at the time her studies were done, smooth muscle antibodies were imperfectly understood. Now at least three types of SMA could be distinguished by immunofluorescence and one of them appeared to be anti-actin. A more detailed study of SMA in early syphilis would be a good subject for the future, since these antibodies appeared transiently in many viral infections, in mycoplasma pneumonia and in various cancers.

Dr Krause asked about the possible role of autoantibodies in the pathogenesis of lesions in secondary syphilis and tertiary syphilis. One possibility was that there were autoantibodies similar to those in lupus erythematosus such as those against nucleic acid. For example it had been shown that skin and kidney lesions in lupus were due to complexes of the autoantibodies and the nucleic acid. He asked whether there was any evidence of such complex deposits in the lesions.

Dr Fulford said that he had recently examined a small number of sections from primary chancres and had found some IgM, IgG and complement. It was in the vessel walls in some cases and diffusely distributed in others. The work was proceeding and there was not yet enough information to present a clear picture.

Dr Robinson (*Chairman*) pointed out the importance of immune complexes in collagen diseases and spoke of the great efforts that were now under way to attempt to block these interactions either through new drugs or immune mechanisms.

Dr Knox said that immune complexes in the skin of the patients with lupus erythematosus were limited to the basement membrane area but that histopathologically there were much broader changes than that one area. Also, immune complexes were found in clinically normal skin of patients with systemic lupus erythematosus. He cautioned that care should be taken not to attribute to the immune complexes the cause of skin lesions. The immune complexes might equally well be the result of the disease. In many inflammatory skin diseases, immune complexes could be found but proof should be established before they were considered to be the specific cause.

Dr Wilkinson pointed out that there had been reports of immune complexes in the kidneys of patients with congenital syphilis.

Dr Fred P Sparling (*North Carolina*) said he was surprised that Dr Knox had not made further comments on atypical neurosyphilis as there had been an increasing number of cases reporting with these manifestations.

Dr Knox agreed and thought that neurologists should still be on the alert so as not to miss neurosyphilis. With the recent increase in the incidence of early syphilis it was important to look out for unusual cases including deafness and blindness.

The Future Direction of Research into Syphilis

Thomas B Turner
*Johns Hopkins University School of Medicine,
Baltimore, Maryland 21205*

At the request of the program committee I have dusted off my crystal ball in an attempt to discern the shape of things to come in research on the treponemal diseases. More often, however, the crystal ball turns out to be nothing more than a reflecting pool, mirroring in slightly distorted form the experiences, hopes, defeats and yearnings of the viewer. Yet as Whitehead (1947) has pointed out, the world of values, which constantly modifies the world of action, comprises both the past and the future. It is in this context that I shall look backward and forward in an attempt to bring some perspective, some values if you will, that might help us with the present.

The most easily documented and perhaps the most encouraging statement to be made is that in each decade of this century significant advances in knowledge of the treponemal diseases have occurred. There is every reason to anticipate, therefore, that succeeding decades will be equally fruitful. Indeed, it is my expectation that in this decade or the next extraordinary developments in this field will occur. I shall suggest the bases for that statement, so embellished by faith. My task is made easier by the perceptive papers by Dr Knox, Professor Doniach and Dr Wilkinson, which really look into the future.

The Projection of History

Let me first adopt the posture of the historian, who may be the best prophet in the long run. Short of the discovery of some ancient manuscripts, it is unlikely that much direct new evidence on the origin of syphilis and the treponemal diseases will be forthcoming. Yet there is plenty of latitude for new interpretations of old facts in the light of the growth of knowledge.

For example, the discovery of treponemal infections in nonhuman primates in the African jungles raises questions of historical import. If syphilis in fact was only indigenous to the Western hemisphere before 1492, is the current situation an example of retrograde evolution whereby five centuries ago the spread of infection was from the Western hemisphere to Europe, to Africa, to the jungles? This seems less likely than that these arboreal diseases are very ancient, possibly even the original reservoir, although it should be noted that nonhuman primate infection has been found only in animals living near foci of human infection, an observation open to various interpretations.

Again, we know enough about the close biological relationship between the yaws and syphilis treponemes to visualize that mutations in either direction might readily have taken place more than once.

The fifteenth century saw great movements of people between Asia and Europe and Africa; overland through Constantinople until the gateway was closed in 1453; across the Sahara, around the Cape of Good Hope, and eventually from along the West coast of Africa – all long before the Western hemisphere was host to Columbus and his men. Hackett (1963) has traced some of these migrations from the viewpoint of the treponemal specialist – fascinating material.

The field of historical evolution is also challenged by recognition of a natural treponemal infection in rabbits, first in England and shortly thereafter in America. A disease now known to be widespread in many areas of the world, it is bacteriologically, immunologically, and therapeutically out of the same package as yaws and syphilis. How many other species harbor natural treponemal infection is not known. Was all this recent on the historical scale, and if so, was the direction of spread among species from higher to lower, or vice versa? If ancient, what are the evolutionary implications? We can only speculate on all these questions, but even tentative answers carry us away from simplistic notions of the origin of syphilis and its prototypes.

Cultivation of Virulent Treponema Pallidum

For fifty years or more cultivation of *T. pallidum* on artificial media has headed the list of priorities in syphilis research. And well it might; for at every turn the investigator of treponemal diseases is frustrated by the lack of this missing link so clearly elucidated by Robert Koch. A renewed research effort is now being mounted in universities, research institutes, and industrial laboratories. Promising murmurings emerge from time to time, but it cannot be documented that we are significantly closer to the goal than before. Yet despite years of disappointment, faith in the processes of intelligent biochemical research permits a degree of optimism on this score. Encouraging is the growing interest of investigators whose competence has been tested in other fields.

It would be presumptuous of me to suggest new approaches with any confidence, although recent work on nutritional immunity (Weinberg 1974, 1975) indicates the complexity of the requirements of many bacterial species for trace metals and other nutrients. Moreover, evidence is accumulating that mutual biological antagonisms occur between such trace metals as zinc, selenium, cadmium and copper (Davies 1974). The rational step by step approach of well trained investigators hopefully will lead to the goal; or else some competent scientist may, like Arthur Koestler's Sleepwalker, blunder on to the key. It seems reasonably certain, however, that unless there are a few laboratories where there is sophisticated knowledge of disease-inducing treponemes, unless there are at least a few individuals who are familiar with the handed-down skills of spirochetal research, opportunities for successful cultivation will scarcely exist.

Therapeutics

It seems unlikely that a better, all-purpose, single therapeutic agent than penicillin will become available; nor would one be needed were it not for well-known biologic clouds that overhang our abandoned drive down the therapeutic speedway.

It is scarcely necessary to dwell upon the high prevalence of penicillin-sensitive individuals found among present populations – now in the order of 20% of older adults. Will this figure increase or decline? Is it a product of the prodigal use of penicillin in the decades immediately following World War II, or is the currently more circumspect use of the drug adequate to maintain this rate? No good cohort studies are available, yet answers would be of practical value in planning for the future.

Another small cloud still only faintly in the distance is the possibility of increasing resistance of *T. pallidum* to penicillin. There is no evidence that this is happening, a heartening sign in the light of the rapid development of resistant strains in many other species of bacteria. Yet enough is known about the development of resistant mutants to leave little room for complacency. The treponeme has shown itself to be a resourceful and versatile adversary, challenging man's ingenuity at every turn. It behooves us to be wary, to respect its capability for survival which may parallel that of the human species.

To revert to the pragmatic, every antimicrobial agent should be tested against *T. pallidum*. Perhaps it would be unrealistic at this time to commit substantial resources to developing new drugs just for syphilis, but the notion should not be buried altogether. Of course, the penicillin-sensitive proportion of the syphilitic population of the world still provides a significant demand for therapeutic agents other than penicillin.

Shall We See Tertiary Syphilis Again?

To my generation of physicians, syphilitic aortic regurgitation, thoracic aneurysm, tabes dorsalis, general paresis and other manifestations of tertiary syphilis were commonplace. Now they are museum pieces. The point in mentioning these earmarks of a bygone age is that they may just come again; not in such profusion to be sure, but often enough to confound the skilled diagnostician and engender embarrassing lost opportunities for therapeutic success.

The evidence is overwhelming that everywhere in western civilization the incidence of syphilis – the new infection rate – declined precipitously in the 1950s. It is pleasant to believe that this was due to measures directed to the control of syphilis. Certainly these helped, but it seems to me more likely that the dramatic decline in syphilis was primarily a product of the widespread use of penicillin. For every fever the word was: treat and think later, and Western populations were blanketed with an overlay of penicillin – "penicillin fallout", as Schamberg termed it.

But with decline in the use of penicillin the new-infection rate has been slowly climbing. Since the most serious manifestations of tertiary syphilis have a lag time of fifteen to twenty years, the low current incidence of these conditions may simply reflect the trough of the new-infection rate. What is ahead? One need not be a Cassandra to expect an increase in tertiary syphilis. Our index of suspicion should be high. Moreover, one should be alert for new syndromes by the "great imitator", e.g. the apparent change in the clinical patterns of neurosyphilis, as described by Smith (1969) and by Hooshmand *et al.* (1972).

Serology

The tangled web of serologic tests for syphilis is likely to snare all but the most sophisticated clinician and epidemiologist whom, it should be remembered, the tests are designed to enlighten. As new tests have been developed over the decades countless studies to assess so-called sensitivity and specificity have been made, most of them without much relation to a clinical base, while certain fundamental yet very practical questions have remained largely unanswered.

The earliest serologic tests for syphilis stemmed from basic immunological investigations of complement fixation and immune flocculation in the first decade of the century. Many modifications of these techniques have been introduced. Later, tests based on immobilization of living treponemes, immune adherence, immunofluorescence and hemagglutination have been added. Out of this serologic Tower of Babel has come some illumination for the clinician, but not much. Indeed, one would have difficulty in stating with assurance that in the realm of serology the knowledgeable physician is much better off today than he was fifty years ago. Of all these tests only the TPI seems to detect a special antibody. This is not to decry the value of this vast investigative effort, but one has the feeling that perhaps the most important questions have not been addressed; that the clinician and the serologist have often not been on the same wavelength.

In broad terms, the clinician and the epidemiologist would like to know whether the individual has ever had syphilis; whether the infection is still present; whether there are reliable indices to the activity of the disease; what can be learned about the immune status of the individual. Most of the studies on sensitivity and specificity have been directed to the first question, but this has been largely on a trial and error basis in which two unknowns are involved. Very little research has been carried out on the biological and immunological basis of positive reactions in the absence of one of the major treponemal diseases. What, for example, is the role of symbiotic infections with saprophytic types of treponemal-like organisms which are universally present in the mouth, gastrointestinal tract and about the anus? It has been known for years that pathogenic and nonpathogenic treponemes share certain common antigens (D'Alessandro *et al.* 1949, D'Alessandro and Dardanoni 1953, Nell and Hardy 1966), but there has been little attempt to assess the serologic role of the nonpathogens. Thus far it appears that only the TPI test qualitatively stands apart as an index of host invasion by pathogenic treponemes, and even here false positives probably occur.

After fifty years the relation of positive serologic tests to persistence of infection is not clear. The question is complicated by recent work suggesting the persistence of treponemes after what is regarded as adequate treatment. It is known, however, that in thoroughly treated rabbits in which infectivity tests are negative, serologic tests may remain positive in low titre. A related question is whether there is a reliable serologic index to the activity of treponemal infections. The evidence from animals strongly suggests that the titre of lipoidal antigen tests is correlated with the degree of tissue reactivity to the treponeme (Turner 1970). In short, it seems likely that high titre tests (8 units or more) indicate active disease. But the scientific base for this statement is inadequate, although the question is an important one and should be actively explored.

Finally, it would be highly advantageous if some information were available on the significance of positive serologic tests in terms of the immune status of the individual. Clearly the results of lipoidal antigen tests shown no correlation (Turner 1970), but the situation as it relates to the TPI antibody and to immunofluorescence is anything but clear. Not only would clarification be desirable from the clinical standpoint, but if the development of treponemal vaccine becomes a reality, such indices of immunity would be most useful.

It is not suggested that the answers to these persistent questions can be obtained easily, but without research directed to them there is little hope that answers will be forthcoming.

Antigenic Composition of Treponemes

Progress has been made in the past two decades in sorting out the antigenic components of treponemes. Beginning with D'Alessandro and his associates in 1949, a number of investigators have identified, in varying degrees of purity, protein, carbohydrate, and lipid fractions (Nell and Hardy 1966, Pillot *et al.* 1973, Pillot and Dupouey 1964, Dupouey 1972). For the most part these studies have dealt with cultivable strains, because of the difficulty of obtaining sufficient quantities of the pathogenic organisms for analytical work. More recently electronmicroscopic and microchemical methods have been used by Ovcinnikov *et al.* (1974) and Hardy *et al.* (1975) to relate antigenic fractions to specific structural components of the treponeme. This type of research is most promising and we may yet see the emergence of serologic tests whose immunologic base is much more specific than anything presently available.

Immunity in Syphilis

The subject of immunity in syphilis is too broad and complex to be summarized in a paragraph. Suffice it to say there is demonstrably enhanced resistance to infection which develops slowly and persists well after all traces of infection have been eliminated, and there are both humoral and cellular expressions of this resistance; but tools for their study are still crude. The more sophisticated techniques for the study of the cellular aspects of resistance have not been widely applied to immune phenomena in the treponemal diseases, although attempts in this direction have been made by, among others, Levene *et al.* (1971), Fulford and Brostoff (1972), Musher *et al.* (1972), Wicher *et al.* (1974), Musher *et al.* (1974) and Metzger and Michalska (1974). Study of the differing roles of human T and B lymphocytes may offer new insights into treponemal immunity. T cells derived from the thymus appear to be involved primarily in cellular immunity, while the bone-marrow-derived B cells play a role in humoral immunity (Bentwich and Kunkel 1973, Fridman *et al.* 1974).

It seems likely that damaging lesions in syphilis are basically an expression of an antigen-antibody reaction at the cellular level (Rodin and Komarovskaya 1972). The practical benefits of a deeper knowledge of this basic phenomenon can scarcely be predicted.

The Dormant Treponeme

All this emphasizes how little is known about the basic relationship between the syphilis treponeme and its human host. When they are in open conflict lesions flare, serology bubbles up, the spirochete can be visualized and the host is often sick. But there comes a time when they lie down together, so to speak, apparently in peace and comfort, often without specific treatment, sometimes after it. It is a problem that needs intensified exploration, for latency in syphilis is shrouded in mystery. Is it basically a continuing antigen-antibody interaction in which the activity of the one component wanes while the other waxes? Or are there hitherto unsuspected factors involved, such as that connoted by the term "nutritional immunity" (Weinberg 1974, 1975)?

It is not necessary to recite in detail the growing evidence pointing to the persistence of still virulent *T. pallidum* in human beings and animal models after treatment to recognize that questions of major import have been raised. When the literature is critically reviewed, however, the hard evidence is meagre. There can be no doubt that treponemes of disease-producing capabilities persist in some persons after what is generally regarded as adequate treatment with penicillin. But in what proportion of cases does it occur and what are the circumstances that lead to this result?

It has been known for many years that despite so-called adequate penicillin treatment for early syphilis there is a small therapeutic failure rate, in some large series up to 5%. What is the explanation? It does not seem to be that the remaining treponemes are penicillin resistant, for transferred to a new host they have been found to be consistently penicillin sensitive. Is it that penicillin acts only on dividing cells, as in other species of bacteria, and that some treponemal cells may have been in a biologically dormant state during the course of penicillin therapy? This view is supported by the studies of Collart (1974) and associates, and appears to be the most likely explanation at present. Or are there areas of the body, the eye or the central nervous system, for example, which are penetrable by treponemes but not readily by penicillin? The facts seem to be determinable but have not been conclusively demonstrated.

One facet of the problem seems abundantly clear, however, which is that in the present state of our technology the mere visualization of a treponemal-like organism, with or without supposedly immunospecific stains, does not provide conclusive evidence that the visualized treponemes are pathogenic *T. pallidum*. Not only are there artifacts that resemble treponemes, but saprophytic treponemes are commonly present in various parts of the body and may well be found in aberrant locations. Expensive and time consuming as it may be, therefore, it seems to me essential that infectivity tests form the anchor to this type of research.

Epidemiological, Behavioral and Sociological Research

These important aspects of syphilis research will not be dwelt upon at length, for they are common to all the venereal diseases and have already received attention in this symposium. A continuing problem in the field of syphilis, however, is measurement of incidence. While the age distribution of new infections might not be changing much, there is growing evidence that profound changes are occurring in the sociological patterns of infection.

Detection of these changes is important in order to focus health educational efforts more sharply. We usually succeed in educating the people who need it least, while the high-risk groups are notoriously difficult to reach; or so it has been. We should make renewed efforts to direct educational efforts to those groups where the problem is greatest.

Even so, the lessons of history are that we change human nature but slowly if at all; the old savage still inhabits the new civilization. By supplying new things — clean water, motor cars, contraceptive pills — we alter the results of what the old savage does; change comes more slowly by just talking to him. This brings me to the ultimate direction in which research into syphilis might go.

Artificial Immunization

Mention the subject of artificial immunization and a host of conditioned reflexes come into play. Our mind jumps forward to visualizing a mishmash of spirochetes being injected into an array of human beings, and we conclude that the notion is foolish. But viewed in the long range the goal may not be so easily dismissible. For taken piece by piece it may be possible to build a usable road to this objective of artificial immunization. Like all the great problems in medicine and health, the immediate goal should be to divide the big problem into smaller ones, each of which might be tackled on a short-range perspective.

I can remember when the "wise ones" said confidently that it was useless to induce antibodies to poliomyelitis because "did not paralysis occur in the presence of high titer antibodies?" Two significant facts were not then appreciated: first, that the crucial event in paralytic polio – viremia – occurred before antibodies developed; second, that a small degree of measurable immunity gave useful protection to a large proportion of human beings. Thus a "rational" approach based on inadequate information was worse than useless – it was inhibitory to progress.

Awe of the practical, therefore, should not deter steps toward the goal of immunization. Clearly, growth of treponemes in bulk is central to this objective. But need we wait for this signal event to investigate other essential elements of the larger question? Can, for example, immunity to syphilis be artificially induced without actual infection? Evidence has been adduced by Miller (1972) and Metzger and Smogor (1969) and their associates that it can be. It is imperative that these observations be confirmed. If they are, steps of major importance have been taken. Never mind at the moment how much immunity, for a little might be of the greatest practical value in terms of preventing infection in man.

Is it possible to identify a particular antigenic component of the treponeme that has immunogenic capacity beyond other components? Never mind how laborious the method or how many treponemes are required for a measurable effect, for these problems can be dealt with when treponemes become available in abundance. If present, is immunity based predominantly on cellular or humoral mechanisms? Can sensitive methods be devised for measuring this immunity? How best can the immunogenic potency of an antigenic fraction of treponemes be determined? Answers to these questions are not only ultimately necessary but they will lay a scientific base for the development of a vaccine against treponemal diseases if such is ever possible.

Concluding Remarks

In respect of syphilis and the other treponemal diseases, we face the future with hope, fortified with the knowledge of a rich background of accomplishment thus far in the twentieth century, and armed with techniques not available even two decades ago. It is not necessary to unleash a major all-out assault on syphilis, as might well be done for some of the greater scourges of mankind. But it is essential that work in the field be kept alive, that a nucleus of well-trained scientists give continuous attention to the field, that we go for quality of performance and dedication to these specific goals.

It might be useful as each decade is turned, to pause for a moment, as has been done in this conference, to take stock of accomplishments, reassess short-range goals, and perhaps gain new insight into long-range objectives.

References

Bentwich, Z. and Kunkel, H. G. (1973). *Transplantation Reviews* **16**, 29-50

Collart, P. (1974). *Semaine des hôpitaux de Paris* **50**, 673-679

D'Alessandro, G., Oddo, F., Comes, R. and Dardanoni, L. (1949). *Rivista dell'Istituto sieroterapico italiano* **24**, 134-166

D'Alessandro, G. and Dardanoni, L. (1953). *American Journal of Syphilis, Gonorrhea and Venereal Diseases* **37**, 137-150

Davies, N. T. (1974). *Proceedings of the Nutrition Society* **33**, 293-298

Dupouey, P. (1972). *Annales de l'Institut Pasteur* **122**, 283-285

Fridman, W. H., Nelson, R. A. and Liabeuf, A. (1974). *Journal of Immunology* **113**, 1008-1016

Fulford, K. W. and Brostoff, J. (1972). *British Journal of Venereal Diseases* **48**, 483-488

Hackett, C. J. (1963). *Bulletin of the World Health Organization* **29**, 7-41

Hardy, P. H. jr., Fredericks, W. R. and Nell, E. E. (1975). *Infection and Immunity* **2**, 380-386

Hooshmand, H., Escobar, M. R. and Kopf, S. W. (1972). *Journal of the American Medical Association* **219**, 726-729

Levene, G. M., Wright, D. J. M. and Turk, J. L. (1971). *Proceedings of the Royal Society of Medicine* **64**, 426-428

Metzger, M. and Michalska, E. (1974). WHO Venereal Diseases and Treponematoses Technical Documents No. 323

Metzger, M. and Smogor, W. (1969). *British Journal of Venereal Diseases* **45**, 308-312

Miller, J. N. (1972). *Medical Clinics of North America* **56**, 1217-1220

Musher, D. M., Izzat, N. N., Min, K. W. and Györkey, F. (1972). *Acta dermato-venereologica* **52**, 349-352

Musher, D. M., Schell, R. F. and Knox, J. M. (1974). *Infection and Immunity* **9**, 654-657

Nell, E. E. and Hardy, P. H. jr. (1966). *Immunochemistry* **3**, 233-245

Ovcinnikov, N. M., Delektorskij, V. V. and Sagdeeva, L. G. (1974). WHO Venereal Diseases and Treponematoses Technical Documents No. 325

Pillot, J., D'Azambuja, S. and Creau, N. (1973). WHO Venereal Diseases and Treponematoses Technical Documents No. 303

Pillot, J. and Dupouey, P. (1964). *Annales de l'Institut Pasteur* **106**, 456-468

Rodin, I. A. and Komarovskaya, V. N. (1972). *Vestnik dermatologii venerologii* **46**, 61-65

Smith, J. L. (1969). "Spirochetes in Late Seronegative Syphilis, Penicillin Notwithstanding". Thomas, Springfield, Ill.

Turner, T. B. (1970). *In* "Infectious Agents and Host Reaction". Ed. S. Mudd. Saunders, Philadelphia; pp 346-390

Weinberg, E. D. (1974). *Science* **184**, 952-956

Weinberg, E. D. (1975). *Journal of the American Medical Association* **231**, 39-41

Whitehead, A. N. (1947). "Essays in Science and Philosophy". Philosophical Library, New York

Wicher, K. J., Wicher, V. and Dabrowski, M. (1974). *British Journal of Venereal Diseases* **50**, 319-320

Discussion

Dr Willcox said that he had very much enjoyed Dr Turner's wide-ranging paper. He was intrigued by his suggestion that research might obliquely reveal data relevant to the origin of syphilis and asked Dr Turner what practical approaches to treponemal research might also provide information on this matter.

Dr Turner replied that he thought research of this sort should be done by old men who had nothing else to do. He thought it was still mostly speculation but he had no doubt that treponemes were widely distributed throughout the world before 1492.

Dr Krause asked about the evidence for a possible role for humoral or cellular immunity in experimental syphilis. He wished to know whether it was possible to transfer serum passively from a rabbit infected with *T. pallidum* to an uninfected rabbit and enhance its resistance to infection.

Dr Turner said there was no doubt that there was humoral immunity but it was relatively feeble and did not seem to be of very much practical value. The evidence suggested that most of the immunity to treponemal disease came from cellular immunity.

Dr Knox said that not infrequently experiments had been planned in his department, but then they looked in Dr Turner's book, and found that he had done it before them. Experiments at Baylor had shown that if enough serum from an infected animal were given, the chancre formation could be delayed, and also, if white blood cells were transferred, this could delay the onset of the disease, but would not stop it completely. Cellular immunity appeared to be the most important factor. His group had shown that if an experimental animal was given syphilis and later listeria was injected, the listeria would be killed, indicating a "turned on" cellular immune system. He believed that further work on cellular immunity was of the utmost importance.

He thought it was essential that somebody confirm the work of Miller who had shown that animals became immune following massive injections of irradiated treponemes, and the results obtained by Metzger, who had immunized rabbits with massive doses of *T. pallidum* kept at 40°C for seven to ten days before injection.

Dr Wiesner said he was worried that there were so very few young investigators interested in syphilis.

Dr Fulford (*London*) said that if Professor J N Miller were present he would probably say that one of the difficulties in this field lay in drawing analogies between rabbits and human beings. For example, if a rabbit were infected with syphilis and treated after the thirteenth week, in the majority of cases the infection was eradicated but the animal was immune to further infection: this was probably not the case in human beings.

Dr W G Henderson (*Hertfordshire*) said he had recently been associated with Dr Hashim Al Samarai of Baghdad in carrying out some experiments on immunization which had demonstrated partial immunity in rabbits with a variety of antigens. His antigens were prepared at 0°C and were stored at –20°C until used. In his view there was no question about the fact that some immunity was produced.

Dr Roberts asked whether it was certain that *T. pallidum* survived and multiplied within human polymorphonuclear leukocytes.

Dr Knox said that there were reports of the treponeme being found inside cells. In his university experts in electronmicroscopy had looked at photographs from Professor Miller's department in Los Angeles showing a monocyte in which they discovered a treponeme. However, there was some doubt as to whether it was actually in the cell or superimposed upon it in some way. To his knowledge, intracellular reproduction had not been established.

Dr Catterall said that Dr Turner had reported that probably about 20% of Americans were sensitive to penicillin but that the comparable figure in the United Kingdom would be about 10%. He drew attention to Dr Wilkinson's statement that the majority of syphilis was now presenting in the latent stage and that this was often difficult to differentiate from the chronic biological false positive reaction. It was very important to make the distinction as people with the chronic false positive reaction were often sensitive to penicillin, and symptoms of collagen disease could be precipitated in them if they were given penicillin in the mistaken belief that they had syphilis.

Dr Robinson asked about the relative incidence of the Herxheimer reaction and said it was interesting that endotoxins produced fever but stimulated the synthesis of prostaglandin E2. He wondered whether this was also involved in the Herxheimer reaction.

Dr Catterall replied that the Herxheimer reaction was commonest in secondary syphilis and was not uncommon in patients with neurosyphilis if there was a high cell count in the cerebrospinal fluid. The incidence of the reaction in cardiovascular syphilis was unknown but a small number of patients were known to have died, probably as a result of a Herxheimer reaction following treatment.

Dr Fulford said that he had been studying the mechanism of the Herxheimer reaction and had found that there were significant changes in complement in the blood. The changes suggested that there was rapid activation of complement by the classical pathway, usually about two to three hours after the injection of penicillin, and that the clinical changes usually started a little later. There was also a fall in the antibody titres in the FTA and TPHA tests. There was no significant change in the titres of TPI antibody or in the VDL antibody. He thought that this might be due to the exposure by penicillin of hidden antigenic determinants resulting in sudden activation of complement.

Dr Knox said that in his clinic they did not pay much attention to the Herxheimer reaction except in cardiovascular syphilis. Clinicians warned patients of the possibility of a reaction but did not take any other measures.

Dr Morton drew attention to the fact that he had recently seen a number of patients with chancres of the cervix of an atypical sort and he recommended that careful assessment of the cervix should be made in all female contacts of men with syphilis.

Dr Turner commented that if the use of penicillin or other antibiotics in the treatment of syphilis or yaws ceased there would be a return of the old-fashioned more classical manifestations of the disease.

Dr Milton Puziss (*Maryland*) commented on the small number of recruits into research work on treponemal diseases. He said that in the United States a programme begun in 1972 had grown rapidly and had now reached a point where there were 58 projects with well over $3 000 000 used to support research. There were four venereal disease research centres and there had also been a great increase in training programmes. There were now 8 fellowships and institutional training grants and a total of 27 investigators being trained in research. Obviously, at the present time, the greatest effort was being made into gonorrhoea, but attempts were being made to stimulate more research into syphilis. There were about 10 people working in this field at present and recently there had been a large symposium on spirochaetes at the University of Minnesota. Attempts were also being made to stimulate more research into the problem of herpes virus and into group B streptococci as a potential sexually transmitted disease.

Responsibility for Education and Prevention Programmes

Chairman
Sir John Stallworthy
President, the Royal Society of Medicine

The Role of Government in Research and Educational Programmes in the UK

Sir Douglas Black
Chief Scientist, Department of Health and Social Security, Alexander Fleming House, London SE1 6BY

It is possible to envisage two kinds of ideal world – one in which research into the causes and prevention of the sexually transmitted diseases (STD) had brought about their disappearance, comparable to that which we may be about to achieve with smallpox; and another in which all members of the public were fully educated in the measures required to prevent them from contracting and transmitting these age-old scourges of mankind. But we live in the actual world of 1975, and for some time to come the major role of Government will still lie in the provision of services to deal with the existing situation. This aspect, so far as the UK is concerned, has already been dealt with by Dr Nicol (p 13) and Dr Catterall (p 61); and the matter of my own brief is of smaller present moment, though not without promise for the future.

Research

There are three main areas of research to be considered – biomedical research in the microbiology and natural history of STD, and improved chemotherapy; research into the provision of services; and research into preventive measures, which leads naturally into the educational aspect. Government has a role in each of these areas, using different agencies in each case, but with overriding responsibility remaining with the Health Departments.

Biomedical Research

The principal agent for this, the most developed area of research related to STD, is the Medical Research Council; but under the new arrangements for Government research and development, outlined in the White Paper (Cmnd 5046, 1972), the funding of this area of research falls largely to the Health Departments, through a Broad Commission placed with the Council. The content of this commission has recently been reviewed by the Panel on Medical Research, which advises the Health Departments on work commissioned from the MRC; and in what follows I am much indebted to an analysis of the commission carried out by Professor R E O Williams, formerly Professor of Bacteriology at St Mary's Hospital Medical School, and now Director of the Public Health Laboratory Service.

The range of work supported within the commission is wide, including studies on the mechanisms by which gonococci become attached to and enter phagocytes; immunological work on gonococci with the ultimate aims of serological diagnosis and vaccine production; and epidemiological studies of gonococcal "typing". One project deals with antibiotic resistance in gonococci. The possible role of Chlamydia and of mycoplasmas in nonspecific urethritis is being studied. Other topics within the commission include an animal model of trichomonad infection; immune responses to *Treponema pallidum*; and the sexual transmission of hepatitis B.

The Panel is, however, very conscious of the need to extend the scope of biomedical research into STD, with particular reference to the etiology of nonspecific urethritis; the epidemiology of STD; the long-term sequelae of gonorrhoea and other STD; and the validation of treatment regimes by controlled trials. They have recommended that in the next five years funding should be increased to above the present level (£62 000 in 1973/4) as opportunity offers. It has to be recognized, however, that the limitation of research in this field has not been so much of funding as of the availability of trained research workers, and of time which can be spared from exacting and expanding service commitments. There are, however, some indications of increased interest in this field of research, both at the level of molecular biology and that of epidemiology.

Health Services Research

The actual provision of services is a function of the National Health Service; but the Health Departments have supported from their own research funds, or indirectly through the locally organized research scheme, work directed to the evaluation of service provisions. For example, the DHSS has directly supported an investigation by Dr R D Catterall of the Middlesex Hospital into the incidence of STD among patients attending family planning clinics; this should yield information on the extent of the problem posed by those who have sustained infection, but who have not sought the help of STD clinics. A more extensive study is planned to determine the incidence of STD in a defined population. Somewhere in the debatable ground between health service research and health service development lies the encouragement by the Department of visits abroad by the medical and nursing staff of STD centres.

Research Related to Prevention

To label STD as "special" is no more helpful than to describe epilepsy as "sacred"; the motivation for such epithets is emotional rather than rational. Like other infectious disorders, STD represents an interaction between a microbial invader and an human host. The biomedical approach is in the main directed against the microbe; in view of the multiplicity of known causal agents, and the existence of syndromes such as nonspecific urethritis whose microbial cause has not been precisely identified, the biomedical approach does not lack complexity; but nor does the human host. We have still much to learn about the social and occupational correlates of STD, and about the determinants of the behaviour on which their transmission is based. Work on this aspect is at an early stage; but the Scottish Home and Health Department is supporting a study in Glasgow into the personality, family dynamics and social background of patients attending STD clinics; and the Middlesex Hospital proposals include attention to behavioural, social and occupational factors.

The present time is not one in which it would be easy to attain a consensus view on what constitutes deviant behaviour; and it would be still more difficult to attempt to control such behaviour, even if identified, by any means other than education – which brings me to the second part of my brief.

Educational Approach to the Control of STD

My own experience in this field of health education is both limited and outdated, being confined to wartime experience of giving "the VD lecture" to troops. But it made me conscious of what still seems to me the essential difficulty in this endeavour, that of combining an idealistic advocacy of continence with a pragmatic detailing of "sensible precautions". Looking around, I somehow fail to discern the fulfilment of the promise that the permissive society would bring us universal happiness and love; but the pursuit is still undeniably with us, and we must at the very least perform our minimum duty of advising our liberated fellow humans how to escape the undesirable physical consequences of their communion. As in other forms of health education, those in most need are often also the hardest to reach — but, on the other hand, they may be the most knowledgeable. There is evidence from a Health Education Council study mounted in Lambeth and Wandsworth that the transition from innocence to experience in teenagers has been associated with a reasonably adequate general level of knowledge of the symptomatology of STD, and of the facilities available for treatment. Such surveys of what is already generally known are clearly one of the necessary bases for planning an educational programme. The same survey identified "at-risk" groups — those in the 18–30 age group with social problems; homosexuals; and recent immigrants.

Although appropriate health education on STD can, and should, be given in the context of biological instruction in schools, and in various clinics, central effort by the Health Departments is mediated through the Health Education Council, an independent body mainly funded by DHSS; and in Scotland by the Health Education Unit. Area Health Authorities and Local Education Authorities also have powers and responsibility in health education. Virtually from its inception in 1968, the Health Education Council has given special attention to education of the public in the nature, detection and facilities for treatment of this important group of communicable diseases. Their chief medical officer, Dr A J Dalzell-Ward, has described (1973) the design of the large-scale survey conducted in the boroughs of Lambeth and Wandsworth, some of whose findings have already been referred to. A notable increase in the number of contacts traced and treated was brought about, and a new record system for patients and contacts was evolved, which is capable of being more widely used. The Council has also designed posters and leaflets for use and distribution by local authorities; the display of posters had to be preceded by a legislative amendment to the Indecent Advertisements Act of 1889, exempting local and public authorities from restrictions on advertisements related to STD being visible from the public highway. Certainly, there are no resources available to compare with the massive expenditure which attempts to associate the consumption of tobacco, alcohol and sweets with sexual prowess; and direct attempts to lessen promiscuity would not command universal acceptance. But by concentrating on providing factual information to identified "at-risk" groups, much can be and is being done in the secondary prevention of STD.

Reference

Dalzell-Ward, A. J. (1973). *British Journal of Venereal Diseases* 49, 171

Discussion

Sir John Stallworthy (*Chairman*): Before calling on Dr Theodore Cooper, who is the Assistant Secretary for Health at the Department of Health, Education and Welfare, USA, I am taking the liberty of departing a little from our programme.

Those of you who were here on the first day will remember that in the discussion there was some considerable reference to the question of health education and educational programmes. We are fortunate to have with us today Dr Dalzell-Ward, a Divisional Director of the Health Education Council, and I have invited him, if he would care to, to speak for five minutes on the policy of his Council.

Dr A J Dalzell-Ward
(*Health Education Council, London WC1A 1AH*):

I am very grateful for the opportunity of removing any misunderstanding which may have arisen as a result of the discussion the day before yesterday, of which I have heard brief accounts.

Sir Douglas Black has indicated some of the recent activity of the Health Education Council in this particular field of public health. Briefly, the Health Education Council's role is to conduct large scale national and regional campaigns based upon research. In this case the research is triple. It is the feasibility decided by epidemiological research, which is not necessarily carried out by ourselves, of course; the communications angle is carried out by communications research, and that involves the design and pretesting of materials of representative groups, the establishment of baselines of knowledge, attitudes and behaviour, and subsequent remeasurement of those at the end of the campaign. The third level of research concerns attitude and behaviour. This kind of work requires very large resources, and although our resources are never large enough, they are relatively large compared with what has been available before.

The Area Health Authority is responsible for local and regional campaigns of its own, but you must not imagine that we are divorced from our colleagues, the Health Education Officers and the Area Medical Officers. We have a system of regular contact through a liaison unit, staffed by a Chief Liaison Officer and two assistants who make regular tours and talk with the Health Education Officers and other health officials, bring back to us any particular problems where we can help, and generally give advice and act as a link which is maintained throughout. Again the materials we produce for national campaigns in the form of posters, leaflets or other devices are available to Health Education Officers and the Area Health Authorities. Therefore, it is a co-ordinating role as well as an initiating role, and I would not like our friends from the United States to think that the Health Education Council was in any way separated in its functions from day to day practical health education which goes on in the areas.

If I might just comment on the result of the Lambeth and Wandsworth experiment, one of the most important things that has emerged is that it seems we have reached the stage where widespread blanket indiscriminate publicity about this group of diseases is no longer valuable, and that we should concentrate on vulnerable groups and aim at particular targets. So much for our role.

Our functions are set out in a DHSS document about health education generally (NHS Reorganization Circular HRC (74) 27).

The Role of Government in Research and Educational Programs Related to the Sexually Transmitted Diseases in the USA

Theodore Cooper
Assistant Secretary for Health,
Department of Health, Education
and Welfare, Washington DC 20201

I propose, with regard to the sexually transmitted diseases, quite briefly to outline the Federal role in: all aspects of research; some of the policy decisions facing Government today; the production of professional manpower; and education of the public.

In the United States, as in most other countries, the Federal Government has assumed a major role in supporting research and educational programs relating to the sexually transmitted diseases. One of the prime reasons that the Government has become involved in this field stems from the need to fill a "vacuum". The sexually transmitted diseases have received much too low a priority from health professionals for many years. In part, this has been due to their social unacceptability by the public in general, the medical profession, and local health agencies. The individual community, while recognizing the need for educational programs aimed at reducing the problems caused by the sexually transmitted diseases, has not been willing to pay the price necessary to institute adequate programs. Research institutions. likewise, have not given the priority to these diseases that they have to the diseases which are considered more important in the eyes of the general public, such as cancer, heart diseases, &c.

The Federal Government entered this area by providing grants designed to expand research, to encourage the development of local case-finding programs and to assist local educational programs aimed at improving public awareness of the problems created by the sexually transmitted diseases.

In the United States, the Federal Government plays the dominant role in supporting research into the sexually transmitted diseases. The National Institute of Allergy and Infectious Diseases (NIAID) and the Center for Disease Control (CDC) are the primary institutional sources of this support. The NIAID works through extramural grant and contract programs which mainly support scientists working outside of Government in basic research. The CDC employs a small research staff of its own, and supports some research through contracts. It is involved in basic as well as in applied research. In Fiscal Year 1972, approximately $2.3 million was spent by the Federal Government in direct support of sexually transmitted disease research. This figure grew to $5.6 million for FY 1974, and is projected at $5.8 million for FY 1976, a two-and-one-half fold increase since 1972. I would like here to describe two basic objectives of that support, the acquisition of additional knowledge and the development of technical competence and capacity in the delivery of clinical care.

It is apparent from the increasing incidence of many of the sexually transmitted diseases that more knowledge is needed in order to strengthen and expand our existing control efforts. Basic biological research is needed to elucidate the pathophysiology of host and pathogen interaction with particular emphasis being placed in the area of host defenses. Applied research is also needed to evaluate alternative uses of preventive and curative approaches already at our disposal. Within the past five years there has been a conscious effort to expand the total Federal resources supporting basic and applied research efforts, and to expand the scope of those efforts to include research on a wider array of pathogens and potential pathogens. Emphasis is also being placed in the area of behavioral research, since human behavior is such a fundamental determinant of risk for these particular diseases and plays such an important part in determining the interactions between patients and health care providers.

One factor which is all too frequently overlooked by those who are involved in research is the social acceptability of one of the end-results for which we are striving. Today's research is moving us closer and closer to the time when vaccines will be available, for both gonorrhea and syphilis. The research which will produce the vaccines is moving us toward a medical solution. The problem, however, which will have to be faced and which will ultimately become one of policy is: "How will we use these vaccines?" I do not profess to have the answer, but I suggest that those of us in the health professions – particularly those dealing at the policy level – will soon have to face the issue realistically. Should we recommend giving a vaccine against gonorrhea and syphilis to children just as we give them DPT, polio, &c.? What sort of reaction would we get from the public if we were to make such a recommendation? I can clearly hear people saying that to vaccinate against these diseases is increasing even further the present-day sexual permissiveness. From the medical point of view, we look at the long-range effects on health caused by these diseases and our conscience dictates that we must strive to prevent their occurrence. Ultimately, a stand will have to be taken to support or deny the use of vaccines against the sexually transmitted diseases. As I said earlier, I do not have a solution, or even a recommendation, but I clearly recognize the need to address the sociologic implications of prevention and treatment of these diseases. In this area, I believe the Federal Government will ultimately have responsibility for establishing the policy.

A conscious effort has also been made to use Federal support in an attempt to improve professional competence and capacity in the delivery of clinical services for patients with sexually transmitted diseases. Some direct support has been, and will continue to be, given to train persons now working in venereal disease clinics and in the private sector. However, the long-range goals of increased professional competence are best accomplished through support of institutions capable of conducting multidisciplinary investigative efforts directed toward many sexually transmitted diseases, and by creating STD research fellowships within such institutions. This approach fosters both institutional development in the field of research and institutional development with respect to teaching and delivery of care for the sexually transmitted diseases. Such centers of excellence for research, training and clinical care for the sexually transmitted diseases are likely to play an increasingly important role in the United States as our health care system continues to evolve toward more payment for medical care by the Federal Government, and toward increasing use of medical standards to evaluate the worth of the care being purchased.

Future successes will depend to a great extent on the young people now in school or even those just contemplating a career in science. When penicillin was first discovered to be effective against gonorrhea, many people felt that our problems with the sexually transmitted diseases were over. The tragic aftermath of this was that venereology, as a specialty, began to decline in the United States. I need hardly mention the differences between our two countries' approaches in training people who will work with the sexually transmitted diseases. In the United Kingdom, venereology is still a specialty in its own right. In the United States, however, venereology is taught in medical schools only as a very small part of the whole field of infectious diseases. We in the Federal Government have a responsibility, I believe, to put further emphasis on training.

With this idea in mind, the National Institutes of Health are now supporting training for research. So far, institutional fellowships have been awarded to the Universities of Indiana, Washington, Virginia and Chicago, and Baylor University has a training grant, all to provide young health scientists and clinicians with opportunities for postdoctoral research in venereal disease. In addition, six individual fellowships have been awarded in this field. A total of 19 post-doctoral scientists are now receiving training supported by the National Institute of Allergy and Infectious Diseases. Such training of new investigators will provide a firm basis for the continuation of venereal disease research for many years.

Health education likewise is being promoted by Government. However, within the schools, in contrast to the situation which exists in the field of research, State and local governments are playing the dominant role and have delegated quite limited authority to the Federal Government. In particular, the contents of the school curriculum are determined at the State and local levels, not at the Federal level.

The Federal Government endorses the position concerning the goals of education in the control of the sexually transmitted diseases which was set forth in a World Health Organization meeting in November 1974: The report of that meeting states:

> Two basic goals of health education in STD control can be distinguished. The first consists in the preparation of the young toward a positive appreciation of their sexuality and correct information about its health related aspects. This involves a long-term approach and is the most realistic possibility for influencing attitudes and behavior with respect to multiple sexual contacts or to casuality in selecting sexual partners. The second goal is based on the elimination of barriers and the improvement of positive factors which will lead to the adoption of a number of basic actions among people at risk, such as the use of individual preventive measures, participation in community prevention, seeking of early diagnosis and treatment, and the cooperation of patients with treatment, including contact tracing.

The Federal role is that of adviser to the various State and local systems with respect to the content of their curricula. Although much of this is done through the Office of Education, within the

Department of Health, Education, and Welfare, the Center for Disease Control also plays a major role. Acting through State and local health departments, it serves as the principal Federal focus for advice. Within the past year, the Center for Disease Control, in cooperation with the Offices of Education and State and local Health and Educational agencies, sponsored a questionnaire sample survey of venereal disease educational programs being conducted at the elementary and secondary school level.

The results indicated that less than half (42%) of the nation's 102 000 elementary and secondary schools provide some form of venereal disease education to their students. Schools which did provide such education were likely to be secondary schools, and/or schools with large populations. Units of venereal disease instruction were typically of one or two weeks' duration, and two-thirds of the schools included them within their health education curriculum. Less than a quarter of the schools which offered units of instruction required instructors to have any special training in venereal disease education. Among the schools which offered no venereal disease education, the major reasons cited were the lack of public interest in and awareness of the problem, and the opinion that no venereal disease problem existed in their school system.

The Center for Disease Control is attempting to develop a mechanism to compare the efficacy of various types of VD educational curricula now in use, and plans to work with State and local governments in expanding the number of schools offering instruction in this area, as well as improving the quality of that instruction.

Education within the school system, however, represents only a portion of the total needs. The Federal Government supports information and education activities, as well as surveillance, case-finding, contact-tracing, and special studies through a program of grants to State and local health departments. Routine diagnostic and treatment services, however, are regarded as being a State and local responsibility. Of the annual Federal appropriation of approximately \$25 million which is allocated in the form of grants, we estimate that about \$3 million is being used to support information and educational activities. The funds are supplemental to State and local funds. They subsidize counselling services provided within public clinics to patients with either syphilis or gonorrhea, as well as community outreach educational programs designed for youth and other high-risk groups. They are also used to subsidize educational programs for the health professionals responsible for diagnosing and treating patients with these diseases, and to promote community organizational efforts whose basic objective is to facilitate attitude change with respect to these diseases.

Conclusion

The Federal Government will continue its support of many programs aimed at the problems associated with the sexually transmitted diseases. This will include support of:

(1) Interdisciplinary centers of excellence, where basic clinical, bacteriologic and immunologic research can be pursued toward the end of vaccine development. A nucleus of dedicated, well-trained young investigators will be generated from these centers.
(2) Epidemiologically based demonstration areas, where established and new control techniques can be evaluated, and where the magnitude of the problem of all sexually transmitted diseases can be assessed.
(3) Professional education and clinical training regarding sexually transmitted diseases, in collaboration with medical schools and medical societies.
(4) The development and evaluation of programs that increase the awareness and knowledge of at-risk populations regarding the seriousness of sexually transmitted diseases and modes of prevention.

Reference

World Health Organization (1974). Report of the Meeting on Health Education in the Control of Sexually Transmitted Diseases, Geneva; p 17

The Role and Responsibility of the Mass Media in the UK

Peter Goodchild
Editor, "Horizon", British Broadcasting Corporation, Kensington House, Richmond Way, London W14 0AX

As my own experience of working in the media has been exclusively in television I shall confine myself to considering how this medium can be employed in an area of public health. What I would like to do in this talk is to define the types of programme that the broadcasting industry readily generates at present, the evidence as to whom they seem most to help, and then in what way they might be improved.

But first let me define certain terms of reference. Just how mass is the media that we are talking about? The highest audience achieved by the BBC recently has been for certain sporting events, like international football and "Miss World", for war films like "The Longest Day" and for "Kojak", all of them achieving audiences between 20 and 25 million. However, public health issues are normally dealt with as documentaries, and the audience for such documentaries at peak viewing on the BBC's first channel is around 5 million viewers. But perhaps of as much interest as the actual size of this audience is its constitution. From time to time our Audience Research Unit produces profiles of audiences for different types of programme. These profiles present a breakdown of the audience according to occupation into groups A, B, C. More than 70% of the entire population is in group C. Now while there are shifts between the social groups watching say a soap opera or a symphony concert, these profiles are far more remarkable overall for their consistency. Most programmes, and these documentaries are no exception, are watched by 55–75% from social group C.

Thus while not completely absolving us from the criticism of preaching only to the converted it does mean that such programmes do stand a chance of penetrating to groups at risk. What is more, this viewing pattern applies to the BBC's second channel as well, a channel which quite falsely has the reputation of being an intellectual ghetto. On this channel documentaries are watched by audiences of on average 3 million.

Such a wide potential audience makes planning a programme or series, in the way an advertising campaign might be handled, almost meaningless. It makes it so difficult in fact that the way programmes are chosen may on the surface seem almost random. The system really relies on individual producers and individual programme editors remaining sufficiently "in touch" and using their judgment. Basically, a producer or editor can only follow his own nose. He will read an article, talk to someone and come across something which interests him. On the basis that what interests him will interest others, he will start to consider what programme possibilities there are. He will use a whole series of cross checks. Is there enough new material for fifty minutes? Has it "been done"? If so, when, and is there a new angle on it?

I think it is fair to say that at this stage when a programme is conceived, it is conceived primarily as journalism, and only secondarily as a public service. Thus anybody confronting the problem of doing such a general programme on sexually transmitted diseases knows that many aspects of the subject, contact chasing, the work of the clinic, the general direction of research, have been covered in previous programmes. The producer has to ask himself if he can, or wishes to, do another programme on the subject which seems on the face of it already familiar.

The answer is more likely to be yes, if there is a new aspect, a new set of statistics. Such a programme starts life angled away from providing just straight information, though such information will amost certainly be provided. In the end the programme will be of general interest, the sort of programme which is invaluable in helping to establish a public awareness of the problem and perhaps a more flexible attitude towards it. And while there are conferences such as this at which interesting research results and new statistics are reported one can predict that every two to three years a producer will consider the time shadow of the previous programme has faded and a new one is due.

Yet in dealing with the groups at risk and providing them with crucial information, such programmes seem to be of only marginal use. In his follow-up study (1973) to his report on "The Sexual Behaviour of Young People" (1965), the sociologist Michael Schofield asked his 370 subjects several questions related to VD. They were asked where they got their information. Parents were mentioned by 2%, 4% mentioned school, and 6% of his group mentioned television as the source. But all these are a much smaller proportion than those mentioning either books or friends (31%). What is more, of the 6% quoting television, not one could describe the symptoms absolutely correctly.

It seems then that the best that can be said of general television programmes in this respect is summed up by one of the BBC's viewing panel, writing about a programme called "VD – Who Cares?": "It should help show people who may have VD that they have nothing to fear from seeking help." The questions of when to seek help, and where, remain at best partly answered.

The immediate thought for a programme maker is whether these programmes' shortcomings, in particular the seemingly small impact on young people, have anything to do with the actual way the programme is made. It could be that we should be making a much more deliberate effort to reach the younger generation. All the BBC-produced documentaries on STD have so far been produced according to well-tried conventions: the use of the authoritative but fairly impersonal narrator: the descriptive scenes shot in labs and clinics and so on. However, two years ago it was decided to show the American prizewinning programme "VD Blues", not the whole of it but excerpts, as much of the original programme was considered too American. I am sure that many of you here have seen it, but for those who have not, "VD Blues" was constructed as a cross between an anthology and a revue. It was linked by a popular American "chat show" chairman, Dick Cavett, and included songs like "Don't give a Dose to the One you Love Most" sung by Dr Hook and the Medicine Men, and sketches, including a very surreal one. This consisted of a chat between two actors in classical garb posing as the gonococcus and the spirochaete sitting in what looked like a papier mâché cave, but represented a cell in the girl's body – and discussing how they were going to subdue their victim. It ended when a puff of smoke appeared through one of the openings in the set and killed them. It was a dose of penicillin, or "penny" as they kept calling it.

There were a doctor and nurse, both non-professional, swapping symptoms. There were more songs, and these excerpts were set in the context of a studio discussion, a phone-in where concerned listeners could talk directly to doctors. The reports which had heralded the show's arrival from the States were mixed. *Variety*, the US show-business newspaper, had described it thus: "The show was not exactly 'VD can be fun' in its format, but it veered enough in that direction to create serious doubts." Alongside such sceptical remarks there were also reports of spot checks on clinics in Gary, Indiana, on the days after it was shown, where more than half the new patients attending were there because of the programme.

So how did this approach go down with viewers? Unfortunately our audience research report is not as full or clear as one would hope but it includes the following comment:

> A sizeable minority of the imported material was considered unnecessarily irritating, even downright rubbish . . . the sketch of two bugs portrayed by actors in classical garb fighting for possession of a girl's body was ridiculous: in fact the overall effect of these inserts was to trivialize the subject and give the impression that it was all a huge joke.

Yet unfortunately the report does not state which group of viewers made up this sizeable minority. Was it mostly the older or younger section of the audience? As part answer what it does do, however, elsewhere, is to measure the audience's appreciation index of the programme by age group. This index is a figure out of 100 which gives a qualitative assessment of viewer's reponses to a programme. For the 15–29 age group this index was 75, a very high figure indeed; for the 50+ age group, it was 66, a mediocre figure. So the programme was more highly valued by this younger age group, and although some of them might have found the sketches silly it is my surmise that they valued the general feel of non-authoritarianism as much as anything.

So, somewhat reluctantly, for I have to admit my personal distaste for "VD Blues", I do see a case for a more populist approach in general programming. I do also agree with *Variety* that such films stand a much greater chance of making VD seem fun, of being accused of encouraging immorality. Also one has to admit that no audience figures exist defining how popular the previous, more conventional, programmes have been with the younger audience. On balance, though, I feel there is a case for trying a more experimental approach.

Up to now I have concentrated on the general programming area, but there are opportunities to get through to the groups at risk through more specialized output like the programmes made for schools. Here the audience is more or less captive and a 20-minute film can form, indeed is designed as, the basis of a 20-minute class discussion. In fact a programme was made three years ago which I would describe as very conventional in programme-making terms but made with sympathy and care. It has been received with great enthusiasm and, so our sales people tell me, has topped the sales records for a single programme. It has been translated into half a dozen languages and sold all over the world. Last month alone Kuwait bought a dozen copies of the film. It carefully spelt out symptoms, it reassured about what would happen in clinics, it emphasized the link between VD and casual sexual contact. It illustrates that where you don't have literally to grab your audience's interest such a straight approach is valuable. With this special audience a straightforward approach has been valued enormously.

But that still leaves an area which broadcasting should be able to help and yet, because of the way the system is structured, does so very rarely. I hope I have shown that most general programmes are conceived primarily as pieces of journalism and only secondarily as public information broadcasts. That means that the programmes may be strong on their reports on new research, but less good in telling concerned people, for instance, where clinics are.

Again to quote Michael Schofield's follow-up report. More than half the group he studied did not know where their local VD clinic was situated. This is not surprising if, as he states, very few of the 200 or so clinics in this country have an entry in the telephone directory, and he also noted some less than practical ideas of how people though they might find out where they were.

At the moment it must be difficult for an anxious person to get information about local facilities, but in Birmingham the local BBC radio station has for the last four years been helping out. Jack Johnstone, the Station Manager, was approached by a local consultant to see if he would help with contact chasing. With some trepidation he agreed and at the end of midday and evening news broadcasts they gave details of cases that had failed to come back for treatment. They mentioned the case number, sex, race, and so on, and where the person should report to. In 1971 they were handling 7 or 8 cases a week. Now, perhaps a measure of success, they are handling only one or two, and there has not been a single complaint about the service. Not only is this useful for the hospital, but indirectly it is familiarizing the public with the disease, and where it can be treated. Early on in the experiment, Radio London were approached to see if they would do the same but they refused on the grounds that being in a port and capital city they could be inundated. Since then, as far as I can discover, no similar service has been established elsewhere. That Birmingham experiment was initiated by a medical practitioner. It could be that similar initiatives would discover completely new uses for the services that such local stations have to offer.

To sum up, the audiences of millions for the general programmes are seductive and in the way they help form general attitudes, important, but there is much that remains unexplored in the use of the public service aspects of local and regional broadcasting in public health.

References

Schofield, M. (1965). "Sexual Behaviour of Young People". Longmans, London
(1973). "Sexual Behaviour of Young Adults". Allen Lane, London

The Role and Responsibility, 1975, of the Mass Media in the USA

Alton Blakeslee
Science Editor,
The Associated Press,
New York, NY 10020

Looking into some newspaper files, I found a story telling of a young woman who had been viciously beaten. She sustained a fractured skull, several broken ribs, mashed nose and broken teeth, and other injuries. But, the story said, "she had not been criminally attacked." That phrase was the general newspaper euphemism at the time for rape, a word which otherwise appeared only on the commodity market.

The year was 1940, when sexually transmitted diseases were mostly still being euphemized in the mass media as "social diseases", causing some concern to puzzled people who inevitably engaged in nonsexual social congress. Indeed, it was a time of some wonderment over what such words really meant. As an example, before the polio vaccine appeared, frustrated epidemiologists were advising that people "avoid intimate contact" during summer months to deny transmission of the polio virus. That led one young married couple into separate bedrooms from June to September.

Those were the days when giving an editor a story about sex or syphilis produced the reaction of a man just handed a live grenade, with the pin pulled. But candor is triumphing. Just a few months ago in the so-called heartland of America, in Missouri, the Columbia Missourian printed a frontpage story which frankly discussed vaginal deodorants. A main point was that such sprays can mask vaginal odors which could be signalling some disease. The story, 1000 words long, was specific throughout.

Let me focus on three elements in my assigned topic. One is the influence of the so-called sexual revolution. Another is how various media are and have been handling information about STD. And lastly, mention of some things, desirable to health officials, that they cannot really expect us to do.

Candid, effective discussion about sex-related diseases has paralleled, to some extent, candid, open discussion about sexuality and sex practices. That latter began, numerous observers believe, with publication in 1953 of the Kinsey Report on sexual behavior of American females. As a story, it received very wide play, with a few newspapers the next day editorially tsk-tsking as though they had been a small boy caught writing dirty words on the back fence. For the first time, to my knowledge, newspapers printed such words as penis, vagina, orgasm, masturbation. But that did not mean that victory for frankness and realism was complete, that everyone fell into lockstep.

Fifteen years later, when I wrote a five-part series on scientific studies of sex, one story began with the anecdote of a college student who asked his roommate for help – because he masturbated. The roommate could only suggest that they kneel and pray. The counselling roommate was Alfred C Kinsey. However, in my story, the word "masturbation" was changed to "a sexual practice". Perhaps because it appeared in the very first paragraph? I never learned.

Another writer only two years ago had the words "pubic hair" eliminated from his story about an obstetrician reporting, at a medical meeting, that the practice of shaving a woman's pubic hair before delivery probably caused more infections than it prevented. But just recently, "pubic hair" survived his editorial desk when he wrote a detailed story about vasectomy, mentioning all male genitalia and nether-regions hair.

One can only chalk such incidents up to individual editors' attitudes and feelings, biases and prejudices too, about sex.

The same individuality and ambivalence applies, I think, to the attitudes of editors and producers of radio and TV concerning our unlamented "social diseases". Further, they may be sensitive to some public attitude that sex is OK – at long last – but that people who get STD should not have been doing what they did, should be punished for having been evil, or for having had fun. Many people in our society just do not want to hear about STD.

The media have opened up now to discuss homosexuality. But it is rare to read or hear word about STD acquired through homosexual practices. Some medical journals only now are writing about it.

Progress comes in inches on these subjects. But we in newspapers and magazines, at least, were frankly referrring to syphilis and gonorrhea in 1936. Dr Thomas Parran forced us into it when he became Surgeon-General of the US Public Health Service – as *Newsweek* magazine in 1936 wrote: Dr Parran has "decided he would put the words syphilis and gonorrhea into the language and people's mouths. Familiarity might breed respect." Dr Parran called, said *Newsweek*, for a campaign against moral "ostrichism". Dr Parran did not quite deliver a mortal blow to euphemisms and lack of candor. But it was a beginning.

My files yield a story from 1938, reporting events at the meeting of the American Public Health Association, which began: "The day has come when gonorrhea, one of the major problem diseases in America, can be completely eradicated, Dr Walter Clarke of New York declared today." Dr Clarke was then director of the American Social Hygiene Association, and was betting – before penicillin – on sulfanilamide as one weapon. That same story, incidentally, warned of adverse health effects from air pollution in cities.

Progress by inches . . . Yes, newspapers and magazines were there, transmitting knowledge of STD to the public before – in some cases – and after Parran and Kinsey. An early story described the first National Social Hygiene Day organized before 1940 by social and civic organizations (and Dr Parran) to discuss prevention of syphilis; pointing to its toll in suffering and death. As they came about, there were the stories about progress in treatment, the search for vaccines, the advent of penicillin, VD in the Armed Forces during World War II, the rise and fall in incidence of syphilis and gonorrhea, the rises again, and so on to the present.

Newspapers and magazines were the first to become candid about STD. *The New York Times*' news index file refers to "syphilis" in a story in 1935, and might well have done so before that date. Radio has become, in general, quite candid now in talking about STD. But just after Dr Parran began his campaign, one nationally-known physician was abruptly cut off the air because he said "syphilis" instead of "social disease".

Our media became, with time, more responsive to the meaning of STD as a health problem of frightening dimensions, and have responded to that. Some critics say it has come about in fits and starts, and that criticism will be mentioned in a moment.

Our magazines, *Time, Newsweek, Cosmopolitan, Playboy* and others, have dealt frankly with STD in lengthy articles. *Newsweek* a few years ago ran a cover story on VD, focused upon the search for a gonorrhea vaccine. It and other magazines, as well as newspapers, gave prominent coverage to the sex research of Masters and Johnson.

The June 2, 1975, issue of *New York Magazine*, a highly respected general circulation publication (not to be confused with *The New Yorker*) carried a half-page advertisement for one brand of condom, which "allows two people sensitivity when using a prophylactic". A footnote in the advertisement says the manufacturer "is making available through your local pharmacist educational material on the value of prophylactics in the prevention of venereal disease".

Some of my colleagues in communications give higher marks to radio than television in conveying solid information on STD, and more credit to local TV stations than to networks. A spokesman for the American Social Health Association says he finds no problem in winning time for awareness programs on radio, and says radio is very responsive to the venereal disease question. Radio stations in the Eastern United States are more responsive than those in ultra-conservative sections of California, for example. TV stations show a similar pattern. Sometimes, he adds, a radio station will carry candid programs about STD while a TV station, owned by the same company, will be reluctant to carry announcements or programs on the subject. Individual or local TV stations seem to befriend the cause of STD much more freely than the networks. Local stations will broadcast anti-VD campaign announcements more than networks will.

One editor for the New York NBC station says he has seen on local TV most pictorial aspects about VD "except for the chancre on the end of a penis". One program displayed the syphilitic result of loss of a nose.

The Public Broadcasting System carried a program, entitled "VD Blues", hosted by entertainer Dick Cavett, combining entertainment and popular singers with solid information about VD. Most of its 233 stations carried it in prime time, 8 pm. In 85 cities, this was followed up by explanations of local VD problems, and where to seek help. Locally, a station in Chicago associated with CBS produced a program on VD and later distributed, for free, a pamphlet on the subject, including addresses of local clinics. Another network, ABC, featured a play starring Cloris Leachman presenting VD as a serious and continuing problem. Some critics called it good entertainment, sensible and adult. Others closer to the problem of STD were unhappy that it contained overtones of a punitive attitude toward the victims of STD. A popular medical-drama program, "Marcus Welby", has dealt with the issues of STD.

As for advertisements or commercials, one on a network concerns a pretty girl saying that a certain disposable douche is valuable for "cleanliness". Another, more on local display, shows a young girl receiving a dismaying telephone call, and then saying, "Then I must have it, too", with the message being to consult a doctor or clinic.

This recital may not sound very impressive. In terms of what some specialists would term effective education, it is not. The basic fact is we have written and spoken a great deal about a serious, menacing health problem, and will continue to do so. But the "mass media" cannot perform this educational task on a regular, scheduled basis, unless health educators find means of making a column or regular story interesting and fresh, fresh with new information.

As one editor of *The New York Times* expresses it, "The Press is not a university". We inform; thereby we educate. But we are not a classroom. We would lose readers and attention if we kept repeating the same thing, about STD, the energy crisis, inflation, political dilemmas. We can be alert to new developments, to the continuing story of how best to deal with STD. The mass media are concerned also with hundreds of other subjects and challenges, which many of their champions regard as more important than STD.

Newspapers by definition deal with news. So do some radio and TV programs, other than those engaged in entertainment. In newspapers, a bridge column will bring you increasing expertise about bridge. Sports pages recount the successes and defeats of favorite athletes. Medical columns deal with health, and frequently with the subjects of STD.

In news columns, newspapers and other media do attempt to deal responsibly with progress on many medical subjects and setbacks of unexpected side-effects from new developments.

And the "mass media" are just that – plural. Radio, television, newspapers, magazines, have different purposes and procedures, different audiences oftentimes, and some are more fearful of offending their audiences than others are.

Because we report mostly new developments, it is true that the mass media deal with STD in a kind of fits and starts or occasional basis, not a daily one. We are looking for things new, informative, constructive in this case, and will be most responsive to physicians and health officials or organizations who tell of new developments, or new ways of tacking old problems. When, in one Pennsylvania county, a 17-year-old boy organized 3700 teenage volunteers to visit every home in a large country and personally deliver pamphlets dealing with VD – that was a news story, an informative and helpful one, carried by all newspapers, radio and TV stations in the county.

The mass media are frequently criticized as being more interested in reporting rapes and abortion, and matters sexual, preferably the sensational occasions, than in STD. That is, overall, likely true. But we are also interested in STD as a health problem, and would like to know of studies which give clues as to how to write about or present such topics most effectively.

The mass media are defeated by those people who cannot or will not read, or who turn off the radio or TV if the subject is one they regard as distasteful or boring.

Sometimes we are accused of issuing false information. One very well-known authority on sexuality says, quite flatly, that *Trichomonas vaginalis* is "just about a specific cause for divorce", because it implies a husband strayed to another woman's bed. Are we to believe and report that? Or are we to believe and report an authority on STD who says that *Trichomonas vaginalis* is not always transmitted sexually by any means?

We are also accused at times, or often, of looking for sensational aspects of the subject of sex and STD, of introducing the idea of punitive attitudes towards STD. One example of this – it was given to us, not conceived by us in the media – is the slogan phrase that "even nice people" contract VD. The Victorian attitude toward sex and sexuality, as publicly expressed, erodes slowly.

STD is and continues to be a source of concern and interest to the mass media, because of its health and social meaning to so many millions of people. Let me cite some very recent published stories: A frank account, written by myself last August, on evidence that more venereal disease is being caused by herpesvirus Type 1, acquired through oral-genital contact; a very responsible account of Georges Causse's article on STD in *World Health*; a *New York Times* story reporting incidence of gonorrhea to be at an all-time high, mentioning also that homosexuality is significant in transmitting syphilis; an advice column, "Dear Abby," discussed the fact some women may develop vaginal infections from dyes in pantyhose.

Prominent display was given to a story about a judge ruling that male customers of female prostitutes in Alameda County, California must also be arrested, jailed, quarantined and tested and treated for VD along with the women; the County is appealing. There were stories also about the possibility that spermatozoa might trigger cervical cancer in the female partner, or prostatic cancer in the male.

There was a story about an explicit comic book from a health educator in San Francisco detailing the facts of life, including venereal disease, through the sexual misadventures of characters named Fertile Fanny, Clarence Crablice and Fat Freddy. "It's a good way to get the message across about VD and birth control", says the book's originator, Lora Fountain. She wants to teach teenagers. She thinks most of them ignore dry formal books and stories, that teenagers must be approached in a new, effective manner. She may well be right. We must consider the idiom, the language and the lifestyle of others if we are to reach them, and not proceed under false assumptions.

Recently, in a little campus newspaper at the University of Missouri, I became aghast over a few items appearing in a "personal" column. One read: "Barbara. Happy VD. John." Another, "Tom. Happy VD. Joan." Were these youthful people *celebrating* the acquisition of venereal disease? Then I noticed the date of publication, February 14: "VD" meant love wishes on St Valentine's Day.

Society's Responses

The Right Reverend Dr J S Habgood
Bishop of Durham

The fact that you have invited an outsider – and a bishop at that – to address you during this last session of your conference is in itself an illustration of the extent to which the sexually transmitted diseases raise much larger issues than purely medical ones. How far these ought to concern you, as medical men, is a question I shall be posing in the course of my remarks. But first of all let me make it clear that in trying to spell out some of society's responses, I cannot give you the kind of information a sociologist might provide; nor can I speak with confidence about people's attitudes in general towards different forms of sexual behaviour. What I hope to do is much more modest, namely to help clarify some of the issues; and in so doing I may perhaps help to identify some rather disquieting features in our present situation. I shall, of course, be speaking about the situation in Britain, which is the only one I know.

Historically there seem to have been three main social attitudes towards the classic venereal diseases, attitudes which reflect in part the state of medical knowledge about them, and in part general assumptions about sexual behaviour. These have in turn influenced the preferred medical approach. I shall call these approaches: (1) Legal compulsion. (2) Moral persuasion. (3) Moral indifference.

Legal Compulsion

I shall deal with this in a very summary way, as I am sure the story is familiar. The modern history of legal compulsion in this country begins with the Contagious Diseases Act of 1866, which provided for the compulsory examination and treatment of prostitutes in certain ports and garrison towns. The assumption behind the Act, which was repealed in 1886, was that the root cause of the spread of the venereal diseases was prostitution, and that preventive measures should be concentrated on those most at risk, i.e. the armed forces. Similar assumptions seem to have underlain Defence Regulation 33B, which was introduced in 1942 and lapsed in 1947, and has been described as a "panic wartime measure", designed to protect servicemen. Like the 1866 Act, this was vigorously resisted on the grounds that it seemed to condone prostitution while taking away some of the prostitutes' rights.

The last attempt to introduce legislation in Britain was in 1968, when a Private Member's Bill sought to revive the wartime powers of compulsory contact-tracing. But by this time the climate was entirely different. Prostitution was scarcely mentioned in the Parliamentary debate. As a subsequent *Times* leader put it, the diseases were now more likely to be "caught from acquaintances rather than prostitutes". The Bill was withdrawn after the Government spokesman had argued that compulsion would be ineffective anyway, and would merely make contact-tracing more difficult.

The lessons to be drawn from this brief history are that compulsion is unlikely to succeed unless there is a relatively restricted class of persons to whom it applies, and in these circumstances it raises serious questions about individual rights. However, if moral opinion were to change so radically that confidentiality was no longer an issue, the objections to compulsion would lose some of their force, and it would be possible to treat the diseases in the same way as any other notifiable condition. I shall return to this point later.

Moral Persuasion

This has traditionally been the main non-medical weapon against the diseases, but there has often been confusion between two distinct motives underlying it. There have been those for whom the moral motive has been primary, and who have regarded the prevalence of the venereal diseases as an index of the moral health of society. Eradicating them by adopting stricter standards of sexual morality has been urged on the grounds that these standards are good in themselves. Sometimes the conclusions have been drawn that it is therefore socially dangerous to remove the deterrent effect of the diseases, but responsible moral opinion has usually managed to avoid overstressing this point. Thus as long ago as 1924 a Commission on Christian Social Morality (Conference on Christian Politics, Economics and Citizenship 1924) dismissed fear as a means of countering sexual promiscuity, and wrote: "What is needed is not a mere unwillingness to perform the act, but a moral repudiation of it . . . To be satisfied with saying 'Avoid this, or you will suffer from it' is to stimulate ingenuity to find a means by which the consequences can be avoided and the act enjoyed."

Prophetic words!

The other motive for using moral persuasion has been medical. It has been argued that the medical problem can only be solved in so far as the social, and by implication the moral, problems underlying it are tackled. There was an interesting example of this approach at a BMA Conference held in 1964 for young people. The overwhelming emphasis in a very wide-ranging discussion was on the need to change behaviour. However, the explicit reason for calling the Conference was not to discuss promiscuity as such, but to consider means of preventing the spread of the diseases.

Both motives, of course, frequently coincide, expecially in educational work. In a paper written in 1970 on "anti-VD education", Dr Dalzell-Ward made the point that "education regarding venereal disease cannot be considered apart from education for mental health and personal relationships". He went on to express the hope that it would be possible to "fashion a new educational policy based on sound scientific principles, rather than upon empiricism or the mere arbitrary application of personal judgment". I find it fascinating that science, empiricism and mere arbitrary judgment should be thought of as the only alternatives. But the whole paper is interesting in that it spells out very clearly the moral dimension of the problem, and wavers between making this primary, and sticking to the safe scientific ground of dealing with proven ills.

Awareness of the dual motivation of the moral approach may have made some doctors increasingly hesitant to use it. Among the general public there are very large numbers who still think of venereal diseases as shameful, more shameful probably than the conduct which spreads them; and there are strong lobbies which still use VD statistics as an index of moral corruption. But the very strength of these feelings may be counter-productive, in that careful professional attempts at moral persuasion can seem to lend weight to moral attitudes of a much more extreme kind.

In 1971 a West Indian nurse was subjected to a routine test after returning from a holiday abroad, was accused of having contracted VD, and was promptly dismissed by the Birmingham Regional Hospital Board. Admittedly the Board apologized when the nurse was subsequently found to be suffering from yaws. But the whole incident seemed to symbolize a condemnatory attitude with which many in the medical profession no longer wish to be associated. And this, I suspect, is one of the reasons underlying the third approach I want to describe – moral indifference.

Moral Indifference

I do not believe that the majority of people professionally concerned with medical and social problems share as a personal attitude the sort of moral indifference expressed by the teenager who said: "I cannot fell guilty or ashamed about having gonorrhoea because I have done something completely natural like just to sleep with somebody . . .". But I want to suggest that professional attitudes have changed radically in the last few years, and that professional moral indifference is a fair description of a very widespread approach.

The Office of Health Economics briefing on the venereal diseases, issued in October 1974, expresses the change very succinctly:

> Attempts to control sexual behaviour, preventing promiscuity and so limiting the chances of infection spreading . . . are unlikely to be successful, and may today be thought absurd by those to whom they are directed. This area is so complex that would-be educators who try to change the population's sexual behaviour may even influence it in a manner which is the reverse of that which they intend.

The handout accompanying a BBC programme for teenagers on VD broadcast in November 1974, illustrates the same tendency. The six-page pamphlet is entirely medical in content, and the only hint that there might be other aspects of this problem is contained in a single sentence at the end:

> Needless to say, the factual approach of both the programme and these notes does not assume that values held by many teachers and students concerning sex before marriage and casual relationships are to be dismissed or rejected.

Some campaigners put it more forcefully. Thus Germaine Greer, in an article in the *Sunday Times* (February 1973) wrote: "It's time VD was socially accepted." And countless teenage magazines spread the gospel of sexual liberation of which VD is an inevitable, but scarcely troubling, side-effect.

Professional moral indifference has great advantages in a social climate where actual moral indifference in sexual matters is becoming more common, and where moral uncertainties are deeply felt even by those who have no liking for promiscuity. Indifference eliminates fear and guilt. In a less guilt-ridden situation the problem of confidentiality would not loom so large, contact-tracing would be easier and, as many now suggest, the venereal diseases could take their place among other genitourinary complaints without any complicating moral overtones. "Stop moral posturing," says the reformer, "and treat the problem as one aspect of everyday personal hygiene. The moral emphasis may have had its value when methods of treatment were less successful, but is irrelevant now."

I hope I have not caricatured this attitude, but it seems to me that it is not confined to the venereal diseases alone. The Family Planning Association has produced fairly blatant examples of moral indifference. Some of its literature seems so obsessed with the single aim of eliminating unwanted babies that virtually any sexual behaviour is condoned provided it is "responsible" in the limited sense of not being reproductive.

I want to suggest to you, however, that moral convictions are not so easily by-passed. Neutrality or indifference are themselves moral attitudes, and what may have been adopted as a professional stance very rapidly becomes interpreted as a personal moral recommendation by those towards whom it is directed. Moral indifference conveys the message that in this sphere moral considerations are of no account.

Since indifference is frequently confused with tolerance, let me spend a moment distinguishing between them. Indifference says "I don't care", whereas tolerance says: "I do care, but I recognize your right to differ." Indifference ceases to use the language of right and wrong. Tolerance uses moral language, but uses it humbly and in a spirit of acceptance. The difference is vital.

The danger I foresee in our present mood of moral indifference is that a medical profession, which for good practical reasons wants to avoid moral complications, may be unconsciously legitimizing all sorts of undesirable social practices, under the guise of being tolerant.

This process whereby one person or group legitimizes another person's behaviour is still not widely appreciated, although there are obvious and well-known examples. Crowd behaviour is a case in point. The crowd in some way gives permission or sanction for acts which in other contexts would clearly be recognized as wrong. A recent American study called "Sanctions for Evil" (Sanford and Comstock 1971) analysed the sort of permissions given by society which led, in full flower, to the atrocities of Vietnam. Moral indifference about VD may seem insignificant by comparison. But my point is that its effects are not neutral; they may be much greater than we think.

Another facet of the same problem is the curious irony whereby, just as the moment when so much of the emphasis in modern medicine is on the treatment not of diseases, but of whole persons in their social context, the moral dimension is in danger of dropping out. Not from medicine as a whole, of course; there has surely never been a time when medical ethics have flourished so profusely, or the medical profession been burdened with so many difficult ethical choices. But the focus of attention has been on the ethical problems which are, as it were, internal to medicine, rather than on the personal moral standards of patients, and the social forces which mould them. I wonder, though, whether a profession which takes seriously its concern for health, in the broadest sense of the word, can afford to remain neutral in matters which deeply affect growth in personal maturity, and which influence prevailing social assumptions about something as central to life as sexual behaviour.

The alternative to moral indifference need not be censoriousness, nor the attempt to apply moral persuasion of a kind whose motives, as I suggested earlier, can be questioned. Personal conviction allied with tolerance is a healthier mixture than either of these; and I therefore very much hope that members of the medical profession will not come to believe that in a puzzled and morally divided society, the right thing to do is to keep quiet.

Convictions expressed with tolerance and understanding create a climate in which there can be honest and open debate, but where nobody doubts the seriousness of what is being discussed. In such an atmosphere, those who look for moral guidance may find it; whereas those who reject it need not be shamed into neglecting the medical help they need.

It would be going too far beyond my brief to try to spell out what kind of convictions might be held, and how in practice they might be expressed. May I suggest as a starting point, however, the phrase used a moment ago — "whole persons in their social context". Morality, as well as medicine, is about wholeness. Moral insight begins as we consider individual actions in relation to a whole life and in the broadest possible context. Religious morality widens and changes the context by the perception of spiritual dimension. But any morality worth the name must point the individual beyond his immediate concerns and gratifications and limited horizons, and help him to see the kind of life he is making for himself and for others.

To open up such questions, even in a medical setting, is the first step towards showing that convictions matter. Nor can it be claimed that to do so is an alien moral intrusion. If my argument in this paper is sound, such questions also have an essential place in good medicine.

References

Conference on Christian Politics, Economics and Citizenship Report (1924). Longmans Green, London; iv, 116

Dalzell-Ward, A. J. (1970). *British Journal of Venereal Diseases* 46, 159

Office of Health Economics (1974). Venereal Disease No. 1. London

Sanford, N. and Comstock, C. (1971). Sanctions for Evil. Josses Bass Inc., San Francisco

Discussion

Mr Alan Hilton said that he was the Area Health Education Officer for Lancashire and had responsibilities for health education. There was often hysterical reaction on the part of some people when considering the problem of sexually transmitted diseases. There was a punishment syndrome in that the public considered that as people enjoyed getting these diseases, there should be pain and punishment involved in getting rid of them. He also asked whether venereologists saw themselves as consultants in the sense of giving advice or as clinicians dealing with a strictly medical problem.

Dr Habgood replied that he had been trying to approach the problem from a wide viewpoint and that he had not wished to be censorious. But to pretend that these larger questions about the whole life-style did not exist would not be helpful. On the second point, he thought that we all retreated into our specialties and put up a barrier around us so that ordinary people found it difficult to get general advice.

Dr Cooper thought that the specialist should be both a consultant and a clinician. Most consulting specialists wanted to go on practising clinical medicine and not just acting as consultants. Patients with sexually transmitted diseases should be seen primarily by general practitioners and private physicians, and he thought that we had gone too far in trying to have every clinical problem treated and solved by a specialist.

Dr Catterall thought specialist clinicians in the United Kingdom regarded their role as being consultative and that they would all welcome approaches from and frequent discussion with their Area Health Education Officers.

He asked Dr Cooper what had been done to improve the undergraduate medical student training in sexually transmitted diseases in the United States since the strong recommendation by the International Travelling Seminar of the World Health Organization and the National Commission on sexually transmitted diseases that undergraduate training in this subject should be improved in quality and increased in quantity.

Dr Catterall also asked Mr Goodchild if any attempts had been made to assess the effects of medical television programmes on the attitudes of the people who saw them.

Dr Cooper agreed that the medical curriculum in many of the United States medical centres was inadequate in this field. He pointed out that the Federal Government did not direct the curriculum but could have an influence on it by applying subtle pressures and by applying carrots in the right place. They could approach accrediting commissions and qualifying boards to ask them why they were not asking the right questions and attempt to convince the examiners of the importance of asking questions on sexually transmitted diseases. He thought it was also possible that in the future there might be some new form of legislation that could help with this problem.

Mr Goodchild said that attempts had been made to assess changes of attitude after programmes but that this had not been done with any of the programmes concerned with sexually transmitted diseases. In general he thought that in sex education the results of changes of attitudes had been disappointing but he pointed out the difficulty in making true assessments on such changes. The machinery was not sophisticated enough, big enough or sensitive enough.

Dr G R C Palmer (*Alberta, Canada*) was concerned, on epidemiological and clinical grounds, about the far reaching side-effects of widespread promiscuity – and the chronic pelvic inflammatory disease patient with intractable pain, discomfort, and infertility, and alternatively, the mentally retarded offspring, result of later consanguinity.

He stated that on the North American continent the public media and sociologists publicized, encouraged and glamourized sexuality, failing to emphasize the concomitant risks of promiscuity and sexually transmitted disease. At the same time, publishers of profiteering propensity joined in to supply pornography in profusion in airports and railroad stations. He questioned how much these factors influenced young people's minds towards promiscuity with all its potential, long-term complications, direct and genetic.

Professor Alexander G Bearn (*New York*) thought there would be no genetic effect at all. The dangers of promiscuity were societal not genetical.

Sir Douglas Black said he was concerned about the relationship of sex to advertising and the commercialization, glamourization and cheapening of sex for financial gain.

Mr Blakeslee asked whether there really had been a sexual revolution and if people really were doing something different, or whether they were just doing the same thing but talking about it more and being more candid about it. His personal view was that the subject had come into the open more, but he was uncertain as to whether this would in the long run affect human behaviour.

Dr Cooper thought the commercialization of sex on news stands was a straight economic affair and persisted because the products could be sold to the public.

Dr Habgood thought that western society was going through an extremely difficult period and that young people in particular were subjected to enormous commercial pressures. It was possible that there might be a puritan type of reaction in the not too distant future. He thought it was important that those who had convictions should say so. The most frightening thing about society was not the concentration on sex but that people had become over-timid about their moral convictions.

Dr Turner said he had much appreciated the Bishop of Durham's sensitive talk. With regard to medical education in the United States on sexually transmitted diseases, a question raised by Dr Catterall, he thought that medical centres could only teach well the things that they did well. The clinics for sexually transmitted diseases in America had been transferred outside the teaching hospitals and he believed that medical students would only be taught satisfactorily about these diseases when the clinics were moved back into the mainstream of the teaching hospitals.

Dr P J Schwartz (*Seattle, Washington*) thought that many of the issues discussed were in the realm of the sociologist. There had been a commission on pornography in the United States which had accumulated a great deal of data and had come to the basic conclusions that pornography on balance did not warp people's minds but that it sometimes had a desensitizing effect. In comparison with violence its effect seemed negligible. Violence was thought to be a much more serious problem. She thought that in medical education too little use was made of sociological, psychological and sexual behavioural studies and she suggested that more should be known about sexuality and various life styles before doctors became counsellors and instructors of patients.

Dr Habgood thought that sensible moral discussions were impossible unless all the data were available for consideration. He thought that morals were a matter for rational discussion which employed a sensitive awareness on many levels of understanding including the scientific. In the United Kingdom over a number of years there had grown up a system of interdisciplinary discussions in which medical students took part. The Church of England had been particularly active in bringing these groups together in order to try to work through as many social and medical problems as possible from a multidisciplinary angle. He pointed out that it took a great deal of patience and goodwill on the part of those participating to be able to learn to speak and understand each other's language, but groups of doctors and clergy were working together in various parts of the world.

Miss Elspeth Robertson said that on the first day of the conference she had asked what the conference required from Health Education Officers and what could be done to further health education. She thought that she had received a partial answer to her question during the last three days and that the most important consideration was rational discussion. She saw her role as talking to parents and young people and to those at teacher traning colleges who would in future be doing the teaching, and approaching the problems from the widest possible angle.

Reflections on the Conference

Dr Ambrose King

The project for this meeting was an imaginative idea which has been carried through most efficiently and effectively. It has been a splendid meeting, and I am sure we shall all go away and think about it, and learn a great deal from what we have heard.

It has been to me a special pleasure, after almost a lifetime spent in the study of these diseases, to be here, and to appreciate that this despised and neglected subject seems to have come of age at last, and that people are beginning to realize how important it is to the public in general, and also to the medical profession.

It has been a privilege to meet so many colleagues from the United States and other countries, and, if I may mention names, two friends of long standing who have made an immense contribution to the subject and added distinction to their profession. I refer to Dr Thomas Turner and Dr Bruce Webster. I hope that these contacts, having been made, will go on, and I see from the programme that there is a scheme whereby the Royal Society of Medicine Foundation can on occasions send medical representatives to be attached to clinics in special subjects. I hope it will be possible in this as well as other subjects.

Coming more specifically to what has gone on here during the last three days, it is well known, and I do not think we need go into the reasons, that for a number of years past the American scene as regards venereology or sexually transmitted disease has been in difficulties because of the absence of trained physicians with special experience in the subject. Dr Turner put his finger on the nub of the matter, pointing out that they do not have departments at their teaching hospitals. They had a magnificent department once at the Johns Hopkins Hospital, but unfortunately it was turned over to other uses. I believe one has seen from this meeting that there are young clinicians coming along who are interested in the subject, and who will I am sure extend their activities and associations and make a contribution. It is absolutely vital to the control of sexually transmitted diseases to have good physicians who are thoroughly trained in the subject. It is the most important method of controlling these diseases. All other methods, including epidemiological methods, are ancillary, and this I am sure should be fully and generally recognized.

As far as the British situation is concerned, I believe it is true that until recent years we dragged our feet in the matter of certain epidemiological methods, including contact tracing. We have learned a great deal from our American colleagues in that respect, and are beginning to catch up. Those of us who study the literature and who have listened in the last few days must be impressed by the contribution which the Americans have made to the control of gonorrhoea by routine testing of women where for other reasons they undergo pelvic examination – in obstetric and gynaecological clinics, family planning clinics and cervical cytology clinics. I regret to say that we have not yet convinced our obstetricians and gynaecologists in this country of their responsibilities in this matter, but I hope we shall continue to try to do so.

I wish also to refer to another matter which came up, a vexed matter that has been with us for quite a while. It is what is called epidemiological treatment. I am sad to hear that it is still recommended and practised in the United States. It is an epidemiological trick, and I think not a good trick. It is a question of treating certain contacts of patients without really submitting them to proper investigation. It is a violation of a fundamental principle in medicine – diagnosis before treatment. I have argued this on a number of occasions and I will not bore you by going through the gamut of reasons. But every venereologist knows that many patients have more than one venereal disease, and that one remedy is not going to be sufficient to cure all the diseases that he or she has. Venereologists know that vital information about their patients can be obtained from examining sexual contacts. We are not dealing with sheep to which we apply sheep dip. We are dealing with complex human minds and bodies, and this seems to me an extremely bad practice which has built up with our American colleagues because of the lack of good clinicians in the subject. I hope they will think it over, and I hope they will come to see our point of view. It is a fact that American medicine has great prestige throughout the world, and there are many people throughout the world who have undertaken this practice, and justified it on the grounds that it is recommended and practised in the United States. So I hope they will agree to think about that.

Those who have listened during the last few days to the admirable work which has been done by serologists, microbiologists, geneticists and others must be very much impressed with the standards of that work, and the enthusiasm that goes into it. The fruits of this are not immediately obvious, but these do provide the seeds of future progress, and this kind of research work should, I am sure, be extended.

I should like to say a little about health education, sex education, call it what you will. It is not a matter on which I could hope to speak as an expert, but it has an important bearing on our work.

The Bishop of Durham spoke to us about morality, and he spoke about moral indifference. It has seemed to me that there is more than moral indifference in attitudes to this matter. The word I should use is "antagonism". There is a section of society which seeks to undermine the morals of our young people, and to encourage them to do things which we and our forefathers thought they should not be encouraged to do. I am concerned about some of the things that are taught to children. It is a fact that in our society words like "virtue" and "morality" have come to be dirty words. After all, morality is a question of right and wrong, and every society, whether it is based on religion or humanism or anything else, has to decide for itself what is right and what is wrong; what is good for it and what is bad. I believe it is wrong to teach the young that there is no harm in indulging in sexual activity providing that they avoid pregnancy and venereal disease. I believe it is right to appeal to their idealism, to try to convince them that self-restraint is essential in this life, and the road to happiness and freedom lies in the ideals of love, marriage and the family.

All of us – venereologists, genitourinary physicians, and others in other disciplines – are extremely grateful to Sir John Stallworthy, to the Royal Society of Medicine and to the Royal Society of Medicine Foundation for sponsoring this meeting which I think has been immensely successful. We are deeply grateful to those who devised and planned the programme, and to those who have carried it through so successfully. We are grateful to the staff of the Royal Society of Medicine, with a special word for Mr R N Thomson and Miss Muriel Mitchell, who have been so generous with their time and care during the last few days. May I conclude by expressing the hope that this will be done again. Where is not for me to suggest. It so happens I live round the corner, but I would go a long way to be present at such a meeting as this if in the future it were to be arranged.

Dr Bruce Webster

First of all, on behalf of this group I should like to express the appreciation of all of us to the Royal Society of Medicine and the Royal Society of Medicine Foundation for setting up this series of meetings. In any meeting of this kind there is always a question whether it will be clinically or research oriented. I think it is essential – and this has been demonstrated here – to have a blending of the two. It is important for the pure investigators to have contact with the clinician in order that he knows what the problems are, and it is important for the clinician to be updated by the investigator.

Further, I think that international meetings are most productive. Throughout the years at the International Union, and at the WHO, I have had the opportunity of exchanging ideas with people interested in sexually transmitted diseases throughout the world, and I think this meeting has accomplished just that. Although the situations differ in each country and the methods of control are different, there is a great deal in common.

As Dr Catterall and other speakers have said, the worldwide situation in sexually transmitted diseases is alarming at the present time. If any other disease were increasing at the rate at which gonorrhoea is advancing today, the populace would panic, yet this increase has been going on for several years, and we find great complacency among legislators and the populace as a whole. The results of our efforts to control this have been disappointing. Obviously, present methods are not effective. Some time ago, in a speech, I made the statement that new tools were needed to combat this rising epidemic. This phrase was picked up by *Playboy* Magazine, and making a play on the word "tools", I was quoted at some length in that magazine.

Some three or four years ago, the Secretary of Health, Education and Welfare set up a national commission, in the United States, and we were charged with making plans and recommending ways and means to stem the rising tide of the sexually transmitted diseases. Dr Turner and Dr Knox were members of this commission, together with a group of distinguished physicians. In the course of the report great emphasis was naturally laid on research. We must interest microbiologists throughout the world in this problem. We must bring in new blood, and I should like to take this opportunity to pay tribute to what has been done by the National Institute of Allergy and Infectious Diseases, particularly by Dr Puziss, in the United States, in selling the problem to microbiologists throughout that country. We recently had a seminar in Minneapolis on the biology of the spirochaete and it was astounding the number of people who were, I think indoctrinated into the importance of this.

Another aspect of reseach which has been neglected is the behavioural sciences and their relationship to the control of sexually transmitted diseases. Some other countries, particularly Denmark, have pioneered in this. We need to know a great deal more, not only about high-risk groups, but also about the sexual habits of the population as a whole. Perhaps these are changing, and again we must always keep in mind that the sexually transmitted diseases are not confined to high-risk groups alone. Some work has been done in profiles, and I think this is a very important factor. However, in our country we have been unable to convince the National Institute of Mental Health that behavioural science plays any role in the control of these diseases.

There has been much discussion of the whole question of public education. Originally it was suggested by the National Commission that a public campaign against sexually transmitted diseases be held. Perhaps we were not right in that recommendation. There is still a question in the United States as to whether or not the public campaign against smoking was successful. We have had an experience quite recently. We got the Advertising Council, which is a voluntary agency which does "do good" public information, one of the best of which is Smokey the Bear against forest fires, to get one of the better advertising agencies to do material for this publicity campaign on television and radio. I think I am only fair in saying that the results have been disappointing. The smaller stations picked it up, but the big national networks were afraid of offending their clients. I think this is interesting in this day and age. Perhaps our approaches have been wrong.

It seems to me there are three groups that we have to reach. We have still, I think, to consider the population as a whole. That comprises the parents and the legislators. Of course we have the high-risk groups, and then there is the question of education in the schools.

I should like to say a word about medical education. This is a very important problem in the United States. A World Health Organization study a number of years ago on venereal disease education of physicians throughout the world, showed that education in the sexually transmitted diseases was badly neglected. I think that this still holds true in our country in spite of the fact that 80% of cases are handled by the practising physician, who is receiving little or no undergraduate instruction in these diseases. In a recent meeting of the WHO in Geneva, and again in the General Assembly, they made the strong recommendation that immediate steps are urgently needed to improve undergraduate medical training and education. The National Commission took an interest in this, and we devoted some time to it and made the recommendation that teaching grants be offered to medical schools. This was done a number of years ago in the case of military medicine and it worked.

I do not think there is any doubt that the promotion of research centres will do a great deal to arouse interest; but I am afraid that may not reach the clinically orientated group. We need the sort of thing that was established many years ago at Johns Hopkins where there is a combination of both investigation and clinical interests. The answer to that, as was brought out today, is in bringing the public clinics into the university hospitals. This I am sure would meet our needs, as Dr Turner has pointed out.

The problem is primarily a financial one. Most university hospitals cannot afford to do this. The travelling seminar sponsored by the International Union and WHO which has been referred to, pointed out this factor in some detail.

We have also the question of postgraduate education. How shall we reach the doctors who are already in practice? In one or two states in our country task forces have been formed consisting of the State Education Department, the State Medical Department, the Parent Teacher Association and youth groups. In two instances with which I am familiar these have been highly successful in improving not only education, but clinical facilities, and many other things.

There is one more aspect, and that is the question of prophylaxis. In World War I they gave credit to prophylaxis for controlling sexually transmitted diseases. We forgot about it for a long time. It is our feeling that perhaps this should be explored more fully. Studies are being done in Sweden and the United States on the use of the condom. Here again, I think we need behavioural science studies as to its acceptability. I am very much impressed with the work that is being done by Dr John Cutler, University of Pittsburgh School of Public Health, on vaginal prophylaxis with some of the birth control products. In certain segments of the population, I think this would appeal. Certainly we need to consider all these new approaches.

In conclusion, I feel that the situation is critical. I think our hope for the future lies in research and the continuation of our efforts in public education. In the meantime we must continue our present methods of control and attempt to improve our clinical facilities.

Closing Remarks

Sir John Stallworthy

The problems we have been discussing vary in intensity from place to place, and are even greater in their social impact in the Third World than they are here.

Dr Nicol spoke of 60 000 new patients with gonococcal infection in this country each year, and many noted the surprise when Dr Knox referred to 18 000 new patients reporting to his own clinic with gonorrhoea and between 500 and 600 with early syphilis, in a city about one-fifth the size of London. It would have been helpful if there had been an opportunity of asking Dr Knox to tell us more. I cannot conceive of a clinic so attractive that it induces people to contract venereal disease! On the other hand many clinics are so unattractive that they do not influence people to seek help. There must be an atmosphere of understanding, compassion and a willingness to help, and no sense of judging people's morals. It would have been interesting to hear a little more about this.

Dr Willcox spoke of high-risk categories. He will probably be misquoted, but I hope not, otherwise he might not be able to leave the country by air! But those of you who have come into Heathrow must have been impressed by the mass of humanity disgorged there almost every hour of the day. People come from different countries, different races and different cultures, sometimes individually, sometimes in groups, and sometimes in hundreds. They come with great hopes but do not know what they are going to do. They hope to stay and make a life here. They know that some people may welcome them, and others will exploit them. It is not a happy situation. Just as it was said a long time ago that no man is an island, so no country is now an island. The roads leading into all the great cities of the world are now roads in the air, and many of the problems which have been considered here have their applications elsewhere. People come with their hopes but bring their problems with them as well. So the situation, difficult as it was some years ago, is even more difficult now, with increasing immigration.

We were fascinated by the account Dr Falkow gave of genetic manipulation and engineering. The hope is that new preparations will be found that are even more effective than the excellent ones now available. When they are developed in research laboratories this knowledge becomes available all over the world. So the impact of a meeting such as this goes far beyond this small hall.

In the meantime, movement of people from one part of the world to the other continues, so we come back to the subject of the final session today: namely the question of educational programmes and communication. If we cannot communicate properly with our own people, there is an even bigger challenge in learning how to communicate with other people living in our midst, whose background, culture and outlook is different. This challenge faces educationalists and clinicians. On several occasions speakers referred to the necessity of the team approach. We all need to be humble about this and to admit that there are great problems and great challenges. No one section has the answer. It may take a long time, even if we combine our resources, before we can make a great impact on this very serious social problem of sexually transmitted disease.

It is terribly distressing when youngsters come along with a completely distorted attitude and have their health and outlook on life permanently impaired because of pressures put upon them. The fact that they have not been properly informed of the repercussions of the sort of life they are encouraged to lead makes them the victims of contemporary society.

Two days ago it was my privilege to bid you welcome. The time has now come for me to bid you farewell. Before doing so, I should like to join with the generous speakers from the United States who have expressed their thanks to all who have made this conference possible. Financial support for the conference was received from many sources; in particular, the National Institutes of Health gave very considerable support by assisting with the travel expenses of some delegates from the USA, and the Wellcome Foundation has promised to meet the cost of providing the printed proceedings of the conference for those who attended.

We pay special tribute to the President of the Royal Society of Medicine Foundation, Dr Harry Robinson; to Professor Alex Bearn and Dr Richard Krause, who came from the United States to help with the planning of this conference; to my two London colleagues, Dr Catterall and Dr Nicol and to the staff of the Royal Society of Medicine who have been responsible for much of the work behind the scenes.

Later you will receive your copy of the report of the conference, and when you do I hope that as you read it it will renew the challenges which I am sure all of us have had. I hope also that it will bring you happy memories of your visit to London.

I bid you farewell, and wish you a safe journey home.